Pulse Diagnosis
A Clinical Guide

Sean Walsh
BHSc (Acupuncture) PhD
Senior Lecturer,
University of Technology, Sydney,
Department of Medical and Molecular Biosciences,
Traditional Chinese Medicine,
Sydney, Australia

Emma King
BSc BHSc (Acupuncture) MSc
Sessional Lecturer and Tutor,
University of Technology, Sydney,
Department of Medical and Molecular Biosciences,
Traditional Chinese Medicine,
Sydney, Australia

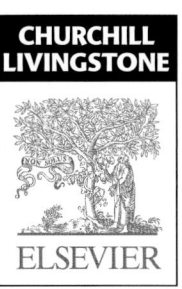

CHURCHILL
LIVINGSTONE

ELSEVIER

EDINBURGH LONDON NEW YORK OXFORD PHILADELPHIA ST LOUIS SYDNEY TORONTO 2008

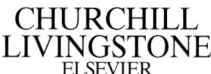

CHURCHILL LIVINGSTONE / SAUNDERS / BAILLIÈRE TINDALL / MOSBY /
BUTTERWORTH-HEINEMANN / BOOKS FOR MIDWIVES / WRIGHT
An imprint of Elsevier Limited

First published 2008

ISBN-13: 978-0-443-10248-6
ISBN-10: 0-443-10248-1

British Library Cataloguing in Publication Data
A catalogue record for this book is available from the British Library

Library of Congress Cataloging in Publication Data
A catalog record for this book is available from the Library of Congress

Notice
Neither the Publisher nor the [Editors/Authors] assume any responsibility for any
loss or injury and/or damage to persons or property arising out of or related to
any use of the material contained in this book. It is the responsibility of the
treating practitioner, relying on independent expertise and knowledge of the
patient, to determine the best treatment and method of application for the
patient.

The Publisher

ELSEVIER your source for books,
journals and multimedia
in the health sciences
www.elsevierhealth.com

The
publisher's
policy is to use
**paper manufactured
from sustainable forests**

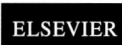

Working together to grow
libraries in developing countries

www.elsevier.com | www.bookaid.org | www.sabre.org

ELSEVIER   BOOK AID
International   Sabre Foundation

Printed in China

Pulse Diagnosis

Commissioning Editors: *Karen Morley, Claire Wilson*
Development Editors: *Kerry McGechie, Alison Turnball*
Project Manager: *Jess Thompson*
Designer: *Stewart Larking*
Illustrators: *David Gardner, Michael Courtney*
Illustration Manager: *Merlyn Harvey*

Contents

Preface   ix

Acknowledgements   xi

Notes for the reader   xiii

**Chapter 1 Contextualising pulse within contemporary
            clinical practice**   1
  1.1 Contextualising the learning environment   1
  1.2 Addressing misconceptions   2
  1.3 Why is a reliable system of pulse taking important? The evidence   3
  1.4 Ongoing practice   4

**Chapter 2 The pulse: its place in contemporary biomedical
            and CM practice**   5
  2.1 The circulatory system   5
  2.2 The pulse   6
  2.3 Blood   10
  2.4 Summary   13
  2.5 The pulse in biomedicine   13
  2.6 The pulse in contemporary CM clinical practice   17

Chapter 3 Historical pulse records and practice   23
  3.1 *Nei Jing*   23
  3.2 *Nan Jing*   25
  3.3 *Mai Jing*   26
  3.4 *Bin Hue Mai Xue*   27
  3.5 Historical perspective: regional pulse assessment and the
              Cun Kou pulse   27
  3.6 Historical problems in contemporary practice   29
  3.7 Pulse classics and contemporary practice   30

Chapter 4 Issues of reliability and validity   33
  4.1 Pulse diagnosis and the need for clear and unambiguous
              terminology   34
  4.2 Pulse diagnosis, subjectivity and the need for reliable assessment
              methods   37
  4.3 Pulse in changing contexts   38
  4.4 The normal pulse   38
  4.5 Reliability and validity of the pulse diagnosis process   39
  4.6 Radial pulse palpation method   42

Chapter 5 Getting started: pulse techniques, procedures and the development of a methodical approach to pulse assessment 45

5.1 Positioning the patient 46
5.2 Locating the radial artery 47
5.3 Locating the pulse positions for assessment 49
5.4 Practitioner positioning 51
5.5 Assessing the parameters 51
5.6 Locating the pulse depth 53
5.7 The normal pulse 56
5.8 Assessing health by the pulse 57
5.9 Channel, organ and levels of depth 58
5.10 Comparison of the overall force of the left and right radial pulse 58
5.11 Pulse method 59
5.12 Other considerations when assessing the pulse and interpreting the findings 61
5.13 Summary 68

Chapter 6 Simple CM pulse qualities and associated pulse parameters 71

6.1 Introduction 72
6.2 The simple pulse parameters 73
6.3 Rate 73
6.4 CM pulses defined by rate 78
    6.4.1 Slow pulse (Chí mài) 78
    6.4.2 Rapid pulse (Shuò mài) 80
    6.4.3 Moderate pulse (Huan mài) 82
6.5 Rhythm 83
6.6 CM pulses defined by rhythm 88
    6.6.1 Skipping pulse (Cù mài) 88
    6.6.2 Bound pulse (Jié mài) 88
    6.6.3 Intermittent pulse (Dài mài) 89
6.7 Depth 91
6.8 CM pulse qualities defined by level of depth 94
    6.8.1 Floating pulse (Fú mài) 94
    6.8.2 Sinking pulse (Chén mài) 96
    6.8.3 Hidden pulse (Fú mài) 98
6.9 Length (longitude) 100
6.10 CM pulse defined by length 101
    6.10.1 Long pulse (Cháng mài) 101
    6.10.2 Short pulse (Duan mài) 102
6.11 Width (latitude) 103
6.12 CM pulse qualities defined by arterial width 109
    6.12.1 Fine pulse (Xì mài) 109
6.13 Summary 112

Chapter 7 Complex CM pulse qualities and associated pulse parameters 115

7.1 Introduction 115
7.2 The complex pulse parameters 115
7.3 Arterial wall tension 116
7.4 Pulse occlusion 120

7.5 CM pulse qualities defined by arterial wall tension and ease of pulse occlusion   123
    7.5.1   Stringlike (Wiry) pulse (Xián mài)   123
    7.5.2   Tight pulse (Jín mài)   127
    7.5.3   Scallion Stalk pulse (Kōu mài)   129
    7.5.4   Drumskin pulse (Gé mài)   133
    7.5.5   Scattered pulse (Sàn mài)   135
7.6 Pulse force   137
7.7 CM pulse qualities defined by pulse force   142
    7.7.1   Replete pulse (Shí mài)   142
    7.7.2   Firm pulse (Láo mài)   144
    7.7.3   Vacuous pulse (Xū mài)   146
    7.7.4   Faint pulse (Wēi mài)   148
    7.7.5   Weak pulse (Ruò mài)   150
    7.7.6   Soggy pulse (Rú mài)   151
7.8 Pulse contour and flow wave   154
7.9 CM pulses defined by pulse contour   158
    7.9.1   Slippery pulse (Huá mài)   158
    7.9.2   Rough pulse (Sè mài)   162
    7.9.3   Surging pulse (Hóng mài)   168
    7.9.4   Stirred pulse (Spinning Bean pulse) (Dòng mài)   169
7.10 Revision of the 27 CM pulse qualities   170
7.11 Using the pulse parameter system   170

Chapter 8 Genesis of pulse qualities   179
    8.1 Same disease different pulse; different pulse, same disease   179
    8.2 External pathogenic attack versus internal dysfunction   179
    8.3 Blood   188
    8.4 Qi   196
    8.5 Yin vacuity   198
    8.6 Yang vacuity   198
    8.7 Health   199
    8.8 The Unusual or Death pulses   200

Chapter 9 Other systems of pulse diagnosis   203
    9.1 Qi and Blood balance   203
    9.2 The Three Jiao   207
    9.3 Eight Principle pulse diagnosis   212
    9.4 Five Phase (Wu Xing) pulse diagnosis   214
    9.5 Nine Continent pulse system   222

Index   227

Preface

It should be self evident: the pulse reflects life, and so the development of an expert knowledge of pulse must be a key task for practitioners in assessing health. It should also come as no surprise that medical practitioners, from all parts of the world and throughout the course of history, have considered the pulse to reflect or infer aspects of an individual's state of health. Information obtained from measurement of the pulse flow wave still plays a role in contemporary biomedical clinical practice but is supplemented, if not superseded, by measurement procedures using sophisticated medical devices developed specifically for measuring these changes. Similarly, Chinese medicine continues to also employ pulse assessment in the clinical examination process. For the practitioner of Oriental medicine, interpretation of the pulse characteristics depends on manual palpatory discrimination of changes in pulse variables and their relation to health and disease. This practice relies on a complex system of theories, developed over the past 1800 years, that link changes in arterial characteristics and blood flow to health and pathology, taking into account circadian rhythms, an individual's environment and personal traits.

In recent years attention has focused on the use of objective measurement techniques to attempt to record the 'CM' pulse objectively and consequently address some of the problems associated with manual pulse assessment. Yet, in spite of the many claims regarding success in this area using various types of electronic apparatus, to date there is no evidence that these measurements are recording the pulse in the same way that it is palpated manually. This means that pulse diagnosis continues to be a subjective process dependent upon a practitioner's palpatory skills and ability to discriminate changes in the pulse contour. Clearly, the application of pulse diagnosis in practice, and the teaching and learning of pulse assessment techniques, require clear detailing of pulse changes to avoid confusion; pulse diagnosis becomes an inherently unreliable assessment tool if this is not so. Without this clarity, it is difficult to learn and apply pulse palpatory technique in practice. Clear, unambiguous instructions are vital.

Needless to say, the body of literature written on pulse palpation as a diagnostic technique is extensive. It expands across centuries and across cultures, from Galenic traditions practiced until recent times in Europe to the theoretical medical constructs of Imperial China and Oriental medicine. Prognostic and diagnostic directions for the use of the information derived from pulse palpation are extensively discussed in the diverse body of pulse literature. The literature on pulse diagnosis is also eclectic. The literature details both diverging and conflicting theoretical constructs for interpreting pulse findings. These coexist side by side within the same and differing medical systems.

Often, then, for the practitioner to embrace the use of the pulse as part of the examination process requires an acceptance of what is written in the literature as clinically relevant. The only alternative often seems to be to reject the literature and pulse diagnosis altogether. Irrespective of which approach is taken, one thing is for certain: interpreting and understanding the literature and mastering of pulse palpation for diagnostic use can be overwhelming for established practitioners as well as for learners.

Therefore, the aim of this book is to discuss, develop and provide guidelines to assist in the reliable application of pulse palpation and interpretation of any findings within the CM diagnostic framework. As such, we shall start by examining the pulse itself, its mechanisms and formation and the essential pulse components 'felt' when palpated. This is the basis of Chapter 2, which provides an overview of 'pulse' and contextualises its use within both biomedicine and CM clinical practice. In addition, Occidental or Greek medical traditions also attributed enormous importance in reading the pulse within the diagnostic process, echoes of which are evident today in modern cardiology units. Because of this, we will briefly examine the importance of pulse taking within the Western traditions and its use within today's biomedical system of practice. In addition to providing comparisons to Oriental medicine, the biomedical traditions bring unique perspectives and mechanical measurement devices which can enrich the practice of pulse-taking within Oriental medicine.

Chapter 3 continues this process, with a focus on CM, discussing four important historical texts as a basis for fostering an understanding of when and how certain pulse assumption systems developed and their related claims to clinical relevance. These texts are an important point of reference for the many difficult issues with the pulse terminology and clinical interpretation of pulse findings affecting the use of pulse diagnosis within a contemporary practice. For these reasons the pulse procedures and terminology used to assess the pulse need to be sufficiently explicit and detailed to ensure that pulse diagnosis is been done correctly. This is termed *reliability*, and how it is achieved and factors that affect it form the central theme of Chapter 4.

Chapter 5 focuses specifically on the pulse diagnosis process itself, detailing the necessary procedures, techniques and methods for undertaking pulse assessment and the relevance of these issues in developing skills in the learner and practitioner.

Chapters 6 and 7 focus extensively on identifying variations in the different pulse aspects, termed *parameters*, and detail instructions on interpreting any per-

ceived changes within a diagnostic context with their related indications. This includes instructions on identifying the 27 traditional pulse qualities (or 28 when the Racing pulse is considered separate from the Rapid pulse). The approach taken is flexible for interpreting pulse findings into a diagnostic framework and is equally applicable whether the pulse presents as a recognisable pulse quality or, as is often the case, when the pulse 'characteristics' do not resemble any of the traditional pulse qualities. The information can still be used to interpret diagnostically relevant information from the pulse.

A clinical complication in the use of pulse diagnosis is that there can be several potentially very different pulse qualities that form in response to apparently the same illness or dysfunction. To address this, Chapter 8 discusses the traditional CM pulse qualities presented in Chapters 6 and 7 in a comparative manner with respect to the pathologies, dysfunction or health states that they reflect.

Chapter 9 concludes the book with a look at other pulse assumption methods used within CM clinical practice and the application of pulse assessment findings to these systems.

Acknowledgements

The seeds of this book were sown many years ago, and it results in no small part from the encouragement we received when we enrolled in the Chinese Medicine (CM) postgraduate program at the University of Technology, Sydney (UTS). Deirdre Cobbin in particular was instrumental in guiding us towards the investigation of the underlying foundations and assumptions of CM theory and its relevance to practise, an essential but often neglected area of research. Our gratitude and thanks go to Deirdre for her effort, dedication, time and support of those engaged in this necessary research.

We would like to thank our colleague, Liz Allison, who played an integral part in the initial development of the pulse parameter system. Karen Bateman and Chris Zaslawski also made early contributions to the series of pulse studies using student research subjects, and special thanks must go to Chris for the further opportunities he provided to implement the pulse parameter system in the teaching curriculum at UTS.

Thanks also to our professional colleagues, the teaching clinics and the CM students (past and present) at UTS who were generous with their support, time and participation in our research projects and who became the sounding board for our pulse parameter system.

Chunlin Zhou was gently patient in providing valuable advice and Cong Xing Yang gave generous assistance with the Chinese characters throughout the book.

Many people outside UTS made valued contributions to the writing of this book in a variety of ways. The work of Michael O'Rourke, Raymond Kelly and Alberto Avolio contributed significantly to our understanding of the arterial pulse. From a CM perspective, while we found inspiration from a wide number of literature sources, both classical and modern, Yubin Lu's approach to pulse diagnosis was particularly relevant.

Our publishers, Elsevier, gave us the opportunity to unleash our work upon a wider audience and their editorial team have made it look good. Thanks go to Stephen Birch for his support of research in Oriental medicine and valuable advice to those engaged in it. Staff at Lush Bucket Café provided us with much needed caffeine and lastly, but certainly not least, we would like to thank our respective partners (Greg and Peter), family and friends for their unending support and patience throughout this project.

Sean Walsh and Emma King

I would like to thank my colleague, Sean Walsh, for his vision, encouragement and depth of knowledge, without which this book would not have reached fruition.

E.K.

I in turn would like to thank Emma King, also for her encouragement and for her attention to detail. The book would not have been without her substantial effort, contribution, knowledge and support.

S.W.

Notes for the reader

Purpose of this book

The purpose of this book is to provide a clinically useful approach to using information about the changes in pulse parameters and the relation of these to health and disease within a CM context. It may be used as a guide when the parameters present as a traditional pulse quality and, equally, when they do not. It provides directions for using pulse palpation findings within different systems and models of acupuncture and CM. Accordingly, the authors assume a solid introductory level of knowledge in health and/or medical sciences and in the foundations of CM and related theoretical concepts, treatment and scope of practice. The main body of the text describes the changes in pulse characteristics and the relation of these to 'patterns' of dysfunction or illness.

Increasingly, CM practitioners find that patients require biomedical investigations, or require communication of presenting problems in a way they can understand. The vast majority of Western patients, and increasingly, Eastern patients are most familiar with biomedical concepts. For this reason, where appropriate, we have attempted to integrate biomedical knowledge with that of the traditional pulse literature to assist in a better understanding of the pulse than is usually gained through CM textbooks alone. All relevant knowledge, whether from a CM source of not, has been considered in writing this book, to inform best practice. Although the book is intended for CM audiences, it also seeks to be relevant to practitioners from other health disciplines who are interested in these investigative techniques.

Terminology

Pinyin and Chinese characters have been used where appropriate to qualify the use of English terms used to describe Chinese medical concepts. This is done to differentiate the translated Chinese medical term from the generic use of the same term in English. Additionally,

this will assist in reconciling differences in English terminology used amongst different CM texts. Where used, translated terms from Wiseman & Ye's *A Practical Dictionary of Chinese Medicine* have been used for consistency. Where a common alternative name is used for pulse terms, this is included in brackets. For example, Wiseman & Ye describe the Stringlike pulse, which is commonly known as the Wiry pulse; we refer to this as the Stringlike (Wiry) pulse. Unfortunately the translated term does not always convey the actual original meaning of the term in a CM framework, so pinyin terms are used to assist understanding. For example the Stringlike (Wiry) pulse is also designated Xián mài. A succinct list of terms and their meanings is also available in the WHO publication: *WHO International Standard Terminologies on Traditional Medicine in the Western Pacific Region*, compiled by WHO Regional Office for the Western Pacific, published 2007.

Content structure

The book has been structured to provide information about the pulse from several different perspectives. This includes overall pulse qualities as well as using simple units of pulse assessment known as parameters. It has been constructed for individuals with a range of knowledge and experience levels. Guidelines are provided for using the information obtained from pulse palpation in several different pulse assumption systems or theoretical models. Thus it is the same pulse, but can be interpreted diagnostically in several ways. Our intention is to be as inclusive as possible of the diverse range of systems of practice that are encompassed within the term Oriental medicine. The authors do not advocate one approach over another.

Clinical best practice and diagnosis

The pulse is one subcategory of one of four categories of information gathering used within CM. The other methods are broadly categorised as questioning, observation and listening. This book has been written within the context that pulse diagnosis will be used as part of a systemised process for information gathering, rather than as a stand-alone or sole technique for diagnosis. Indeed, each of the diagnostic tools has a unique usefulness and appropriateness depending upon the type of injury or illness and the constitution of the individual presenting in clinical practice. It is the combination of these examination approaches rather than the use of a stand-alone technique that provides the depth and breadth of information required to make an informed diagnosis and formulate an appropriate treatment response. This is best practice. Best practice in relation to pulse diagnosis also encompasses the appropriate use of the approach within a broader assessment process rather than relying solely upon the use of the technique. This includes recognising the individual's knowledge and educational limitations in addition to the limitations of a modality for treating certain conditions best treated by referral to another health professional.

Pulse parameters

In writing this book and developing the pulse qualities within a parameter framework, we consulted over 20 CM texts in order to compile an appropriate methodology. Information pertaining to the location of the three pulse positions on each wrist, finger positioning and the examination of the individual depths at each position was also derived from many sources, to assist in the development of a consistent method of pulse assessment. These methods are clearly detailed in Chapters 5–7. Additionally, the compilation of CM indications and designation has been developed from a combination of a wide range of sources of material including the varying experiences of CM practitioners.

Contextualising pulse within contemporary clinical practice

1

Chapter contents

1.1 Contextualising the learning environment 1
1.2 Addressing misconceptions 2
1.3 Why is a reliable system of pulse taking important? The evidence 3
1.4 Ongoing practice 4

1.1 Contextualising the learning environment

Pulse diagnosis knowledge and its teaching is sometimes written about in nostalgic terms when referring to the traditional methods of learning Chinese medicine (CM) within the master – apprentice system. In this system a student would indenture themselves to a practitioner in exchange for learning CM. This has been termed a 'craft' method of learning, not dissimilar to the European craft system or apprenticeship model (Higgs & Edwards 1999, Swart et al 2005):

> Apprentices learn in the workplace setting, by studying the 'master's art', from simple, highly supervised tasks to more complex and independent tasks, until they become independent practitioners and finally masters themselves. The focus of the apprenticeship system was on the practical knowledge, craft and art of the practice role of a health care worker. At its best, this model offered individual tuition, direct demonstration and supervision at the hands of an expert role model. At worst, this process incorporated poor role models, limited quality control, limited knowledge of the field and lack of foundation in relevant biomedical, clinical and human sciences
> *(Higgs & Edwards 1999: p. 11).*

Traditional apprentice systems also have a tendency to focus on traditions to the exclusion of new innovations. Knowledge associated with the rapid and ongoing development in both CM and biomedical fields of health may additionally be excluded from such systems of training. Thus, as a sole model of education, it is probably unsuitable for providing the basic foundational training required of CM practitioners in the modern context. This is because the contemporary or modern practitioner requires knowledge attained from the biomedical system, in addition to the CM system, in order to practice within an increasingly regulated environment. Such knowledge and regulatory requirements for individuals entering the CM profession today render the traditional apprenticeship model of training as either an adjunct to structured degree courses, or suitable for neophyte practitioners as a postgraduate study stream.

Within the modern context of CM education, most practitioners receive their foundational training from attending structured tertiary courses rather than the craft or apprenticeship system. There are a number of reasons for this. Primarily, there are relatively large numbers of individuals entering the profession with too few established practitioners willing to participate in the training of neophyte practitioners. For example, the British Medical Association noted a 36% increase in acupuncture practitioners and a 51% increase in allied health practitioners using acupuncture from 1998 to the year 2000 (BMA 2000). Such an increase in practitioner numbers within a short time frame could never have been catered for by established CM practitioners using traditional apprenticeship training methods (assuming that the 'new' practitioners were all appropriately trained).

Courses have been created to meet the demand for CM education in many countries, with sound programs structured to produce competent CM health professionals. In some educational sectors, this has meant developing courses and course content to meet specific criteria developed by regulatory or accreditation bodies. For example, the Australian state of Victoria has a Chinese Medicine Registration Board that requires benchmarks in knowledge and associated skills to be met by graduates from university and other tertiary programs in acupuncture and CM in that state in order to practise in that state. The process for developing such courses is not solely driven by educators but is often in response to CM industry directives. For example, a joint working party representing educators and industry bodies developed guidelines for education of primary CM practitioners in Australia, making reference to similar documentation prepared by the World Health Organization (NASC 2001, WHO 1999). In the US the Acupuncture Examining Committee and the National Commission for the Certification of Acupuncturists (NCCA) set industry entry exam requirements for those wishing to be licensed to practice (BMA 2000). Other countries have set minimum competency benchmarks for the safe and knowledgeable practice of acupuncture, such as New Zealand's National Diploma of Acupuncture. In addition to educational requirements, many countries are moving to a regulatory model for the practice of CM and acupuncture on concerns of potential risks of harm to patient health and safety.

Accordingly, this book addresses knowledge and skill guidelines for developing a solid foundation in pulse diagnosis. It is as relevant for those from a range of training methods as it is for those from academia.

It is a flexible modulated guide to pulse diagnosis and is relevant to regulatory requirements for CM education in pulse diagnosis. It is also an appropriate basis for further learning in other systems of pulse diagnosis such as the family lineage teachings or for further study of other complex systems of pulse diagnosis such as described in the *Mai Jing* (Wang, Yang (trans) 1997).

1.2 Addressing misconceptions

A misconception about the use of pulse diagnosis is that it was never intended to be used as the sole method of diagnosis. Ideally, the pulse should be appropriately used in conjunction with other diagnostic practices and this was detailed in several classic literature sources. Yet other classical texts such as the *Nan Jing* clearly emphasised the opposite, noting within its opening chapter that the pulse can be used as the sole diagnostic technique. However, scepticism about such a claim led many commentators over subsequent centuries to question the validity of this claim, warning of the dangers of relying upon a single diagnostic process. The dissent between historical literature sources sets the scene for the perceived usefulness of pulse diagnosis within contemporary practice. While pulse contributes unique information to the clinical diagnostic process, other diagnostic techniques complement this information. Sometimes, pulse diagnosis is not the most suitable diagnostic or most appropriate means of investigation. For example, assessment of the pulse of a patient presenting with an acute sprained ankle would arguably offer little information regarding the extent of the injury sustained to the ligaments. Similarly, Clavey (2003) notes diagnosis should not be dependent solely on the use of pulse for identifying damp/phlegm conditions (p. 296). A systemic condition of damp may not always manifest a damp pulse due to other underlying factors and variables that are present. It is telling that the classical texts on pulse such as the *Mai Jing* also contain information on using pulse diagnosis with other assessment methods. A motivated, highly trained practitioner uses pulse diagnosis as part of the diagnostic process, and when it is appropriate, but does not always diagnose exclusively by it.

Lay and less experienced practitioners may complicate pulse taking by attributing a mystique to pulse palpation, enshrouding the technique in deliberate obscurity. The notion that pulse diagnosis in the hands of an expert practitioner is unparalleled in the diagnosis of illness, in some literature sources, does nothing to discourage such associations. Veith, in translating the *Nei Jing* highlights the emphasis placed on pulse diagnosis in that 'all other methods of determining disease are only subsidiary to palpation and used mainly in connection with it' (p. 42)

Hence it is said: Those who wish to know the inner body feel the pulse and have thus the fundamentals for diagnosis. Those who wish to know the exterior of the body observe death and birth. Of the six (the pulse and the five colors) the feeling of the pulse is the most important medium of diagnosis
(Veith 1972: p. 163).

The Veith translation, first published in 1965, was the first widely available translation of any classical CM text in English. Considering the dearth of information on the practice of CM at the time, and China's closed-door policy, it was widely read and the contents of the book soon integrated into teaching curriculum. Clearly, the Veith translation of the *Nei Jing* soon gripped the imagination of the neophyte professional group emerging in non-Asian countries at this time. Combined with concepts of Eastern spiritualism and the unique nature of acupuncture as the flagship technique that espoused CM, it was not inconceivable for this diagnostic technique to be soon valued over the other methods of clinical examinations by some practitioners. Ironically, in spite of the distinct dichotomy that some proponents of CM pursue between the biomedical and CM systems of health, this view of pulse diagnosis was not dissimilar to that held by practitioners of Western medicine throughout the early modern period and into the late nineteenth century.

In spite of the publishing and refinement of pulse theory over time, theories that have been shown to have little application within the CM framework for over 1000 years continue to be reiterated as the practice of CM has moved beyond its original cultural, demographical and environmental location. Whether through reiteration of previous pulse literature or derived from clinicians' need or desire to conform to traditional theoretical constructs even though they have had little basis in the diagnosis or treatment of illness, such information has been retained in the pulse diagnostic framework. Here research is required to illuminate clinically useful information on pulse diagnosis from clinically irrelevant information. However, research and ready enquiry of the pulse assumptions and theories should be tempered with respect for a body of accumulated learning and knowledge acquired through clinical observation and empirical practice: just because something is old doesn't mean it is outdated. It would be folly to disregard valid empirical knowledge. Conversely, however, because something is simply old doesn't mean it is necessarily clinically useful. A balance needs to attained – the grain sorted from the chaff.

In this context, this book seeks to address some misconceptions about pulse, and its practice within CM, through examination of the available literature and evidence. The book also seeks to provide a clear guide to the practical use of pulse assessment and diagnostic techniques. To this end, we have attempted to use unambiguous terms, define obscure concepts as we use them and provide instruction on pulse diagnosis as a component of the diagnosis approach for best practice outcomes. This book seeks to promote critical appraisal skills useful in differentiating clinically relevant knowledge from non-clinically relevant claims within the literature.

1.3 Why is a reliable system of pulse taking important? The evidence

Although the historical importance of pulse palpation and its crucial role in the diagnostic process continues to be reiterated in many contemporary CM texts, the underlying assumptions and concepts that underpin pulse as a clinically useful technique have not been substantiated in studies that have used reliable research methods. The paucity of evidence means that long-held and untested assumptions are taken as clinical fact even though no independent evidence has been gathered to either support or refute their validity. For example:

- Are there differences in the pulse characteristics between the three radial arterial pulse positions Cun, Guan, and Chi?
- Are practitioners capable of discerning the minute features of quality that are said to be present in the arterial pulses?
- Can practitioners reliably discern these changes and agree with each other in their interpretation of the pulse?

It is the last of these questions that most notably impacts on the legitimacy of pulse palpation as a valid examination technique. Reliability is important in establishing whether the findings are valid, and for purposes of communication. That is, is the practitioner interpreting changes in the pulse validly as representing a particular disease? Is the practitioner consistently reliable in measuring these changes? For any examination technique, establishing that there are high levels of inter-rater reliability underpins the usefulness of the approach. In relation to pulse diagnosis, this takes on extra importance because of the inherent subjectivity of pulse taking.

In light of the subjective nature of pulse diagnosis, Dharmananda (2000) in his essay on the modern practice of pulse diagnosis claims that there is always the danger of practitioners 'fantasising' that the pulse being felt is providing diagnostically valuable information. That is, reading or interpreting something in the pulse when in actual fact there is nothing there.

3

Conversely, and equally dangerous, the practitioner may fail to recognise the presentation of a diagnostically distinct pulse quality or a change in a particular aspect of the pulse which should be used for diagnosis. Both situations may occur from either poor education or poor observational skills. It is also common for experienced practitioners to disregard pulse findings simply because these did not correlate with findings from the other methods of diagnosis. In all situations, diagnoses and hence appropriate treatment may be compromised and practice will consequently suffer.

Because of the subjective nature of pulse assessment using manual techniques this book proposes the 'pulse parameter' system of pulse identification that has been previously shown to have reliability yet retains relevance within the CM diagnostic framework.

1.4 Ongoing practice

Although modern practice has doubtlessly been improved by the introduction of new aids, it seems certain that the average physician's ability to feel and to interpret the pulse has declined
(O'Rourke et al 1992: p. 9).

It is anticipated that the information presented in this book will assist in reversing this trend. To understand any field of medicine one needs to understand its composite parts and the relationship of each to the examination process. Pulse palpation in CM contributes to this process. In CM pulse diagnosis sits within the four examination categories as part of the palpation rubric. The other categories are questioning, listening and observation. Each, including pulse diagnosis, has its strengths and weakness. Some are more appropriate to use for different conditions, situations or with different patients, yet each contributes information for arriving at a diagnosis or understanding of the individual's condition. Too often however, the practitioner may favour one approach over another or set greater store on one technique above all else. Pulse diagnosis is too often viewed in such a fashion. It is eschewed by some for its subjectivity, yet favoured by others as being the technique with almost mystical properties. Little has been written on the practical application of this technique, and less is recorded on the intricate system of haemo-

dynamics that is the pulse. To truly appreciate and understand pulse diagnosis one needs to understand the vessels, the blood, pressure waves and flow waves and the interaction of these in the presence of illness and health. In this book we will examine in detail what the ancient Chinese practitioner termed the *mài*, the 'vessels' or 'pulse' and explore the anatomical basis of the arterial system and the complex formation that is the pulse. Biomedical knowledge contributes to our understanding of pulse and will be included when relevant in tandem with information from the CM pulse literature. Together they will provide a firm foundation for the reliable and ongoing practice of pulse diagnosis.

References

BMA 2000 Acupuncture: efficacy, safety and practice. British Medical Association report. Harwood Academic Publishers, London

Clavey S 2003 Fluid physiology and pathology in traditional Chinese medicine, 2nd edn. Churchill Livingstone, Edinburgh

Dharmananda S 2000 The significance of traditional pulse diagnosis in the modern practice of Chinese medicine. Institute for Traditional Medicine, Portland, OR. Online. Available: <http://www.itmonline.org/arts/pulse>

Higgs J, Edwards H 1999 Educating beginning practitioners: challenges for health professional education. Butterworth Heinemann, Oxford

NASC 2001 National Academic Standards Committee for Traditional Chinese Medicine. The Australian guidelines for traditional Chinese medicine education. AACMA, Brisbane

O'Rourke M, Kelly R, Avolio A 1992 The arterial pulse. Lea & Febiger, Philadelphia

Scheid V 2002 Chinese medicine in contemporary China. Duke University Press, London

Swart J, Mann C, Brown S et al 2005 Human resource development. Butterworth Heinemann, Oxford

Unschuld P (translator) 1986 Nan-Ching: the classic of difficult issues. University of California Press, Berkeley

Veith I (translator) 1972 The Yellow Emperor's classic of internal medicine. University of California Press, Berkeley

Wang SH, Yang S (translator) 1997 The pulse classic: a translation of the Mai Jing. Blue Poppy Press, Boulder, CO

WHO 1999 Guidelines on basic training and safety in acupuncture. World Health Organization, Geneva

The pulse:
its place in contemporary biomedical and CM practice

2

Chapter contents

2.1 The circulatory system 5
2.2 The pulse 6
2.3 Blood 10
2.4 Summary 13
2.5 The pulse in biomedicine 13
2.6 The pulse in contemporary CM clinical practice 17

This chapter introduces the concepts of blood flow and pressure waves, and looks at the radial artery and its essential features, and its relationship to pulse diagnosis. The chapter is intended as a brief summary of a complex and diverse body of literature that is available on the topic, and is presented here to support further discussions on CM pulse diagnosis presented later in this book. It should not be considered definitive but may be used as a basis for further investigations into understanding the physiological basis of the pulse from other literature sources.

2.1 The circulatory system

The circulatory system functions as a transportation system. It distributes the nutrients and substances required for healthy metabolism to tissue cells and organs while removing metabolic waste from those same cells and organs. According to Berne & Levy (1981: p. 1) the components of the circulatory system can in their simplest form be reduced to a pump moving fluids through a distributing network of tubes. Yet this analogy of the circulatory system is overly simplistic when the circulatory system is considered within the context of health. Rather than the passive distributing network implied in the analogy, it is actually a dynamic regulatory system assisting in the maintaining body temperature; regulate volume flow of blood; and act as a communication network between different body regions. These functions of the circulatory system depend on controlled changes in the width of blood vessels (vasoconstriction and vasodilatation) and the pump-like action of the heart to cause blood flow. These functions are all mediated through an innate biofeedback system which helps maintain homeostasis and organ function. For example, by reducing the blood vessel diameter (vasoconstriction), the surface area of the blood vessel exposed to the environment also decreases and body heat is retained while concurrently reducing blood flow to the superficial and peripheral regions of the body. Increasing blood vessel diameter (vasodilatation) increases the surface area of the blood vessel, thus increasing the rate at which body heat is lost to the environment. The supply of nutrients circulating to the tissue cells is regulated by this same vasodilatation/vasoconstriction mechanism. Chemical transmitters, hormones and other chemical markers produced by the body and required for regulating homeostasis are similarly distributed in this manner.

The body's organs and tissues have varying nutritional and blood flow requirements for their health and normal functioning. Such requirements also vary depending on the time of day and level of activity. This is reflected in the differing density and type of blood vessels found in different regions of the body. For example, the skin has small requirements for copious blood flow and so the capillary network is fine but densely distributed; useful in times of tissue repair due to trauma or for dispersing body heat during exercise. On the other hand, the brain has a high and constant requirement for blood flow and several large arteries serve this purpose by maintaining a continuous supply of blood flow to the organ, while the lungs are rich in small capillary beds to assist in the transfer of metabolic waste for oxygen. Similarly, other organs vary in both the density of blood vessels present and anatomical structure of the vessels depending on function and purpose. The kidneys in particular have a unique circulation, using specialised arterial structures to increase partial blood pressures to filter toxins from the blood.

These concentrations of blood vessels that serve such a specialised function can be termed a microcirculation. Berne & Levy have noted that some chemicals, whether intrinsic or introduced by therapeutic interventions, may have differing affects on the microcirculation and on arterial smooth muscle:

In studies on this interesting and important type of muscle, great care should be taken in extrapolating results from one tissue to another or from the same tissue under different physiological conditions. For example, some agents elicit vasodilation in some vascular beds and vasoconstriction in others (1981: p. 124).

In the context of health assessment, it is logical to conclude that dysfunction or increased demands on an organ, whether in response to neural, hormonal or chemical stimulus, should mean that the circulatory requirements, and hence the microcirculation of that organ, would be affected.

Extrapolating about Chinese medical ideas then, it is not inconceivable to link such microcirculatory changes posited by Berne and Levy to Chinese medical ideas on pulse diagnosis. In this sense, it can be that such microcirculatory changes when applying CM theory, are detectable elsewhere in the body, and in particular in the radial artery, via signals carried in the haemodynamic pulse wave. Dai et al (1985) hypothe-

sised and demonstrated that disturbances in the arterial blood flow in one region of the body can be detected elsewhere in the body using the arterial pulse wave. They did this through intermittent occlusion of blood flow in the right leg, showing a corresponding reduction in the force level of the pulse in both left and right radial arteries (using pressure transducer measurements). Therefore, it is not illogical to state that changes in an organ's microcirculation would similarly affect arterial haemodynamics detectable elsewhere in the circulatory system.

At any given point in time, the pulse should reflect the circulatory system's ability to undertake the distributing and regulatory functions described above. What is described as a 'pulse' in the clinical context is foremost, and always, a product of the circulatory system, generated by pressure changes which occur with heart movement. In this context, pulse diagnosis is used to assess heart movement, measuring the rate or frequency of pulse occurrence and whether this is occurring in a rhythmic fashion. From the assessment of pulse movement, it is inferred that the heart is moving and functioning in a particular fashion. Yet these two 'movement' characteristics, rate and rhythm, do not adequately explain or describe the range of information that CM literature, or indeed biomedicine, claim as being able to obtain from assessment of the pulse. Thus, in addition to pulse rate and rhythm, there are several other characteristics of the pulse that are assessed. (These are discussed in Chapters 6 and 7.) In a CM diagnostic framework, each is used to infer the function of a particular aspect of the body via the degree of change occurring in each of the pulse characteristics. The practitioner aims to determine whether the perceived changes in the pulse have arisen due to internal organ function, compromised blood flow, or external conditions such as viruses, bacteria or other environmental factors. It is the body's response to these factors or attempt to maintain homeostasis or balance which is of interest in the process termed 'pulse diagnosis'. Investigation and observation of changes in the pulse and their attribution to health is the aim of pulse diagnosis. This leads us to the next question – exactly what is the pulse?

2.2 The pulse

The pulse is a physiological phenomenon propagated throughout the arterial system. It is generally viewed as a travelling pressure wave caused by the rhythmic contraction and relaxation of the heart. Thus the pulse can be described in terms of systole, when the pulse amplitude increases or the heart contracts; and diastole, when the amplitude decreases or the heart relaxes (Box 2.1). A pulse can also be thought of in terms of any regular movement or change in differential pressure that manifests as a rise and fall of fluid in a vessel.

Box 2.1

Some definitions

- Systole: The period when the left ventricle of the heart is in contraction forcing blood into the aorta. *Systolic pressure* is the maximal pressure exerted in the arteries by the heart during systole.
- Diastole: The period when the left ventricle of the heart is in relaxation following systole, when it is refilling with blood. *Diastolic pressure* is the baseline or resting pressure during diastole, when the heart is at rest. Diastole is the constant pressure that is always present in the artery.
- Blood pressure: The pressure exerted on the walls of the blood vessels. Blood pressure measurements describe the maximal systolic pressure over the resting basal diastolic pressure. Pressure is measured in millimetres of mercury (mmHg). Average blood pressure is 120/80 mmHg.

In terms of clinical practice, a 'pulse' is usually associated with a palpable pressure movement. For example, the radial artery, located at the wrist overlying the radius, is a major site at which to feel the pulse.

The pressure wave produced with heart movement is often considered the 'pulse', but for purposes of pulse diagnosis using manual palpation the pulse encompasses more than the pressure wave alone. In addition to pressure waves, O'Rourke et al. (1992) note the pulse also encompasses flow waves; the actual movement of blood. They note there is even a third type of wave called diameter waves produced with vessel diameter changes, but these waves are very similar to the pressure wave (O'Rourke et al 1992: p. 17) and, as such, will not be discussed any further in this book. Each of these waves is distinctly different when looking at objective measurements of their contours. Therefore, what is regarded as a single 'pulse wave' is in fact a composite of at least two different types of waves. There is the pressure wave, the actual force caused by heart movement, and there is the flow wave, determined by how the pressure wave acts on the actual flow movement of blood. How each contributes to the overall pulse formation probably determines the spectrum of diverse pulse qualities in the CM literature.

In the context of health, it is important to understand that the pulse wave is not a static artefact of heart movement, nor does the pulse remain in constant shape as it moves through the arterial system. It is rather in a constant state of change, acted on by the characteristics of the vessel conduit, the functional state of the organs and tissue and the quality of blood itself, which is in turn determined by the state of health of the individual. It is the cumulative effect of the whole range of these factors that moulds the pulse wave into the pulse that eventually arrives at the radial artery as

felt by practitioners. Therefore, the essential characteristics of how the pulse presents to the practitioner when palpating the pulse infer the nature of illness and an individual's state of health, an intimate 'record' of the bodily environment. Pressure waves, flow waves and blood are discussed in further detail below.

2.2.1 Pressure waves

Heart movement produces pressure which causes arterial blood to flow. Pressure waves are generated by the expulsion of blood with heart contraction into the aorta, causing dilatation of that vessel (Guyton and Hall 2006). Thus the greater the blood volume expelled, the greater the pressure wave produced, assuming the aorta's elastic characteristics remain constant. Blood flows in a closed system of vessels. Any generated pressure therefore affects the entire system. As the pressure wave rises and falls with heart movement, so the blood movement ebbs and flows. In this closed system of pressure and flow, the pressure wave always precedes the actual blood flow, moving considerably faster than its causative affect on the movement of blood (Berne & Levy 1981: p. 105).

The pressure wave has two distinctive components. The first or systolic component has a rise to maximum pressure, followed by a slow decline with a notch or slight increase in pressure from aortic valve closure when the backflow of blood in the aorta overcomes the expulsion force of blood from the heart (Fig. 2.1). According to O'Rourke et al. (1992: p. 40) the second component of pulse formation is due to the phenomenon of wave reflection. Reflective waves are an echo of the initial primary wave that travels from the heart to the periphery. As the arteries narrow in the periphery this results in increased arterial resistance, which causes the pulse wave to rebound, causing a reflective wave to move back towards the heart. Reflective waves occur from the lower and upper body regions. Because the blood vessels of the lower body are larger, the reflective wave affect is also larger than the reflective wave resulting from arterial narrowing in the upper limb. However, both the lower and upper reflective waves have systemic effects and are not confined to the limb in which they were generated. In this way, reflective waves from the lower body interact with the pressure waves in the upper part of the body.

Reflective waves are visualised as a secondary pressure peak in the pulse pressure wave, usually occurring in the diastolic component of the pulse period. Depending on the degree of arterial stiffness, reflective waves can augment the initial primary pressure wave, moving from diastole into the systole component due to arterial hardening (Fig. 2.2). When this occurs the reflective wave merges with the primary pressure wave moving away from the heart, resulting in a greater and longer

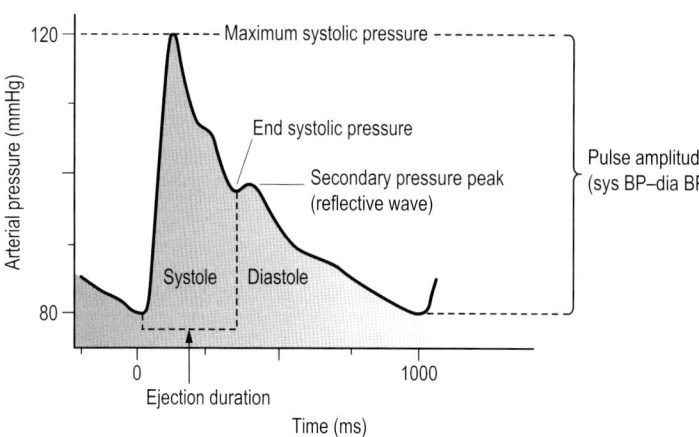

Figure 2.1
Features of the radial arterial pulse wave.

Box 2.2

Sphygmography

Diagrammatic representations of pressure waves called **sphygmograms** or **sphygmographs** are easy to obtain using pressure sensors. Many CM texts on pulse diagnosis use representation of these graphs to attempt to illustrate different pulse types. Although a useful educative tool, they are limited in their use to represent changes in the pulse wave that occur with different illnesses and caution should be used when looking at these, or mistaking them for the 'pulse'. This is because many of the CM pulse qualities are not solely dependent for their formation on pressure variations or pressure waves, which are the sole purpose of this form of measurement.

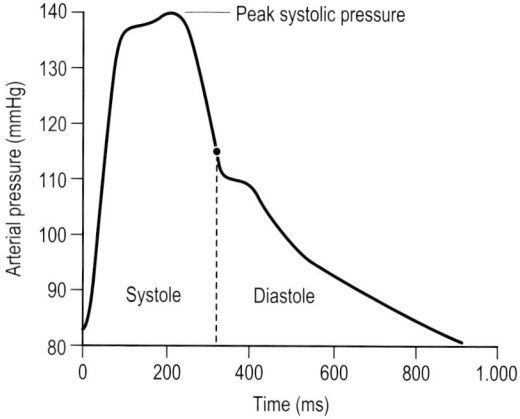

Figure 2.2
The radial arterial pulse wave and augmentation by reflective waves. (After Fig. 3.3.1 in AtCor Medical 2006, A clinical guide: pulse wave analysis, with permission of AtCor Medical Pty.)

duration of pressure during systole than would normally be seen. This often occurs in individuals with illness and conditions in which the arteries become stiff or inflexible. This causes a maximal systolic blood pressure rise above the usual pressure range regarded as healthy for that individual's age. (An increase in arterial tension also increases the overall flow rate of blood through the arteries).

Figure 2.1 illustrates the pressure wave contour typically measured at the radial artery. This is considerably different from the same pressure wave if measured in another part of the circulatory system such as the carotid artery (Fig. 2.3). This is because the anatomy of the arteries varies throughout the circulatory system and this in turn impacts on how the pulse moves through the artery. For example, some arteries are more elastic than others, so their rate of expansion is greater under pressure. This difference is noticeable with palpation when comparing the pulse in the carotid

artery in the neck with the pulse in the radial artery in the wrist. The carotid artery has a broader expansive movement because it is more elastic than the radial artery, which has a more distinct arterial wall because it has a large proportion of smooth muscle and thus is not as expansive. The arteries' capacity to expand with pressure is termed capacitance. The capacitance of a blood vessel is not constant.

Capacitance varies under different conditions, such as differing levels of physical or psychological stress causing a corresponding increase in vessel hardening or vasoconstriction. In this situation capacitance decreases. In addition to capacitance, the pressure wave is also dependent on the stroke volume or amount of blood ejected from the heart with heart contraction. An increased volume of blood gives an increased expansion of the arterial wall, and decreasing blood volume

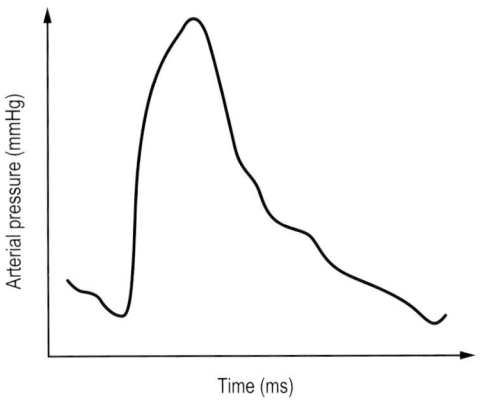

Figure 2.3
Features of the carotid arterial pulse wave. Note the rounded contour of the peak pulse pressure due to the carotid elastic properties and relative large diameter.

has the reverse effect (assuming the arterial width remains constant).

The major blood vessels are elastic and relatively wide contributing to smooth and unimpeded flow of blood (Stettler *et al.* 1986). This means the pressure wave remains similar to that at the aorta and throughout all major arteries until the periphery. At the periphery, the arteries begin to narrow. A decreasing arterial width means the force of the pressure and blood flow are compacted together and the pressure exerted from within the artery increases. This is evident in blood pressure measurements between peripheral vessels such as the brachial and radial arteries and the aorta. Maximal pressure in the peripheral arteries such as the radial artery can be 30% greater than maximal pressures in the aorta. However, the force exerted by the pulse pressure wave on the blood vessels falls substantially on entering the smaller capillaries and other vessels beyond the radial and other arteries. Here, Guyton and Hall (2000) note the combined diameter of all these small vessels is greater than that of the arteries and so the force exerted by the pressure wave decreases because of the relative increase in surface area, and the force of the pressure wave is diluted. It should be noted that it is the pressure differential between the aorta and these small capillary networks which causes blood flow; blood flows from an area of high pressure into an area of low pressure (Guyton & Hall 2000).

In CM it is often said that the 'Qi moves the Blood, and the Blood follows the Qi'. That is, function acts on the blood and the blood responds. In this sense, the pressure wave causes the blood to flow and the blood flow responds accordingly, producing a tidal flow through the vessels. This tidal flow is termed a flow wave and is quite distinctly separate from the pressure wave.

2.2.2 Flow waves

Flow waves refer to the longitudinal movement of blood through the vessel and are the second major component of the pulse wave. Flow waves depend on there being a sufficient volume of blood. It is obvious that if blood volume becomes insufficient then there would be no flow wave. Flow wave formation also depends on the nature of the essential constituents of the fluid. For example, imagine applying a pressure wave to a container of water, and a similar pressure wave to a container of honey. Because of the innate difference in the 'thickness' or viscosity of the two fluids, each pressure wave would have a different impact in the creation of the flow wave. The water would transmit the pressure wave into a flow wave easily, with a noticeable surface movement. Because of the thickness of the honey this would not be as noticeable, most likely producing only sluggish movement. In this way, blood can also vary, becoming more viscous or fluid depending on the relative ratio of cells and fluid that make up the blood. However, assuming sufficient blood volume and appropriate viscosity flow waves are determined by two additional factors. These are ventricular contraction and mechanical characteristics of the arterial wall.

Ventricular contraction determines the amount of momentum imparted into the blood forcing it to flow through the vessel. The strength of ventricular contraction also has a relationship to the volume and speed at which blood is expelled from the left ventricle of the heart during systole (Opie 2004). For example, if the heart were to contract strongly, and assuming sufficient time and blood volume for the heart to have refilled during diastole, then the peak systolic pressure would be achieved more rapidly resulting in a sharper incline to the peak if recorded by a sphygmogram. This would cause a greater volume of blood to flow into the aorta at a given point in time. This volume output is referred to as stroke volume (SV) (see Box 2.3). Obviously, if blood volume is diminished or heart contraction slowed then the flow wave would be similarly affected.

The second additional factor in flow wave formation involves mechanical properties of the arterial wall. When the heart contracts, a pressure wave moves into the aorta causing it to expand. When the pressure is removed during heart relaxation (diastole) the aorta returns or recoils to its normal shape. The recoil releases this potential energy stored during expansion back into the blood, causing the blood to flow forward. In conditions in which the elasticity of the arteries is compromised, recoil is diminished and the blood flow becomes retarded, which compromises circulation and the associated functions of the circulatory system. For example, if the arteries were relatively stiff, then a secondary fluctuation or reflective wave would move from diastole into systole, augmenting the initial flow wave,

Box 2.3

Cardiac output

The total volume of blood flow in 1 minute is termed **cardiac output** (CO). CO depends on the blood volume expelled by the heart during systole of each heartbeat, termed **stroke volume** (SV), and the total number of heartbeats per minute or **heart rate** (HR). Thus:

$$CO \text{ (ml/min)} = SV \text{ (ml/beat)} \times HR \text{ (beats/min)}$$

This relationship is commonly used in biomedical practice for determining the heart's pump function in maintaining adequate blood flow for tissue perfusion. Blood pressure and resistance to blood flow also have a direct bearing on cardiac output.

whereas a relaxed or elastic artery would not produce augmentation of the initial wave. Conditions affecting the arterial wall affect the flow wave. This relationship between arterial properties and characteristic of ventricular contraction is described as vascular impedance.

2.3 Blood

Blood is an important component of the formation of the pulse. It is a complex fluid, composed of a plasma liquid base and several formed particles, the most prominent of which are red blood cells, which make up 99% of all particle types found in blood. Other components include:

- White blood cells
- Platelets
- Proteins (albumins, globulins, fibrinogen) dissolved in the plasma.

For these reasons blood is referred to as a liquid tissue. Blood is the medium in which the pulse wave propagates from the heart to the periphery. Therefore, changes in the blood medium – that is, changes in any of the ratio of its components – will affect the propagation of the pulse wave. Changes can occur in a number of ways. They can arise due to illness, from trauma producing blood loss, or from diet where an individual's inadequate intake of appropriate food groups adversely affects the quality and quantity of the blood. In this way, the ratio of the different cell components of blood can vary between people and can vary within the same individual over time. Blood may consequently 'thicken' or 'thin'. The relative degree of 'thickness' is termed *viscosity*.

Blood viscosity depends on the ratio of cells to plasma in the blood. The higher the proportion of cells, the denser or more viscous is blood. This means that blood becomes more difficult to move through the blood vessels as resistance to its smooth flow increases. For example, polycythemia is a state in which the red blood cell ratio is raised, causing blood to become more viscous. In this state blood flow fluidity is affected, flow velocity slows and blood pressure becomes raised due to increased resistance to its flow in the vessels. Chronic smoking, athletic training and high altitudes can all cause an increase in the ratio of red blood cells. An increased demand for oxygen by the body causes an increased number of red blood cells to assist with oxygen transportation. The concentration of red blood cells can also increase when fluid is lost from the blood plasma through dehydration or burns. Alternatively, dietary intake of iron may fluctuate depending on food sources. Eventually, this also affects blood through changes in the red blood cell ratio and changes in blood viscosity, and changes in the pulse wave will consequently also occur. For example, the decreasing iron levels and haemoglobin associated with anaemia are often accompanied by regulatory changes in blood pressure via vasodilatory mechanisms in an attempt to maintain homeostasis as red blood cell 'quality' and ratio decrease. This in turn affects the propagation of the pressure wave and resultant flow wave. Additionally, sudden loss of blood volume due to haemorrhage (cells and fluid) also affects pressure and flow waves. Interestingly, blood volume can also decrease when fluid moves out of the blood plasma, as occurs in dehydration.

2.3.1 Velocity of blood flow

As hinted at in the description of pressure waves, the speed or velocity at which blood moves through the vessels is not constant. There are a number of variables that affect this. The first and most obvious is heart rate. As pressure exerted by the heart increases during systole, blood flow increases under the influence of the pressure wave; as the heart relaxes, so blood flow slows. Any change in pulse rate frequency, or strength at which the heart contracts during systole, will affect blood velocity. Blood flow velocity is measured in centimetres per second (cm/s).

The velocity of blood flow also depends on arterial width. When an artery is wide the blood velocity slows in comparison to blood flow in a narrow artery, in which the velocity hastens. The velocity of blood flow is inversely related to arterial width. Tortora & Grabowski (1996) state:

> This means that blood flows slowest where the cross-sectional area is greatest, just as a river flows more slowly as it becomes broader. Each time an artery branches, the total cross-sectional area (diameter) of all its branches is greater than that of the original vessel. On the other hand, when branches combine,

for example, as venules merge to form veins, the total cross-sectional area becomes smaller . . . Thus the velocity of blood flow decreases as it flows from the aorta to arteries to arterioles then capillaries and increases as it leaves capillaries and returns to the heart (p. 620).

For pulse diagnosis purposes the relative degree of arterial wall tension also influences blood flow velocity (arterial wall tension can increase without arterial narrowing). Blood velocity hastens because the artery resists the pressure being exerted by the pulse wave, no longer expanding as it usually would. Consequently, this energy is redirected back into the forward movement of blood. This is likely to be seen in conditions where arterial tension increases via the contraction of the arterial muscle layer (the tunica media), as in cases of psychological or physical stress ('fright, flight or fight' response). It is hypothesised that the Stringlike (Wiry) pulse may be attributed partly to this action and the consequent change in blood velocity and resultant diminishing of pulse wave contour. Additionally, pulses which have a distinct amplitude/contour or shape, such as the Slippery pulse, could be associated with a decrease in arterial hardening in which the pressure pulse easily expands the vessel wall, shaping it to the flow wave, assuming there is sufficient blood volume for this to occur.

2.3.2 Arteries

The two primary subdivisions of the arteries are the *central* and *peripheral* subdivisions. The central subdivision encompasses all arteries in the region of the torso. Circulatory activity in this region is collectively referred to as the central haemodynamics. The arteries located in the central region are wide and relatively elastic, to deal with the high volume flows and the relatively large pressures that are exerted from within. Examples of central arteries are the carotid artery and the aorta. Their elastic properties also assist in the propagation of the pulse signal further along the arterial trunk to the peripheral blood vessels.

The peripheral subdivision encompasses all arteries located in the limbs. Circulatory activity in this region is collectively referred to as the peripheral haemodynamics. Examples of peripheral arteries include the brachial and radial arteries. The arteries in the periphery are described as muscular arteries, having a greater proportion of smooth muscle relative to elastic fibres in the inner layer of the blood vessels. Consequently, Tortora and Grabowski (1996) note the peripheral arteries have a greater vasodilatory and vasoconstricting function than is found with centrally located arteries such as the aorta (see Box 2.4).

Box 2.4

Elastic and muscular properties of arteries

Differences in the elastic qualities versus the muscular properties of the central and peripheral arteries can be felt by comparing the carotid arterial pulse with the radial arterial pulse. The **carotid artery** is located lateral to the larynx, medial to the sternocleidomastoid muscle. By gently palpating one of the arteries it can be felt that the carotid arterial pulse has a noticeably larger amplitude from the base pressure to the maximum pressure. In comparison, it will be found that the radial artery has noticeably less amplitude difference and is not as expansive across the fingers. Note also that the difference in width between the carotid and radial artery also influences how the pulse feels when palpated.

2.3.3 The radial artery

The radial artery is classified as a peripheral artery. It is a prime area for palpating pulse, and is unique for use in clinical practice as the 'vascular properties in the upper limbs are less affected by ageing, arterial pressure, or various manoeuvres as compared to vessels in the trunk and lower limbs' (Chen et al 1997: p. 1834). This means that the radial pulse probably reflects disease-related changes irrespective of an individual's age. This makes it an ideal area for pulse assessment, and it is the primary site used in both the biomedical and CM systems.

The radial artery commences at the bifurcation of the brachial artery, just distal to the elbow crease, following the lateral portions of the forearm into the hand (Strandring et al 2005). It is the wrist portion of the radial artery, approximately 3–5 cm in length, which is often used for pulse assessment. At this region the radial artery sits superficially, supported by the styloid process of the radius and local tendons such as the brachioradialis. The radial artery is covered by a thin layer of collagen fibres, fat and keratinised cells which form the dermal and epidermal fasciae (Lanir 1986). The radial artery forms two distinct arterial branches. The first is the dorsal carpal branch which meets the ulna dorsal carpal branch and forms the dorsal carpal network that eventually feeds to the middle, ring and little fingers. The second branch is the first dorsal metacarpal artery which supplies blood to the thumb and index finger (Strandring et al 2005) (Fig. 2.4).

All arteries consist of three layers (Fig. 2.5):

11

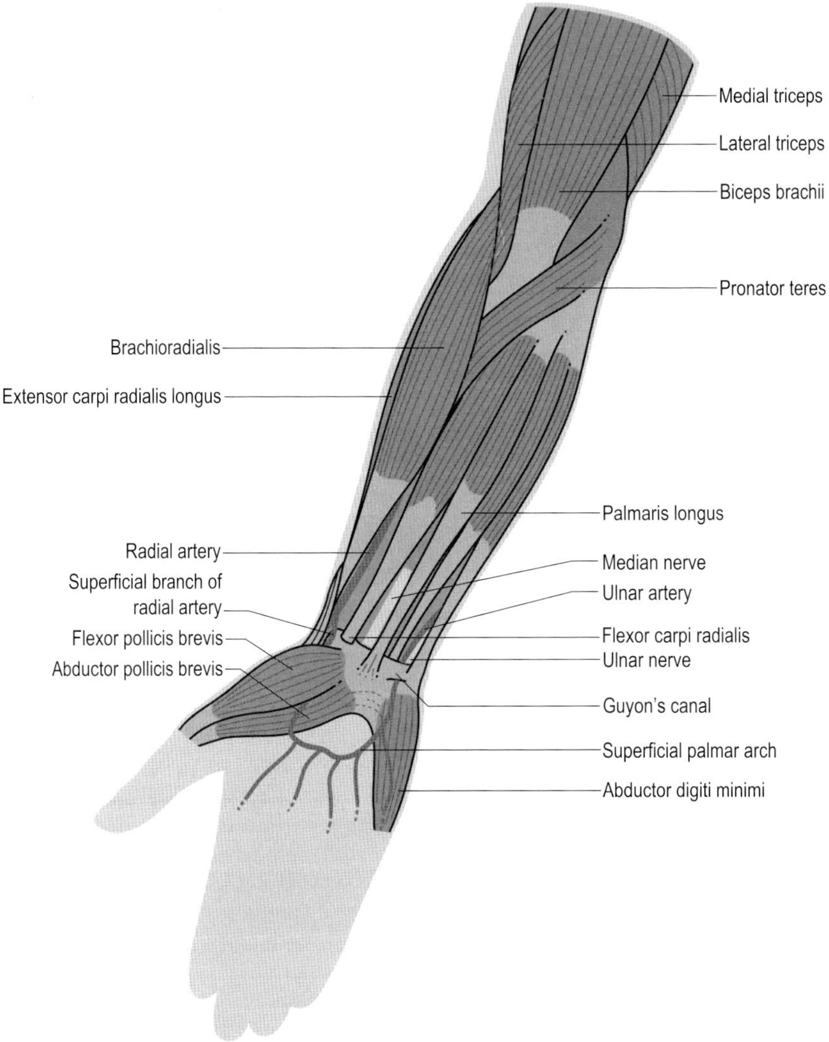

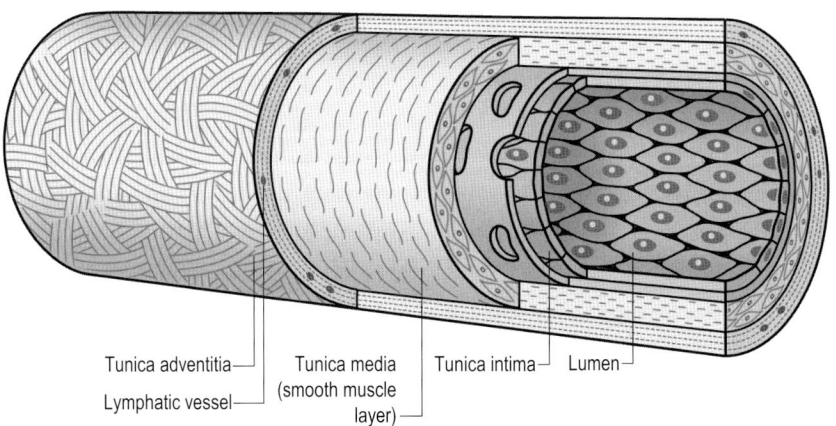

Medial triceps
Lateral triceps
Biceps brachii
Pronator teres
Brachioradialis
Extensor carpi radialis longus
Palmaris longus
Radial artery
Median nerve
Superficial branch of radial artery
Ulnar artery
Flexor pollicis brevis
Flexor carpi radialis
Abductor pollicis brevis
Ulnar nerve
Guyon's canal
Superficial palmar arch
Abductor digiti minimi

12

Figure 2.4
Position of the radial artery relative to other structures of the forearm.

Tunica adventitia
Lymphatic vessel
Tunica media (smooth muscle layer)
Tunica intima
Lumen

Figure 2.5
Structural layers of the radial artery. (After Fig. 7.4 in Gray's anatomy: the anatomical basis of clinical practice, 39th edn, with permission of Elsevier.)

- Tunica externa: The external connective tissue which supports the vessel
- Tunica media: The middle smooth muscle layer that constricts and dilates arterial width
- Tunica intima: The internal elastic layer and thick layer of endothelial cells in contact with the blood. This elastic layer makes the vessel wall smooth for frictionless blood flow and stretches with pulsatile flow during systole and diastole.

The relative proportions of the three wall layers differ depending on the location and associated function that the artery undertakes. For example, the radial artery has a relatively greater proportion of smooth muscle (tunica media layer) than centrally located arteries, such as the aorta, to assist in its distribution and regulation of blood flow.

For the practitioner, it is important to understand that each vessel layer can contribute its own unique 'signature' to the presentation of the pulse wave and how it is felt when palpated at an arterial site. The tunica media and tunica intima are particularly important in the practice of pulse diagnosis. These distinct arterial composites of the arterial wall are identifiers of disease and are just as important as the actual pulse movement. A loss of the smooth internal wall through plaque formation in arteriosclerosis will also affect blood flow. This in turn may activate platelet aggregation and formation of clots, or simply affect the smooth flow of blood causing turbulence. In this way, pulse diagnosis is not simply just about the 'pulse', it also encompasses the assessment of the blood vessel wall.

2.4 Summary

The pulse is a physiological phenomenon propagated throughout the arterial system and can be viewed as an indication of the circulatory system's capacity to undertake the distribution of essential substances required for metabolism to body tissue and organs. In the context of health, the pulse is a complex physiological sign and can be described in terms of systole and diastole. It is primarily composed of pressure waves (including reflective waves), and flow waves.

Once produced, a pulse wave undergoes a series of changes as it moves from the heart or central regions of the body into the peripheral blood vessels of the arms and legs. By the time the pulse wave arrives at the radial artery it may have a distinctly different shape and contour than it had when initially produced by the heart. Variables that influence the presentation of the pulse as felt with palpation at the radial artery include:

- Anatomical structure of the blood vessel
  - Arterial width
  - Arterial tension
  - Ratio of elastic versus muscular tissue
- Viscosity or density of blood
- Blood volume
- Stroke volume of blood flow
- Region of the body the pulse is being palpated
- Heart function.

These, in turn, are influenced by the neural, hormonal and chemoregulatory systems for blood pressure and maintaining blood flow for purposes of homeostasis or balance in health and illness. A change in health status affects homeostasis balance, which in turn affects the pulse.

2.5 The pulse in biomedicine

The procedure of pulse palpation is termed *sphygmology*, literally meaning 'the study of the pulse'. The term *sphygmos* derives from Greek meaning literally a pulse or throb. In contemporary biomedical practice the pulse is used in the assessment of several conditions mainly affecting circulation and reflecting heart function. The pulse is primarily viewed as a product of the heart and compliance of the vascular system, and is highly dependent on the use of sophisticated devices able to record and measure variables quantitatively. Accordingly, the term *pulse palpation* is largely used with reference to the determinant of pulsatile strength, heart rate and heart rhythm by manual palpation. Yet pulse palpation has not always been used in this manner within biomedicine; it once had an equally broad application for identifying 'qualitative' changes in the pulse, as is still claimed in CM.

The principles of sphygmology are derived from the works of ancient Greek physicians, in particular Galen (131–199 CE) (Naqvi & Blaufox 1998), but can be traced back even further to Hippocrates (approximately 450–350 BCE). Other important historical figures in the development of pulse in the health assessment process included Aegimius, whose writings founded the concept of pulse as a diagnostic technique; Rufus of Ephesus and his treatise *Synopsis on Pulses*; and Herophilus of Alexandria, the reputed founder of sphygmology (Bedford 1951, Hsu 2005, Kuriyama 1999, Lloyd 1996). But it was Galen's prolific discourse on the use of pulse in assessing health, including commentaries on the pulse writings of his predecessors, which meant his thinking on pulse would dominant the practice of pulse by subsequent occidental medical healers.

Galen's interpretations and descriptions of pulse characteristics have more in common with the CM view of the pulse than with modern biomedical principles. They include differentiating pulse speed, length, width and depth to the body's homeostasis, and describing them in terms of excess or deficiency depending on the presenting pathology. Variables affecting the pulse presentation were listed as including age, seasons, food, pregnancy and the environment. The pulse was also referred to in terms of organic pulses; authors later interpreted organic pulses as an extension 'by which each organ imparted its personality to the pulse' (Bedford 1951: p. 428). That is, specific pulse types were specifically seen as arising from different organs.

Pulse diagnosis in the intervening centuries since Galen's time remained largely dependent on his books on the pulse, even in times when a more 'scientific' or physiologic basis for circulation of the pulse was described by Harvey in the 16th century. For example, Naqvi & Blaufox (1998: p. 24) note Theophile Bordeu (1722–1776) in his 1756 publication *Recherches sur le pouls* describing the 'gastric pulse', 'renal pulse' and 'uterine pulse' as arising specifically from the organs. Unfortunately, Galen's extensive writings were plagued with descriptive anomalies which meant clinical interpretation was variably successful with physicians just as often disagreeing on the meaning of a pulse as agreeing (Kuriyama 1999).

As an aside, with reference to Chinese medicine, Hsu notes that the language of pulse remained descriptive, even in later centuries as pulse knowledge accumulated. Pulse qualities continued to be likened to descriptive imagery; practitioners associated pulse sensations to what they saw in the environment around them (Hsu 2005). Such an observation regarding the descriptive use of language in Chinese medicine is equally applicable to pulse terminology in the Western traditions and even into contemporary times. For example, the Steel Hammer pulse is compared to the resounding ring of a hammer blow. This perhaps describes the lack of expansion of the artery on pulsation and the resonance felt by the practitioner's palpating fingers. These descriptions used by these classical occidental practitioners to describe the various presentations of the

radial pulse would have had a resonance for contemporary CM practitioners. For example, terms such as tense, wiry and thready were variously used to describe different qualitative aspects of the pulse (Table 2.1). Some of these pulse terms continue to be used in modern cardiology units and for general health assessment.

From the 16th/17th centuries, the traditional practice of pulse diagnosis, still based on Galen's work, was radically challenged in two ways. The first was the emerging understanding of blood flow as a single circulatory system, as established by Harvey in the early 17th century. The second was the increasing experimentation of recording pulse waves objectively using mechanical devices. Objective measurements were free from the observer's personal bias; this meant a recording of the pulse wave could be simultaneously observed and discussed by several practitioners, thereby removing the ambiguity of pulse interpretation that had plagued the technique in past centuries.

By the late 19th century the arterial wave form was being regularly recorded using sphygmograms. For example, Figure 2.6 illustrates such a recording originally published in 1906. Such recordings of the radial arterial waveform were made by mechanisms attached to the wrist region over the radial artery. The pulsations would displace these mechanisms and produce tracings, which were referred to as *sphygmographs*. In the context of clinical practice, the physician concentrated on deciphering the sphygmograph and its relationship to a patient's health and any disease present.

Yet while objective pulse measurements were obtainable using these mechanical devices, quantitative measurement was not the primary purpose of these recordings. Rather the measurements were obtained to visualise the contour of the pulse waveform being palpated (Fig. 2.6).

However, at the end of the 19th century, the pulse and its use in clinical practice was radically changed when Riva-Rocci introduced into clinical practice the

Table 2.1 ● Examples of pulse descriptions for five pulse types from the Western literature as noted in Chapter VII of Amber & Babey-Brooke (1993)

Pulse name	Pulse description	Page number
Jarring	Jerky and sharp	139
Steel Hammer	Abrupt and energetic as the rebound of a blacksmith's hammer; observed in arteries near a joint in rheumatism	142
Tense	When artery resembles a cord fixed at each extremity, a hard full pulse. When it feels still harder and smaller, it is called wiry	142
Thready	A scarcely appreciable one as observed in syncope. Rate is rapid; wave appears quickly, is small, and disappears quickly	142
Trigeminal	Three regular beats followed by a pause	142

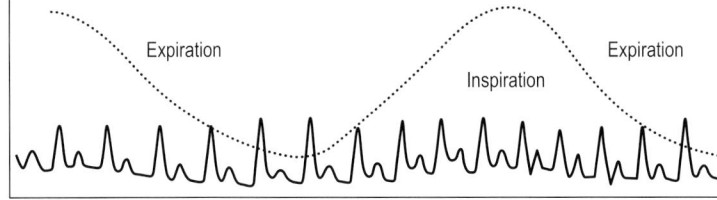

Figure 2.6
A sphygmograph trace recorded by Lewis showing the interaction of respiration in a subject with a dicrotic pulse (After Figure 1, p. 415 in Lewis 1906.)

indirect method by which arterial blood pressure was objectively measured. This involved using a mercury manometer, the forerunner of the present-day brachial cuff sphygmomanometer (Naqvi & Blaufox 1998). Eventually, the focus on the sphygmomanometer, as described by O'Rourke et al (1992), saw the descriptive terms *diastolic* and *systolic* supplant a range of 'qualitative' variables that, until that time, had had high clinical significance placed on them.

This changed perception of the significance and relevance of the pulse wave qualities in clinical diagnosis was not so surprising, according to Kuriyama (1999), since there had always been doubt within the medical fraternity concerning the use of pulse diagnosis to inform diagnosis. The subjective nature of pulse diagnosis, and the inability of the physicians to agree on pulse interpretation, were clearly seen as reasons for this.

2.5.1 Mechanical measurement

In contemporary practice, the benefit of mechanical measurement has been to standardise the system of pulse assessment and to provide a system of accurate record keeping. However, the interpretation of the pulse has largely remained focused on the investigation of the relationship of the heart to systolic pressure, diastolic pressure, heart rate and rhythm. This is evident in the interpretation of sophisticated measurements of the cardiac system back to these basic values. For example, the electrocardiogram (ECG) is primarily interpreted in terms of its presence, rate and pressure values. O'Rourke et al (1992), described this as 'high-tech recording' being linked to 'low-tech interpretation' (p. 25). Little or no attention is paid to the details of the arterial wave formation, and according to O'Rourke et al (1992)

> one would have to concede that basic information presently available on the arterial pulse not only is sparse but also confusing and contradictory. It is surprising that so little is known about the arterial pulse, given the sophisticated knowledge of other bodily functions (p. vii).

It is noteworthy that although objective measurements of the pulse do provide quantitatively derived and standardised values, the interpretation of such

values is still very much dependent on the diagnostic theory and principles underlying the associated medical system. This is particularly evident in biomedicine, with a number of apparently 'abnormal' pulses also having been recorded in people who are, in all respects, apparently 'healthy'. O'Rourke et al (1992) additionally note that it is not unusual for different authoritative texts to give conflicting explanations and indications for the same pulse type, even when it presents in someone who is apparently healthy.

This discrepancy in pulse classification in the biomedical model may be explained by the focus of biomedicine on cardiac and arterial health as the central variable in the origin of pulse formation. That is, if arterial compliance and cardiac competence are not compromised then the pulse wave is often classified as healthy, irrespective of pathology occurring elsewhere in the body.

2.5.2 The process of pulse palpation in contemporary biomedical practice

2.5.2.1 Arterial pulsations and thrills

Biomedicine makes use of several arterial sites throughout the body, including the dorsalis pedis, femoral, brachial and carotid arteries (Fig. 2.7), but the radial artery remains the primary site of manual palpation for most encounters. The others are used for primary or secondary diagnosis of conditions. For example, carotid arterial pulsations are used for assessing cardiac conditions. The dorsalis pedis pulse, in contrast, is used in addition to other pulse sites for assessing strength of peripheral blood flow to the lower limb.

In addition to arterial pulsations, the jugular venous pulse is examined. The jugular venous pulse is synchronous with pressure changes in the right atrium (which receives blood from the vena cava). In this way, it is used as an indicator of heart and lung function. Variations in the usual contour and strength of the jugular pulse indicate that the right atrium is contracting against increased resistance associated with tricuspid stenosis, pulmonary hypertension or pulmonary stenosis.

Additionally, the clinician attempts to identify 'thrills' or vibrations associated with heart murmurs. O'Rourke & Braunwald (2001) state:

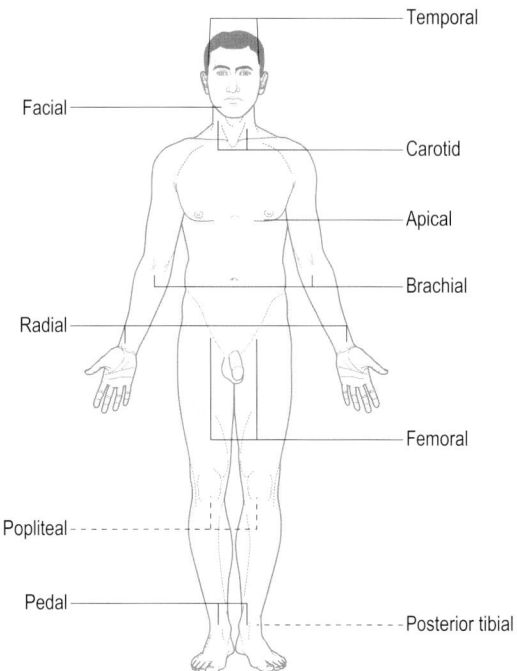

Temporal

Facial

Carotid

Apical

Brachial

Radial

Femoral

Popliteal

Pedal

Posterior tibial

Figure 2.7
Location of the pulse sites. (From Funnell et al 2005, Tabner's nursing care: theory and practice, 4th edn, with permission of Elsevier.)

16

The systolic murmur of mitral regurgitation may be palpated at the cardiac apex. When the palm of the hand is placed over the precordium, the thrill of aortic stenosis crosses the palm toward the right side of the neck, while the thrill of pulmonic stenosis radiates more often to the left side of the neck. The thrill due to a ventricular septal defect is usually located in the third and fourth intercostal spaces near the left sternal border (p. 1257).

2.5.2.2 Finger placement

Using varying increments of pressure, the index and middle fingers are most often used to palpate the pulse at the radial artery. For example, Harvey (1994) asserts that only light pressure is needed to detect pulsus alternans; heavy pressure would occlude it. Some clinicians also suggest the use of the upper palm, where the fingers join, for palpating pulsation through the abdomen and chest as this region of the hand is more sensitive than the finger tips (Harvey 1994). This region of the palm is likely to be used in assessment of thrills at the precordium.

The point at which the pulse is felt most strongly usually dictates the arterial site used for palpation within a given segment of artery. Anatomically, this may very from person to person or within the same person, from day to day. For the radial artery, it is generally the region situated between the wrist crease and medial to the styloid process.

2.5.2.3 Positioning of patient and practitioner

Sometimes, the patient needs to have the arm placed in a certain position to detect specific pulse changes. An example is the detection of the Water Hammer or Collapsing pulse. This is a pulse that occurs in the presence of aortic valve insufficiency in which the aortic valve between the heart and aorta does not close properly. This causes blood to regurgitate or flow back into the left ventricle in the resting or diastole phase rather than continuing forward to the periphery. Therefore, when palpating the pulse during systole the pulse wave increases as usual then suddenly disappears or collapses during diastole. This is particularly noticeable when the patient's arm is raised above their head. At other times the patient may be reclined at a 45° angle for detection of carotid and jugular pulsations. When examining the carotid pulse, the sternocleidomastoid muscle is placed in a state of rest by slightly turning the patient's head towards the practitioner. For the brachial artery, the subject's arm is maintained in a relaxed position, ideally being supported by the practitioner's arm and using the forefinger to palpate the pulse.

Once the pulse is located, the practitioner uses different increments of pressure to assess the diastolic and systolic components of the pulse pressure wave, assessing variations in pulse contour and pulse strength. This includes assessing the strength of cardiac contraction and consequent pulse pressure rise and amplitude during systole, the duration of the maximum pulse amplitude and the downward diastolic slope. For the radial pulse there is often no strict rule for positioning of the patient and palpation can occur at any time during the examination process. As with the brachial arterial pulse, a similar range of contour variables would probably be assessed in addition to rate and rhythm.

2.5.2.4 The pulse in biomedical clinical practice

Although manual pulse assessment alone is still used to assist in the detection of several conditions, it is often performed in conjunction with auscultation by stethoscope. The stethoscope provides auditory information regarding the heart function and smoothness of blood flow. Uncharacteristic sounds arising from blood flow or heart function are distinctly diagnostic of certain types of dysfunction.

Conditions where pulse assessment alone provides an important diagnostic tool include heart disease, aortic coarctation, hypertrophic cardiomyopathy and aortic regurgitation (Tortora & Grabowski 1996). Funnel et al state that the pulse is assessed primarily on three factors: pulse rate, rhythm and volume (2005: p. 267). These three factors inform about peripheral perfusion and cardiac function. For example, comparative assessment of the strength of the radial and femoral pulses can identify aortic coarctation and is also used as a general assessment of circulatory blood flow to the periphery. Pulse rate identifies conditions involving bradycardia and tachycardia, and the ease of occlusion can identify anaemia. Occasionally, the pulse is examined for blood flow and can be useful in detecting aortic regurgitation as with the Corrigan's or Water Hammer pulse (see Box 2.5). The arterial structure may also be assessed for plaques, imperfections or abnormalities affecting blood flow.

Drzewiecki et al (1986) assert that manual palpation cannot detect diastolic pressure – the constant, baseline pressure in the blood vessels that is always there – but can be used 'to determine systolic pressure as long as a palpable pulse is present. Thus it finds application where other occlusive cuff methods fail, e.g., in children, with patients in shock, or with hypotensive patients' (p. 2). In most cases, however, the pulse is viewed as an extension of heart function and used for obtaining measurements of heart rate.

2.6 The pulse in contemporary CM clinical practice

In CM, the process of pulse diagnosis is termed *qie mai*. *Mai* derives from a Chinese character meaning a vessel and can equally be applied to blood vessels and acupuncture channels. *Qie* refers to the process of feeling. Kuriyama (1999) interprets the term *qiemai* as referring to 'streams of blood' (p. 51). In CM, the term *pulse diagnosis* primarily refers to palpation of the radial arteries at both the left and right arms. It also includes Nine Continent pulses, a seldom–used system that involves palpating several arterial sites situated throughout the body, including the head, torso and legs. In contemporary CM practice, pulse diagnosis is believed to provide both specific and general clinical information (Maciocia 2004):

> . . . apart from giving us indications about prevailing disharmonies, it also reflects the constitution of a person; . . . pulse diagnosis can give us a very detailed and accurate picture of the state of Qi in all organs and all parts of the body (p. 457).

A wide range of views regarding the importance of pulse in clinical practice is expressed by various authors.

Contrary to the emphasis placed on pulse in the diagnostic process by some modern CM authors (Hammer 2001, Maciocia 2004, Porkert 1983), its importance in the modern CM clinic appears to be changing. Some practitioners regularly take the patient's pulse throughout the treatment session when administering acupuncture in order to gauge the effect of treatment on the patient, and this will influence the duration of needling, the points needled and the degree of needle manipulation. In this case, treatment would continue until the pulse characteristics presented in a desired formation (Birch & Felt 1999). For other practitioners, the pulse is relegated to playing a 'minor, confirmatory role' (Flaws 1997: p. 7).

In the experience of two modern CM authors (Flaws 1997, Hammer 1993), the use of pulse as a diagnostic skill has been declining worldwide and particularly in China. In Flaws' experience as a student in China as long ago as the 1980s, the pulse was examined only briefly, utilising fewer than 10 of the basic CM qualities, such as slow, fast or deep, and rarely discussed in terms of pulse positions. In his opinion, the low importance placed on the pulse in the diagnostic process appeared to stem from the fact that pulse was unable to be validated from a Western physiological perspective, at a time when the focus appeared to be on scientific validation of CM theories.

The changing role of pulse diagnosis was also evident in the results of a questionnaire completed by a selection of Australian university CM students, which evaluated the use of pulse diagnosis by student practitioners (Smith 1996). The study found that while 82% of the students surveyed rated the pulse as 'important' or 'very important' in formulating a diagnosis, in practice they often used pulse solely as a confirmatory tool and not to establish diagnosis.

In spite of this apparent change in the role of pulse diagnosis observed in students, an Australian survey of CM practitioners found that traditional diagnostic methods are seemingly still being utilised in clinical practice. In 1996 the Victoria State Department of Human Services commissioned a review of the practice of CM in Australia, resulting in a published report called *Towards a Safer Choice* (Bensoussan & Myers 1996). The authors noted that in a survey of both non-medical and medical practitioners who use CM, 90% of those practitioners who identified CM as their major form of practice said that they relied mainly on CM theory for diagnostic purposes.

Therefore, it can be seen that, amongst the numerous practitioners who utilise CM, there seem to be wide ranging differences in the emphasis placed on the use of traditional theory, such as pulse or tongue diagnosis, in clinical practice. The duration of CM education appears to play some role in determining the importance that allied health practitioners (who incorporated CM practices such as acupuncture into their

Box 2.5

Examples of some distinct pulse types recorded in the biomedical literature

- Pulsus tardus: Has a slow rate of climb to the systolic pressure peak, thus a late systolic peak and a similar slow pressure decline. Due to left ventricular ejection obstruction; blood flow is impeded from the left ventricle to the aorta.
- Hyperkinetic pulse: has an increased systolic stroke volume and large pulse amplitude. The peripheral blood vessels are dilated. It is seen during exercise, fever and anxiety.
- Hypokinetic pulse: The opposite of the hyperkinetic pulse, it has a decreased stroke volume with a pressure wave lacking strength.

- Bisferiens pulse: A pulse that has two palpable peaks during systole. It can occur in any condition affecting heart contractility.
- Bigeminal pulse: A variation of the previous pulse, but occurs regularly and is due to premature ventricular contraction following a regular heartbeat. Manifests as, one strong beat, a weak beat, then a strong beat.
- Dicrotic pulse: Two pulse waves for each heartbeat: a pressure wave from the heart during systole and a reflective pulse wave from the limbs detected during diastole.

Pulsus tardus

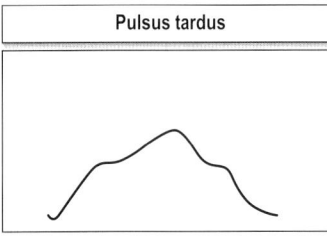

Hyperkinetic pulse

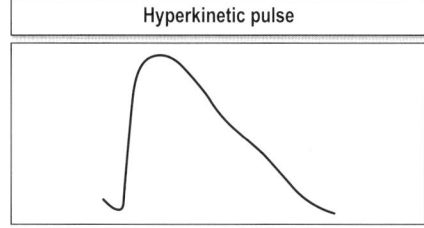

Bisferiens pulse

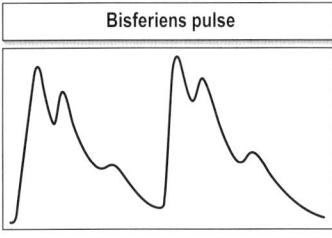

Pulsus alternans

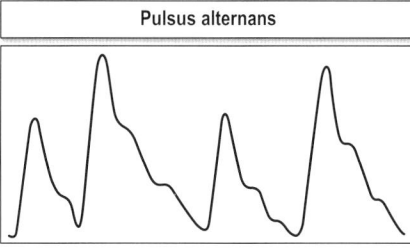

Dicrotic pulse

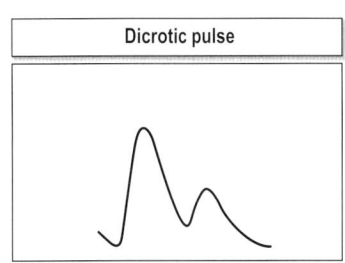

(Descriptions derived from Amber & Babey-Brooke 1996, O'Rourke & Baunwald 2001a, O'Rourke et al 1992).

treatments) give to the traditional theoretical framework. A survey of physiotherapists in the United Kingdom who utilised acupuncture found that:

> Respondents who had undertaken long acupuncture courses were more likely ($p < 0.001$) to use pulse diagnosis, tongue diagnosis and five element theory when compared with those who had not. They placed more importance on traditional diagnosis ($p < 0.001$) and less on Western diagnosis ($p = 0.004$).
> *(Alltree 1993: p. 34)*

2.6.1 The process of pulse palpation in contemporary CM practice: a preliminary introduction

2.6.1.1 Finger positioning

Examination of the radial pulse takes place on both arms at the skin region proximal to the wrist crease, directly above the pulsation of the radial artery. This area is divided into three sections referred to as the three pulse positions: *Cun* (closest to the wrist crease), *Guan* (medial to the styloid process of the radius) and *Chi* (furthermost from the wrist crease) in a region approximately 5 cm in length (Fig. 2.8). Each pulse site can be further divided into two levels (superficial and deep) or three levels of depth (superficial, middle and deep). During assessment the wrist is always placed at the level of the heart to avoid pressure variations that may distort the pulse wave. (Pulse assessment techniques and method are discussed in detail in Chapter 5.)

Various theoretical systems may be used in the interpretation of the radial pulse information obtained during palpation. (These theoretical systems are termed pulse assumption systems.) For example, each of the positions can be considered as a reflection of the flow of energy through specific pathways in the body (known as channels or meridians), or each position may be associated with a particular internal organ. Alternatively, the Cun, Guan and Chi positions may be seen to reflect the upper, middle and lower regions of the trunk of the body respectively (Maciocia 2004). Birch & Felt (1999) describe a number of other interpretations: for example, Worsley's traditional acupuncture system in which the relative strength of each pulse position is classified, the Japanese keiraku chiryo system which only uses the 6 deep positions to identify 4 general patterns of weakness and lastly, the use of specific pulse qualities that attempt to classify the pulse in terms of the 27 or so traditional pathological pulse types.

2.6.1.2 The pulse in CM clinical practice

The pulse as a diagnostic technique is incorporated into clinical practice in the four examinations: the basic structure from which a practitioner garners information from patients. The four examinations consist of observation, listening/smelling, asking and palpation. The last category, palpation, usually involves applying pressure to sensitive acupuncture points and tender

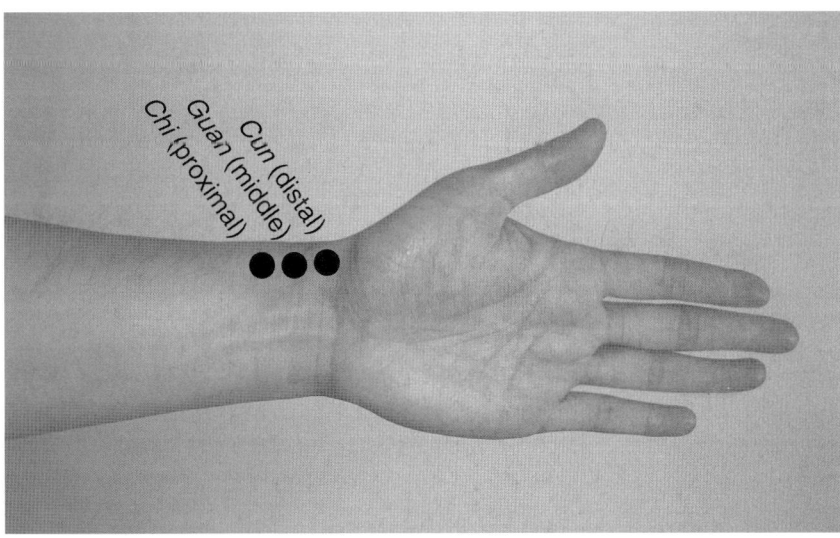

Figure 2.8
Finger placement at the three pulse positions. The distal placement corresponds to Cun, the middle to Guan and proximal to Chi.

muscles around the body as well as examination of the pulse.

The three distinct finger positions at the radial pulse have an important diagnostic value. Each position has a theoretical connection to an internal organ structure and therefore each position reflects the relative health or function of that organ. This idea of function permeates all aspects of CM. The concept's origins can be traced back to the *Nei Jing*, the earliest extant book on Chinese medical theory. In reference to health, the book emphasises the individual as being in direct influence with their surrounding environment and of that environment being reflected within that individual's physiology. This micro/macrocosmic dichotomy formed an important foundation for the development of present-day CM diagnostic principles, with disease categorisation based on functional relationships and interactions in addition to actual organic pathology.

Contemporary theories explain this relationship in terms of fluid dynamic principles. The position of each organ in the body is situated at a specific distance from the wrist. Subsequently, this imparts a distinct signature or harmonic to the overall haemodynamic flow wave, which through amplification in the long arteries of the arm can be uniquely palpated distinctly at each of the three positions (Dai et al 1985, Xue & Fung 1989a, Xue & Fung 1989b).

2.6.1.3 Characteristics and qualities

A theoretical assumption of pulse diagnosis is that each position provides different information on body function, which a practitioner uses to arrive at a diagnosis or prognosis. Diagnosis or prognosis is dependent on the variability of each pulse characteristic such as pulse rate. A slow pulse rate (<60 bpm) can indicate hypometabolic activity, as in the case of hypothyroidism, while an increase in pulse rate above that what is normally expected (>90 bpm) can indicate hyperactivity, as in the case of febrile conditions. These characteristics form the foundation of the specific pulse qualities; a distinctive set of pulse characteristics that occur simultaneously with specific disease states. These are discussed extensively in Chapters 6 and 7.

In addition to disease states, there are several variables that are traditionally assumed to influence the pulse, including age, gender, weight, seasons, circadian cycles, personal traits and environmental conditions. These are explored further in Chapter 5.

References

Alltree J 1993 Physiotherapy and acupuncture: practice in the UK. Complementary Therapies in Medicine 1:34–41

Amber R, Babey-Brooke A 1993 Pulse diagnosis: detailed interpretations for eastern and western holistic treatments. Aurora Press, Santa Fe, NM

Bedford D E 1951 The ancient art of feeling the pulse. British Heart Journal 13:423–427

Bensoussan A, Myers S 1996 Towards a safer choice: the practice of traditional Chinese medicine in Australia. UWS, Sydney

Berne R, Levy M 1981 Cardiovascular physiology, 4th edn. Mosby, St Louis

Birch S, Felt R 1999 Understanding acupuncture. Harcourt Brace, London

Bordeu T 1756 Recherches sur le pouls par rapport aux crises. In: Naqvi N H, Blaufox M D 1998 Blood pressure measurement: an illustrated history. Pantheon, New York

Chen C, Nevo E, Fetics B et al 1997 Estimation of central aortic pressure waveform by mathematical transformation of radial tonometry pressure: validation of generalized transfer function. Circulation 95(7):1827–1836

Dai K, Xue H, Dou R et al 1985 On the detection of messages carried in arterial pulse waves. Journal of Biomechanical Engineering 107:268–273

Drzewiecki G, Melbin J, Noordergraaf A 1986 Noninvasive blood pressure recording and the genesis of korotkof sound. In: Skalak R, Chien. S. Handbook of Bioengineering. McGraw-Hill, New York, Ch 8

Flaws B 1997 The secret of Chinese pulse diagnosis, 2nd edn. Blue Poppy Press, Boulder, CO

Funnell R, Koutoukidis G, Larence K 2005 Tabner's nursing care: theory and practice, 4th edn. Elsevier, Sydney

Guyton A, Hall J 2006 Textbook of medical physiology, 11th edn. Elsevier, Philadelphia

Hammer L 1993 Contemporary pulse diagnosis: introduction to an evolving method for learning an ancient art – part 1. American Journal of Acupuncture 21(2):123–139

Hammer L 2001 Chinese pulse diagnosis: a contemporary approach. Eastland Press, Seattle

Harvey W P 1994 Cardiac pearls. Disease-a-month XL(2):43–113

Hsu E 2005 Tactility and the body in early Chinese medicine. Science in Context 18(1):7–34

Kuriyama S 1999 The expressiveness of the body and the divergence of Greek and Chinese medicine. Zone Books, New York

Lanir Y 1986 Skin mechanics. In: Skalak R, Chien S (eds) Handbook of bioengineering. McGraw-Hill, New York, Ch 11

Lewis T 1906 The factors influencing the prominence of the dicrotic wave. Journal of Physiology 34:414–429

Lloyd G 1996 Aristotelian explorations. Cambridge University Press, Cambridge

Maciocia G 2004 Diagnosis in Chinese medicine: a comprehensive guide. Churchill Livingstone, Edinburgh

Naqvi N H, Blaufox M D 1998 Blood pressure measurement: an illustrated history. Pantheon, New York

Opie L 2004 Heart physiology: from cell to circulation, 4th edn. Lippincott, Philadelphia

O'Rourke R A, Braunwald E 2001 Physical examination of the cardiovascular system. In: Braunwald E, Fauci A, Kasper D et al (eds) Harrison's principles of internal medicine, Volume 1, 15th edn. McGraw-Hill, New York, Ch 225

O'Rourke M, Kelly R, Avolio A 1992 The arterial pulse. Lea & Febiger, Pennsylvania

Porkert, M 1983 The essentials of Chinese diagnostics. Acta Medicinae Sinensis Chinese Medicine Publications, Zurich

Smith W 1996 Pulse diagnosis at UTS and VUT colleges of acupuncture student clinics [BAppSc]. University of Technology Sydney, Sydney

Stettler J C, Neiderer P, Anliker M 1986 Nonlinear mathematical models of the arterial system: effects of bifurcations, wall viscoeleasticity, stenoses, and counterpulsation on pressure and flow waves. In: Skalak R, Chien S (eds) Handbook of bioenginnering. McGraw-Hill, New York, Ch 17

Strandring S et al (eds) 2005 Gray's anatomy: the anatomical basis of clinical practice, 38th edn. Churchill Livingstone, Edinburgh

Tortora G, Grabowski S 1996 Principles of anatomy and physiology, 8th edn. HarperCollins, New York

Xue H, Fung Y 1989a What Nei Jing and Mai Jing say about arterial pulse waves and our attempt to illustrate some of their statements. Journal of Biomechanical Engineering 111:88–91

Xue H, Fung Y 1989b Persistence of asymmetry in nonaxisymmetric entry flow in a circular cylindrical tube and its relevance to arterial pulse wave diagnosis. Journal of Biomedical Engineering 111:37–41

Historical pulse records and practice

3

Chapter contents

3.1 *Nei Jing* 23
3.2 *Nan Jing* 25
3.3 *Mai Jing* 26
3.4 *Bin Hue Mai Xue* 27
3.5 Historical perspective: regional pulse assessment and the Cun Kou pulse 27
3.6 Historical problems in contemporary practice 29
3.7 Pulse classics and contemporary practice 30

The development of CM theory generally is reflected in the development of pulse theory. This is clearly seen in the *Nan Jing*, which documented the further development of pulse knowledge but which reflects the broader change in treatment generally, justifying why stimulation of an acupuncture point on the foot has systemic effects on the circulation.

The classics constitute an important source of information for our understanding of when and how certain pulse assumption systems developed and their related claims to clinical relevancy. They equally provide an important point of reference for the many difficult issues that affect the use of pulse diagnosis in the contemporary context: indeed, the information they contain may be seen as directly contributing to these issues (discussed in Chapter 4). This is because, unlike contemporary biomedical practices, where new ideas and developments supersede the outdated or disproved theories, in CM, both the old and new are retained. In the words of Unschuld, the new is seen as merely adding to the old. This means that the contemporary practice of pulse diagnosis often remains linked with its literary past.

There are four major literary texts available in English which document the development and use of pulse diagnosis in Chinese medicine:

- *Nei Jing*
- *Nan Jing*
- *Mai Jing*
- *Bin Hue Mai Xue*.

3.1 *Nei Jing*

One of the earliest references to pulse palpation in CM as a systemised diagnosis technique emerges from the *The Yellow Emperor's Classic of Medicine* or *Nei Jing*, one of the oldest and additionally described as one of the most important Chinese medical texts, compiled in 300–100 BCE. The *Nei Jing* is arranged as two distinct books, the *Suwen* and the *Lingshu*, the former being the primary source of information on pulse diagnosis. The

Box 3.1

Nei Jing

- Collated between 300 and 100 BCE
- Incorporates the 'vessel texts' from the Mawangdui scrolls
- Details the medicine of systematic correspondences
- Introduced the concept of discrete circulations associated with both Qi and Blood influences, and discussed the normal pulse
- Documents a range of different arterial pulse sites linked with different systems of pulse assessment including:
  - Cun Kou (wrist), Ren Ying and Fu Yang pulses
  - channel/artery assessment
  - Nine Continent pulse diagnosis.

Nei Jing is seen as an eclectic book of writings, representing the collation of knowledge representative of a range of different lineage medical teachings extant at its time of writing, and in particular that of systematic correspondences (Hsu 2005) (Box 3.1).

In the context of the radial artery and pulse assessment, the sites of the radial artery were briefly discussed in Chapter 17 of the *Nei Jing*, described as three positions located above the radial artery, used to 'detect [the] subtle quality of pulse patterns' (*Lingshu*, treatise 74: Ni (trans) 1995: p. 68). These positions, situated at the wrist, adjacent to the radial styloid process and proximal to it, were named Cun, Guan and Chi respectively and were divided into deep and superficial levels of depth. These positions were viewed as representing different regions of the body and some of the positions were linked to specific organs. This meant that a change in the pulse character at the site meant a corresponding change occurring in the related organ.

For using the pulse diagnostically, the *Nei Jing* introduced two important concepts; that of *circulation* and the *normal pulse*. The first of these concepts, circulation, was described as the movement of substances (a vapour called Qi, in various forms, and Blood) throughout the body in 12 linking vessels, located in different regions of the body (Unschuld 1986). The concept of the 'normal' pulse was also introduced and this was used as a standard with which to compare the features of an abnormal pulse.

For example in reference to pulse rate the normal pulse was described as:

> In man,
> during one exhalation, the vessels exhibit two movements.
> During one inhalation, the vessels exhibit two movements too.
> Exhalation and inhalation constitute one standard breathing period.

> If the vessels exhibit five movements,
> this is an intercalation [of a fifth movement]
> because of a deep breathing.
> That is called a 'normal person'.
> *Suwen (Unschuld 2003: p. 257)*

Therefore distinguishing health by the pulse required comparison of the patient's pulse with the normal pulse frequency, deviation in the patient's rate from the normal rate representing illness.

Even this oldest of CM texts borrowed from yet older writings incorporating two distinctly recognisable manuscripts termed the 'vessel texts' from the *Mawangdui* scrolls (Harper 1998, Hsu 2005). These texts include a series of case studies compiled by Chunyu Yi, a Chinese physician, in which Hsu notes in her study of the scrolls that there is 'sufficient detail to recognize in them a particular form of pulse diagnostics, a form that in many aspects was later discontinued' (2005: p. 11). In particular, Hsu mentions Chapter 10 of the *Lingshu* as recording the vessel texts 'in a strongly modified form, yet in places also verbatim'.

Further evidence of the *Nei Jing* as a compilation of writings, rather than as a discrete text, is seen in the reference to the use of pulse diagnosis in various forms, including:

- Nine Continent pulse diagnosis: Pulse sites on the head, lower and upper limb
- Channel assessment by regional pulses: Arterial pulses congruent with each of the channel pathways occurring in all regions of the body
- Heaven, Humanity and Earth: Three permanent pulses located at the carotid, radial and dorsalis pedis arteries.

In this sense, pulse assessment in the *Nei Jing* was undertaken from a range of anatomical regions and not exclusively from the wrist.

3.1.1 Nine Continent pulse diagnosis

The Nine Continent system is specifically named for the use of nine arterial sites: three arteries located in the upper region (the head), three in the central region (upper limb) and three in the lower region (lower limb) of the body. The system is premised on the microcosmic arrangement of the macrocosm reflected within the body with components of Heaven, Earth and Humanity simultaneously assigned to the upper, middle and lower regions. The Nine Continent system provided information about:

- The region of the body that was affected
- Generic information about replete (excess) and vacuous (deficient) conditions, but not necessarily information about the specific nature of the illness

The Nine Continent system of pulse diagnosis, is discussed further in Chapter 9.

3.1.2 Channel assessment by regional pulses

This system of pulse assessment was based on the physiological association between superficial arterial pulses occurring in the same anatomical region in which an acupuncture channel transgressed. In this way, each of the channels was linked to an artery so the pulsation in the related artery came to reflect the strength of the associated channel. For example, the popliteal artery located behind the knee was linked with the Bladder channel (*Zu Tai Yang*). Changes in the presence and strength of the popliteal artery meant a change in the functional strength of the bladder channel.

The *Nei Jing* notes each of the channels as having movement; a distinct pulse associated with its location. In this sense, the coursing movement of the artery was inseparable from the path of the channel: the artery, the pulse and the channel were as one (a linked vessel); an interdependent relationship of function and form, embodied in the concepts of Qi and Blood. Hence, the assessment of the pulse or form reflected the state of the channels or function. For the early Chinese medical practitioner the axiom *Qi leads the Blood and Blood nourishes the Qi* was clearly apparent in the coupling and movement of the pulse sites and channel locations. In this way, each artery/channel was viewed as having a discrete circulation.

3.1.3 The three constant pulses

The three pulse sites were unique amongst all other pulse sites mentioned in the *Nei Jing* in that a pulsation could always be felt in these locations, irrespective of the presence of illness. What this means for the other regional pulse sites is that their related pulses were not always necessarily present – they were in fact, transient. Indeed, it is this factor that allowed the ancient Chinese medical practitioner to use the regional arterial pulses for diagnostic/medical purposes. (The nascent recognition of a united circulation could be seen arising from the three permanent pulse sites. Thus, the *Nan Jing*'s argument for a single site for assessment was an obvious conclusion.)

Wiseman & Ye (1998: p. 470) term these three sites as:

- Rén yíng (man's prognosis): The carotid artery located in the neck – associated with the stomach channel (stomach Qi, sea of grain)
- Cùn kŏu (inch opening): The radial artery located in the wrist and reflects the lung Qi (rules the Qi)

- Fū yáng (instep Yang): Dorsalis pedis artery in the feet (could also be the tibial artery according to p. 85 of the *Jia Ji Jing*) (penetrating vessel, sea of blood).

However, although the *Nei Jing* incorporated pulse palpation into the diagnostic framework, the pulse characteristics and qualities were described in obscure and difficult concepts that had little clinical relevancy for diagnosing disease (Unschuld 1986). It was in this environment that the central message of the *Nan Jing*'s approach to pulse diagnosis was delivered.

3.2 *Nan Jing*

The *Nan Jing*, translated as *The Classic of Difficult Issues*, was produced in response to the 'difficult issues' raised, or left unanswered, in the *Nei Jing*, so constituting an important text in the development of CM diagnostic theory (Box 3.2).

Collated some time in the 1st or 2nd century CE, the first 22 chapters provide instructions on the practical application of pulse assessment, describing a number of palpatory techniques and methods of assessment. The *Nan Jing* author(s) introduced innovative conceptual ideas for applying the pulse techniques, noting two extraordinary divergences from preceding pulse knowledge. The first was that the circuitous route or cyclic ebb and flow of the 'Qi and Blood influences' in the individual channels/vessels logically inferred that these were in fact a single linked circulatory system rather than several discrete circulatory systems as noted in the *Nei Jing*. Further, if the Qi and Blood flow were linked, then it was only necessary to examine movement at one area along the flow (Unschuld 1985). The 'inch-opening' or *Cun Kou* pulse in the radial artery at the wrist was chosen as the site for assessment because it was thought to be the point at which all the vessels intersected. These ideas were profound to the thinking of Chinese medical practitioners as the time, as noted by Unschuld:

> The message offered by the Nan-ching must have been quite convincing in at least one

---

Box 3.2

Nan Jing

- Collated in the 1st or 2nd century CE
- Introduced the concept of a single linked circulatory system
- Focuses solely on the use of a single pulse position: the Cun Kou position on the wrist
- Associated the Zang and Fu organs with a particular pulse position and level of depth.

Table 3.1 ● Association of the pulse positions and two levels of depth with the organs

Left Superficial	Left Deep		Right Deep	Right Superficial	Jiao	Torso region
Small intestine	Heart	Cun	Lung	Large Intestine	Upper Jiao	Thoracic cavity
Gallbladder	Liver	Guan	Spleen	Stomach	Middle Jiao	Abdominal cavity
Bladder	Kidney	Chi	Pericardium	Triple Heater	Lower Jiao	Pelvic cavity

respect. Vessel diagnosis concentrating on the wrists was adopted not only by many physicians (who were criticized by Chang Chi – or by a later commentator to his preface – for an all too simplistic practice both of diagnosis in general and of wrist diagnosis as well) but also by the leading pre-Sung authors of medical works with sections on diagnosis that have been transmitted to us from pre-Sung times *(Unschuld 1986: p. 35).*

With the publication of the *Nan Jing* in the 2nd century CE, the regional assessment of the pulse/channel, described extensively in the *Nei Jing*, was radically challenged with the novel concept of a single or linked circulatory system embodied in the wrist pulse site posited in the book's 'first difficult issue'. In doing this, the *Nan Jing* discussed various methods of examining the pulse at the radial artery. One method of assessment involved each wrist division, Cun, Guan and Chi, divided into two levels of depth, superficial and deep, for the left and right arm radial arterial pulses. This gave 12 pulse positions in total. An acupuncture channel was associated with each of these positions: Yin and Yang organs of each phase respectively associated with the deep and superficial levels of the pulse. Collectively, the 12 pulse positions and 'pulses' were termed the Cun Kou or 'inch opening'. The name and channel arrangement at the pulse positions, and the two depths developed at this time, remain in use (Table 3.1).

Another method of pulse depth examination described in the *Nan Jing* involved assessing three levels of depth at a single position on the wrist, while another system identified five different levels. The pulse positions were also attributed to different regions of the torso. For example, the Cun positions of the left and right wrist respectively related to the heart and lung. As each of these organs occurred in the thoracic cavity, the upper Jiao, then the Cun positions could be used alternatively to infer the function of the upper Jiao. In this way, one pulse assumption system was overlaid on another.

3.3 *Mai Jing*

The *Mai Jing*, translated as the *Pulse Classic* (Wang, Yang (trans) 1997), is the oldest extant Chinese medical

---

Box 3.3

Mai Jing

- Written by Wang Shu-He in the 2nd century CE
- Names 24 specific pulse qualities and associated the formation of each with the simultaneous changes in several pulse characteristics
- Provides lengthy commentary on the clinical significance of the occurrence of 24 pulse qualities occurring across the three Cun Kou pulse positions, as well as occurring at each specific Cun, Guan and Chi pulse position.

---

text devoted solely to the study of the pulse, written in the Jin dynasty sometime in the 2nd to 3rd century CE by Wang Shu-he (Box 3.3). The book symbolizes the apparent flourishing of pulse diagnosis in CM occurring at this time, detailing comprehensive coverage of many aspects of the assessment of the radial pulse, including:

- Methodology of pulse taking
- Types of abnormal pulses
- Prognosis according to pulses
- Advice on treatment protocols according to the presentation of the pulse.

An interesting development in pulse terminology occurred in the *Mai Jing*. Wiseman and Ye (1999) note that Wang applied a specific pulse 'name' to a collective group of descriptive terms, recognising that it is different characteristic features of the pulse such as depth, rhythm, rate, width and length that combine to produce a particular pulse quality. For example, rather than 'sinking and frail, and one can palpate it only deeply' (Ni 1995: p. 74) found in the *Nei Jing*, the *Mai Jing* attributed this group of descriptive terms to the Weak pulse *(ruò mài)*. With the introduction of specific pulse names, this meant that the identification of a specific pulse quality now hinged on the recognition of all aspects of the pulse (Wiseman & Ye 1998).

The *Mai Jing* details 24 specific pulse qualities and the description of pulse qualities associated with specific disease states. Variations of strength, rhythm,

Table 3.2 ● Variation in the diagnostic meaning of pulse qualities relative to their presentation at different pulse positions, as stated in the *Mai Jing*

Position	Floating pulse	Tight pulse	Rapid pulse
Cun	Fever and headaches	Cold damage	Vomiting
Guan	Abdominal fullness	Fullness below the heart/pain	Stomach heat
Chi	Difficult urination	Pain due to cold	Aversion to wind, cold below umbilicus

speed and contour of the presenting pulse are discussed in terms of organ function and in terms of the channel system.

The *Mai Jing* is particularly well regarded for its lengthy commentary on the interpretation of these pulse qualities relating to pathology. There is an extensive discussion of the clinical significance of abnormal pulse qualities occurring in each of the specific pulse positions of Cun, Guan and Chi and the symptoms accompanying them. For example, Vacuity and Repletion patterns affecting the Lungs were diagnosed by the simultaneous increase or decrease in strength at the Lung position of the pulse (this being the deep level of depth at the Cun position on the right wrist). Additionally, the 24 pulse qualities had different diagnostic meaning when occurring at the individual pulse positions. For example, a Floating pulse at the right Cun position meant fever and headaches, the Tight pulse meant cold damage and the Rapid pulse meant vomiting (Table 3.2). At the Guan position, the Floating pulse meant there was abdominal fullness and no appetite, the Tight pulse meant fullness below the heart with acute pain and the Rapid pulse meant guest heat in the stomach. Floating pulse in the Chi position meant wind heat in the lower Jiao with difficult urination, Taut pulse meant pain due to cold and the Rapid pulse here meant aversion to cold and wind and pain below the umbilicus. In this way, Wang Shu-He constructed a comprehensive and detailed approach to the clinical interpretation of pulse. From the time of the *Mai Jing* throughout the centuries till today, authors continue to reiterate the definitions of the pulse as stated in this book.

3.4 *Bin Hue Mai Xue*

The *Bin Hue Mai Xue* was written by Li Shi Zhen in 1564 CE. The book used the Cun Kou or three radial arterial sites method of pulse diagnosis in combination with the overall pulse qualities introduced in the *Mai Jing* with positional and pulse depth dimensions. Consequently the book is a collation of older literature on the pulse and so descriptions from the *Nei Jing* are found alongside information from the *Mai Jing* and other texts such as the *Pulse Knacks* (Li, Flaws (trans) 1998). The author also introduced several more pulse qualities into

Box 3.4

Bin Hue Mai Xue
- Written by Li Shi Zhen in 1564 CE
- A collated summation of all pulse knowledge extant at the time of its writing
- Written in a rhyming form meant for memorization
- An educational text still used in contemporary times

the general CM nomenclature and provided commentary on comparative differences of each pulse type (Box 3.4).

The book was meant for memorisation, so it was written in a series of rhymes, detailing the pulse description and related indications. These rhymes would also have doubled as a mnemonic in clinical practice; the practitioner would feel the pulse and recite the rhymes, so identifying the pulse type being felt.

The book is significant in the history of pulse diagnosis in that it was collated as a summation of all pulse knowledge extant at the time of its writing. Li Shi Zhen organised this knowledge into a comprehensible and accessible format. The book has been an important educational tool and a guide for CM students learning pulse in China since the 16th century and is still used today.

3.5 Historical perspective: regional pulse assessment and the Cun Kou pulse

Although the supremacy of wrist diagnosis is argued clearly in the historical record of CM with the *Nan Jing*, the theoretical and logical argument presented was counter to the notion that the circulatory system serves more than just the organs. The circulatory system distributes blood and fluid to the muscles, skin, tissue and into the periphery in addition to the organs; both localized and systemic requirements are placed on the circulation. In this sense it is logical that pulses in other regions of the body should also play a vital role in the

Box 3.5

Common features unifying the regional pulse sites

- Superficially located arteries
- The arteries have firm foundational support provided by bone or ligament
- Located in regions easily accessible to the practitioner

assessment of an individual's health, and historically, this is what happened.

In the early centuries of the first millennium CE, pulse assessment encompassed examination of the pulse at numerous regions throughout the body. This was the basis of what is termed *regional pulse assessment*: the assessment of arterial pulse sites that occurred in regions of the body other than the Cun Kou. In the *Nei Jing* and other CM literature classics, there is reference to at least three distinct groupings of regional pulses. There are the three permanent pulses, of which the Cun Kou is one; the pulse sites linked with the actual anatomical location of each of the channels; and the Nine Continent pulses. Of the three groupings it is the only the Nine Continent system that is still regularly covered in contemporary CM literature, as the system provides clinically relevant information not gained from the Cun Kou system (Box 3.5).

Interestingly, Kuriyama (1999) notes that in spite of the *Nan Jing*, the use of other regional/anatomical pulses other than that of the wrist was never totally discarded by ancient Chinese practitioners. Vestiges of the regional assessment system of pulse were retained in the *Shan Han Lun*, *Mai Jing* and *Jin Gui Yao Lue* (Kuriyama 1999: p. 45). For example, the *Jia Ji Jing* (Systematic classic of acupuncture and moxibustion), which was written approximately two centuries after the *Nan Jing*, incorporated segments of the *Nei Jing* (*Lingshu*, Chapter 9) speaking specifically of using the assessment of different pulses around the body from the regional pulse sites to assess health through the similarity of pulse strength occurring at all these sites. The *Jia Yi Jing* clearly states that the Mai Kou and Ren Ying pulses are used to determine the presence of 'surplus' or 'insufficiency' of Yin and Yang and determine balance or imbalance (p. 301: in a postscript note from the translators, the chapter was derived from Chapter 9 of the *Lingshu*):

> Those who are considered normal are without disease. Those who are without disease are characterised by a congruity of their mai kou and ren ying pulses with the four seasons and by congruity (between the pulses) in the upper

and lower parts of the body which are synchronous with one another (p. 301).

Additionally, the *Mai Jing*, another text postdating the *Nan Jing's* discussion on the use of a single arterial site for pulse assessment, also incorporated regional pulse assessment. Chapter 28 of the *Mai Jing* states:

> When a person is ill, if the Cun opening pulse and the ren ying pulse are the same in terms of their size and depth, the disease is difficult to cure.

(The translator's note to this chapter points out that ordinarily the wrist and carotid pulses should vary in strength, size. For these to be congruent represents serious disturbances to the Qi and blood flow.)

There are two explanations as to why the authors of the *Mai Jing* and *Jia Ji Jing* included regional pulse site assessment. The first is they did this through reverence of the older text. The second is that the regional pulse sites did in fact provide clinically useful information, probably information that could not be obtained or provided by the assessment of the Cun Kou pulse alone.

It is also apparent that the regional channel/pulse assessment system lingered into later centuries with commentators of the *Nan Jing*, Lu Kuang (3rd century CE) and Yang Hsuan-ts'ao (7th/8th century CE), linking the channels with regional pulses located in anatomical regions other than the wrist. That is, the knowledge was still extant. For example, in their commentaries on the first difficult issue, they state:

> These are the twelve vessels of the conduits in the hands and feet. The movement of the foot-great-Yang [conduit can be felt] in the bend [of the knee]. The movement of the foot-minor-Yang [conduit can be felt] in front of the ear.
> *(Lu Kuang, in Unschuld 1986: p. 66).*

> This is the ch'ung-Yang hole which is located above the instep, hence its name. [This conduit's] movement can also [be felt] in the neck at the jen-Ying [hole] and also the ta-Ying [hole].
> *(Yang, in Unschuld 1986: p. 66).*

Lu and Yang respectively refer to the popliteal, temple(?), dorsalis pedis (ch'ung), carotid (jen-Ying) arteries in addition to the radial artery (ta-Ying). All sites were distinct from other anatomical regions as having a movement present. In this sense, there were several circulatory pathways.

Yet, as Unschuld noted, the argument presented by the *Nan Jing* was convincing, for by the 11th century the *Nan Jing* commentaries distinctly changed, with only minor references to the regional pulses in the text mainly in 'gentle' condemnation of antecedent medical scholars' comments (Yu Shu, in Unschuld 1986: p. 96). It appears these later medical scholars accorded little value to the region pulse system, beyond interest as a curious historical artefact. Additionally, rather than the assessment of arterial segments these authors linked these pulse sites with discrete points or sites. These were increasingly being cited as acupuncture points rather than the channel artery coupling located in the holes or grooves provided by the anatomy. For example, the tibial arterial pulse was discretely located at KD 3 (Taixi). Interestingly, the commentaries of the *Nan Jing* as compiled by Unschuld chart the fracturing relationship between the arterial pulses and the channels with the course of the channel being separated from that of an associated arterial segment.

What is certainly apparent in the commentaries of the *Nan Jing* and reflected in the classics generally, is the temporal change in authors' attitudes to the regional pulse system: from a necessary skill in the time of the *Nei Jing* to a historical relic by the end of the first millennium and finally forgotten by the time of the European Renaissance in the 16th century. In the *Bin Hue Mai Xue*, published in 1564, there is no reference to the regional pulse system in spite of the book being a summation of historical pulse literature.

In some ways, the loss of regional pulse assessment according to Hsu (2005) probably reflects the integration of philosophical doctrines of Confucian ideology into Chinese society in the first millennium, where modesty constraints meant body palpation, whether pulse or anatomically related, was condoned only within the confines of discrete, and socially acceptable, anatomical regions (Hsu 2005). In contemporary times, the societal context of the practise of CM means minor surgical procedures once associated with the practice of acupuncture, in which regional pulse assessment probably served an important purpose, are no longer carried out.

3.6 Historical problems in contemporary practice

Besides being a historical record of the development of pulse diagnosis, the classics highlight the conceptual variation and conflict apparent in the practice of pulse diagnosis through the centuries and up to the present day. This can be seen in the change in pulse position and organ correlation. For example, the *Bin Hue Mai Xue* mentioned only five Yin organs. The superficial Yang organs were seen simply as an extension of these, and are not mentioned. In contrast, the *Mai Jing* listed all 12 organs as distinct and separate entities with each given a distinct pulse depth and position. Theoretical preconceptions shaped the development of pulse taking and were in turn shaped by practice. In the *Bin Hue Mai Xue* the Pericardium, Bladder and Triple Heater organs

were theoretically connected to the Kidneys via internal channel pathways and subsequently were seen as an extension of the Kidneys. For the purposes of pulse taking, this meant the division of the Chi positions into two subcategories; Kidney Yang and Kidney Yin. The Pericardium, Bladder and Triple Heater were not specifically mentioned.

There are also major differences in the division of the variable depth between texts. For example, the *Nei Jing* mentioned only two pulse depths, superficial and deep, while the *Mai Jing* and *Bin Hue Mai Xue* listed three, with the addition of a middle level of depth. The *Nan Jing* listed anywhere from three to five levels of depth; individual organs, organ systems and body substances such as Blood were simultaneously assigned to each position. Alternatively, the Cun, Guan and Chi pulse positions may be seen to reflect the upper, middle and lower (Heaters) portions of the torso (Maciocia 2004, Ho & Lisowski 1997) or may reflect individual organs (Flaws 1997). The positions can be used to assess overall pulse qualities or used individually for specific organ characteristics.

According to Birch (1998) the apparent conflicts in the classics stem from the historical (and contemporary) diversity of CM practice and the conceptual systems they reflect. This reflects the syncretistic tendency, throughout the history of CM thought, for many different theories, often conflicting, to exist side by side (Unschuld 1985). Accordingly, this meant the reconciliation of opposing ideas rather than a resolution of the contradictory views. This is apparent in assumption systems used to interpret radial pulse information and in the specific pulse terminology itself. Unschuld, in his commentaries on the *Nan Jing*, perhaps best describes the coexistence of theoretical variation:

> The reasons for the great degree of conceptual confusion and for the absence of a stringent, technical terminology . . . are to be seen in the fact that at no time in the first or second millennium did more recent conceptual insights replace older views for good . . . When an author introduced a new meaning of an ancient term, this meaning did not eventually replace the older meaning(s) but was merely adding to the existing range of meanings (p. 283).

Unschuld's view has been borne out by the attempts of some commentators on the CM literature to reconcile the 'occasional' conflicting information contained in different texts through tenuous theoretical linkages rather than direct questioning of theoretical foundations. Others have refuted it altogether, maintaining their conservative views in relation to the original source texts. However, the old is often retained with the new, to the point of conflict. This is demonstrated by Unschuld's translation of the commentaries of Hsu

Ta-ch'un, an influential physician scholar and medical writer of the 18th century CE. Unschuld notes that while Hsu's commentaries focused extensively on the *Nan Jing*, he did not acknowledge the book's ideas and contribution to the development of pulse diagnosis. Instead he criticised the *Nan Jing* in favour of the ideas originally presented 200 years earlier in the *Nei Jing*, not because they were more clinically relevant (in fact they were very ambiguous), but rather because they were simply 'older' (Unschuld 1990). This resolution of theoretical differences has never been a strong point of CM theoreticians.

In contemporary CM practice, not much has changed. Today, a number of different systems are still used to interpret variations in the pulse, and they invariably incorporate a number of untested assumptions from the classics concerning the normal presentation of the pulse. Some of these systems are related, and so the interpretation and understanding of the theory can be reconciled. Other pulse assumption systems appear quite contradictory, and reconciling the opposing interpretation is difficult if not impossible. Further complication arises from the development of new and novel pulse systems in recent years. Old problems thus continue to appear in the modern context.

3.7 Pulse classics and contemporary practice

Nowadays there are additional problems to contend with. The first is the assumption that knowledge documented in the classical literature is based on empirical evidence gathered from a broad range of experiences. However, there is no clear evidence of this and so some of the knowledge could be derived from a single case study based on an individual's observation, as is the nature of empirical observation. This makes extrapolation of the knowledge within these books to a broader population base a fraught process. Secondly, pulse diagnosis also largely continues to be reliant on information first presented nearly 2000 years ago and so it is also necessary to contextualise the temporal authorship of the content material in the classics. For example, there are whole chapters in the classical literature devoted to prognosis of impending death. Such knowledge needs to be tempered with the realization that developments in emergency medicine mean that the physiologic impairment to organ structures causing these pulses to form may now be addressed with surgical intervention, dialysis or other forms of therapy now available. Hammer (2002) best summarises this:

> Currently, pulse diagnosis relies on information gathered in a largely agrarian culture expressed in a largely archaic language almost incomprehensible to the 20th century

practitioner. What is available today is material passed down 1900 years from civilizations whose daily life is so variant from our own that the information is often no longer clinically relevant (p. 67).

In contemporary practice, academics and practitioners continue to consult the classics. It is rare to find any writings about the pulse without some 'validation' through direct or overt inferences and connections to these books. However, it can be conjectured that the classics have possibly hindered the development of CM pulse diagnosis as much as they have preserved it. This is best illustrated by comparing two treatises on the use of pulse in medicine published at similar times, both important for pulse diagnosis but for different reasons. The first is Li's *Bin Hue Mai Xue*. The second is Harvey's *Exercitatio Anatomica de Motu Cordis et Sanguinis in Animalibus* [Anatomical Essay on the Movement of the Heart and Blood in Animals] (1624). The texts were published in the late 16th and early 17th century CE respectively and were deemed important works by the authors at those times. Harvey proved the circulation of blood and described the pulsations as the impulse or pressure flow of blood, an event of cardiac contraction (Naqvi & Blaufox 1998). Li focused on collating and annotating earlier CM texts relating to pulse diagnosis, providing a summary of extant works of his time and expanding on some specific pulse qualities. However, although both these works concentrate on the pulse they are starkly contrasted in one very important way. Where Harvey endeavoured to inform practice of pulse diagnosis through ongoing exploration of the underlying principles of pulse, Li Shi-Zhen revisited the books of earlier scholars and reinforced classical methods of pulse diagnosis. Li Shi-Zhen's writing was in effect the embodiment of a culture that revered and respected its past, while Harvey's embodied the deducted logic of practice based on cause and effect that was to become the defining element of biomedical practice.

Interestingly, although there were conceptual links between the heart and vessels described in the CM classics such as the *Nei Jing*, the pulse continued to be viewed in terms of the flow of *Qi* influences; 'there is no indication as to a conceptualisation of either the heart or the lung as fulfilling any kind of a pump like or bellow like function in the classics' (Unschuld 1985: p. 76).

Overall, and in spite of the conflicting views, CM has maintained throughout its history and into contemporary practice a focus on the significance of each individual radial pulse site as being reflective of a specific part of the body. The Cun, Guan and Chi pulse sites are associated with information unique to its location within a given segment of artery. Theoretically, this is associated with palpatory differences in the pulse characteristics between the three pulse positions for each arm. This is in contrast to ancient Greek diagnosticians such as Galen, and even modern biomedical practices that envisage no difference in the pulse and the information obtained when feeling it at different places on the same arterial segment.

References

Birch S 1998 Diversity and acupuncture: acupuncture is not a coherent or historically stable tradition. In: Vickers A (ed) Examining complementary medicine: the sceptical holist. Stanley Thornes, Cheltenham: pp. 45–62

Flaws B 1997 The secret of Chinese pulse diagnosis, 2nd edn. Blue Poppy Press, Boulder, CO.

Li S Z, Flaws B (trans) 1998 The lakeside master's study of the pulse. Blue Poppy Press, Boulder, CO.

Hammer 2002 Tradition and revision. Clinical Acupuncture and Oriental Medicine 3:59–71

Harper D 1998 Early Chinese medical literature: the Mawangdui medical manuscripts. Kegan Paul International, London

Harvey H 1624 An anatomical essay on the movement of the heart and blood in animals. In: Naqvi N & Blaufox M D 1998 Blood pressure measurement: an illustrated history. Pantheon, New York

Ho P, Lisowski F 1997 A brief history of Chinese medicine, 2nd edn. World Scientific Publishing, Singapore

Hsu E 2005 Tactility and the body in early Chinese medicine. Science in Context 18(1):7–34

Kuriyama S 1999 The expressiveness of the body and the divergence of Greek and Chinese medicine. Zone Books, New York

Maciocia G 2004 Diagnosis in Chinese medicine: a comprehensive guide. Churchill Livingstone, Edinburgh

Mi H F, Yang S & Chance C (trans) 1994 The systematic classic of acupuncture and moxibustion. Blue Poppy Press, Boulder

Naqvi N H, Blaufox M D 1998 Blood pressure measurement: an illustrated history. Pantheon, New York

Ni M S (trans) 1995 The Yellow Emperor's classic of medicine (Huang di nei jing su wen ling shu). Shambhala, Boston

Unschuld P 1985 Medicine in China: a history of ideas. University of California Press, Berkeley

Unschuld P (trans) 1986 Nan-Ching: the classic of difficult issues. University of California Press, Berkeley

Unschuld P (trans) 1990 Forgotten traditions of ancient Chinese medicine: a Chinese view from the eighteenth century (I-hsueh yuan liu lun of 1757 by Hsu Ta-ch'un). Paradigm, Brookline, MA

Unschuld P 2003 Huang di nei jing su wen. University of California Press, Berkeley

Wang S H, Yang S (trans) 1997 The pulse classic: a translation of the mai jing. Boulder, Blue Poppy Press

Wiseman N, Ye F 1998 A practical dictionary of Chinese medicine, 2nd edn. Paradigm, Brookline, MA

Wiseman N, Ye F 1999 Translation of Chinese medical pulse terms: taking account of the historical dimension. Clinical Acupuncture and Oriental Medicine 1:55–60

Issues of reliability and validity*

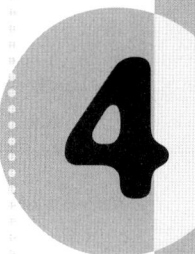

4

Chapter contents

4.1 Pulse diagnosis and the need for clear and unambiguous terminology 34
4.2 Pulse diagnosis, subjectivity and the need for reliable assessment methods 37
4.3 Pulse in changing contexts 38
4.4 The normal pulse 38
4.5 Reliability and validity of the pulse diagnosis process 39
4.6 Radial pulse palpation method 42

In their guidelines for providers of CM education, the World Health Organization (WHO 1999) regarded pulse diagnosis as a core component of the CM diagnostic framework and integral to the curriculum of quality degree programs in acupuncture and Chinese herbal medicine. This view is similarly reflected in curriculum guidelines by accreditation and regulation authorities in various countries (BAC 2000, BMA 2000, NASC 2001). These recommendations are largely founded on the premise that pulse assessment is a clinically reliable diagnostic technique. The antiquity of the use of the technique and historical roots are seen as proof of this; if a technique has been in use for so long, then who is to question the practice of pulse diagnosis? Unfortunately, a ready acceptance of what is written in the classics and contemporary texts, combined with the diversity of CM practices, means the pedagogical framework for using pulse diagnostically is readily compromised, so questioning its reliability for this task (Birch 1998, Hammer 2001, King et al 2002, Wiseman & Ye 1999).

At the core of this problem is the actual nature of pulse diagnosis: it is dependent first and foremost on touch. Consequently, the literature and descriptions of the pulse qualities are enshrouded by tactile imagery constructed from a range of literary devices including analogies, similes and metaphors. For example, Wang Shu-he describes the Tight pulse (*Jiu/Jing Mai*) as being 'an inflexible pulse like a tensely drawn rope' (1997: p. 3). At times, writing involved prose as a learning aid. Notably, Li Shi-Zhen's *Bin Hue Mai Xue* is written entirely in rhyming format. Yet it is this very use of descriptive imagery that makes pulse diagnosis a doubly difficult technique to apply in a clinical context. Not only is pulse diagnosis dependent on an individual's perception of touch, but there are no clear and unambiguous guidelines for interpreting these literary images in a practical sense.

With these factors in mind, a reliance on the practitioner's skills to discriminate between pulses means pulse diagnosis is often regarded as highly subjective.

---

* Some of the information in this chapter is adapted from King (2001) and Walsh (2003).

When the pulse diagnosis process is viewed objectively, the lack of sound scientific evidence to support it can be seen as contributing to its questionable validity, if not complicit in perpetuating the aura of mystification often associated with the technique. It is for this very reason that the pulse procedures and terminology used to assess the pulse need to be explicit and detailed enough to ensure that the diagnosis is done correctly. This is termed *reliability*. How this is achieved, and the factors that affect it, is the central theme of this chapter.

4.1 Pulse diagnosis and the need for clear and unambiguous terminology

Formulating terminology to describe the different pulse types only happened after implementation of pulse in the CM diagnosis process itself (Wiseman and Ye 1999). Originally, pulses were defined descriptively, often using metaphors with particular relevance to everyday life at the time of their development. For example:

> When man is sick the pulse of the liver moves more fully, and it is large and long and slightly tense, felt on both light and heavy pressure; but it is also slippery like the sound of many long bamboo rods strung together, then one can speak of a sick liver.

> At the point of death the pulse of the liver moves with increased speed and strength, like a new long bow of a musical instrument – and then one can speak of the death of the liver.

> When man is tranquil and healthy the pulse of the spleen flows softly, coming together and falling apart like a chicken treading the earth – and then one can speak of a healthy spleen
> *(Veith 1972: p. 174).*

Yet, despite recognition of the need for more detailed and informative definitions of pulse qualities as undertaken in *Mai Jing*, the old descriptive terms remained in subsequent writings. For example, in his classic text on pulse diagnosis, Li Shi-zhen describes the Rough (choppy) pulse (Sè mài) with descriptive terms in addition to more informative details from the *Mai Jing*:

> Fine and slow, going and coming difficult, short and scattered.

> Possibly one stop and again comes [description from the *Mai Jing*].

> Uneven, not regular [description from the *Su Wen*].

> Like a light knife scraping bamboo [description from the *Mai Jue* (Pulse Knacks)].

> Like rain wetting sand.

> Like a diseased silkworm eating a leaf.
> *(Li, Flaws (trans) 1998: p. 79).*

Wiseman and Ye (1999) note interpreting pulse qualities is not helped by complications arising from authors over the centuries attempting to expand and further define the pulse types listed in older CM texts and adding their own interpretations while doing so. A further complicating factor with the use of pulse terminology derived from a different cultural context, and indeed, a temporal context as well, is that it is difficult to determine the exact definition and context of the original author's use of a pulse word or term. Agdal (2005) notes the 'Language is not a neutral tool describing realities but is embedded with cultural meaning; it is a formative principle which constitutes objects as much as it describes them' (p. S-68). According to Manaka, Itaya and Birch (1995) this problem is further accentuated when authors do not reference the sources from which they obtained the pulse terminology used, so negating the benefits of a standard system of terminology.

Confusion also arises when terminology is used in a descriptive manner but also to identify specific CM pulse qualities. The Replete pulse is a good example of this dichotomy. The term 'replete' is often used in the CM literature to convey the idea of excess, and thus is used as a general descriptor of any pulse that hits the finger with considerable strength on palpation. However, the term is also used to name one of the specific CM pulse types, the Replete pulse (Shí mài), traditionally meaning a pulse that 'arrives dynamically, it is hard and full, and its movement is large and long. With light touch it remains; with heavy pressure it has force. Its arrival and departure are both exuberant, and it can be perceived at all three levels' (Deng 1999: p. 125). Further adding to this confusion is the existence of a number of different definitions for the same stated pulse quality, while there may be differently named pulse qualities with the same pulse definition (see Tables 4.1 and 4.2).

Although the traditional pulse qualities have been named for the distinct set of features or characteristics that manifest in the pulse, the names of these specific pulse qualities are sometimes used as general descriptive terms. This arises because the changes in the pulse characteristics cluster in such a way that when a pulse quality 'appears' to occur as described in the literature, it may be further complicated by an additional change in another pulse characteristic, and so does not satisfactorily fit the usual description of a particular CM pulse. For example, Maciocia (2004: p. 485) describes a possible formation of a Stringlike (Wiry) (xián mài)

Table 4.1 ● Comparison of pulse names for the Skipping, Rough and Stirred pulses

Author and source	Skipping pulse (Cù mài)	Rough pulse (Sè mài)	Stirred pulse (Dòng mài)
Cheung & Belluomini (trans) (1982)	Accelerated	Difficult	Agitated
Deng (1999)	Skipping	Rough	Stirred
Flaws (1997)	Skipping, rapidly, irregularly interrupted	Choppy	Stirring
Kaptchuk (2000)	Hurried	Choppy	Spinning Bean
Li (Huynh, trans) (1981)	Hasty	Choppy	Moving
Lu (1996)	Running	Choppy	Tremulous
Maciocia (2004)	Hurried	Choppy	Moving
O'Connor & Bensky (trans and ed) (1981)	Hasty	Rough	Not mentioned
Porkert (1995)	Agitated	Grating	Mobile
Morant (1994)	Accelerated	Hesitant Astringent Rough	Turbulent
Wiseman & Ellis (1996)	Skipping Interrupted	Uneven	Stirred

Table 4.2 ● Comparison of pulse quality definitions for the Replete pulse (Shí mài)

Author and source	Definition	Page no.
Deng (1999)	A replete pulse . . . arrives dynamically, it is hard and full, and its movement is large and long. With light touch it remains; with heavy pressure it has force. Its arrival and departure are both exuberant, and it can be perceived at all three levels	125
Guanzhou Chinese Medicine College (1991)	Felt at Cun, Guan and Chi forceful, long and large, on both light and heavy pressure	18
Li (Huynh, trans) (1981)	Sinking, firmer than the firm pulse, and has a strong beat	15
	When a pulse is felt both superficially and deeply, and has big, long, wiry, strong beats	73
Kaptchuk T (2000)	Is big and also strong, pounding hard against the fingers at all three depths	199
Maciocia (2004)	The Full pulse feels hard, full and rather long; it is felt easily at all levels and it has a springy quality resistant to finger pressure' Also notes the term as a description of a 'broad range of full pulses . . .'	475
Porkert (1995)	Strong pulse manifesting on at least two levels. Still, the pulse shows its greatest strength and deployment on one particular level, 'its specific level'	38
Wiseman & Ellis (1996)	Similar to the forceful except it is forceful on both rising and falling	120

and Slippery pulse (Huà mài) occurring with Full Liver pattern and Phlegm, which appears quite contradictory. That is, the Stringlike (Wiry) pulse is defined by the tension in the arterial wall which constrains the arterial contour from manifesting, whereas the Slippery pulse is defined by the arterial contour deforming the arterial wall, which is quite distinctly rounded as it moves under the fingers, and it is the relative lack of arterial tension which allows the pulse wave to form in this way. (There are additional changes in other pulse characteristics that further differentiate the two pulses.) So the question is, why have these two distinctly different terms been used in this way?

The answer is that they have been used in this way because the focus has been on the most apparent or distinctive change occurring in the pulse, rather than on all the information available. By focusing on the apparent changes, the increased arterial tension has been termed the Stringlike (Wiry) pulse. Yet, the classical definition of the Stringlike (Wiry) pulse notes this pulse without a distinct contour, and so by definition the pulse described by Maciocia is not *the* Stringlike (Wiry) pulse. Similarly, the pulse described is not *the* Slippery pulse either, despite the presence of Phlegm.

Yet in undertaking the process of pulse diagnosis it is hard for the practitioner not to think of the terminology of the traditional pulse qualities, if only because they have dominated any discourse of pulse diagnosis in Chinese medicine for so many years. However, it soon becomes apparent that there are limitations to the use of the pulse names when used in this way, as evidenced in the example above.

The pulse diagnosis process is further complicated when the traditional pulse names are used to discretely classify the pulse when this is not warranted (that is, when the pulse is categorised or termed as one of the traditional CM pulse qualities but not all aspects or characteristics of its presentation actually fit the traditional definition). In doing so, the other pulse characteristic changes, which do not match the traditional description of the pulse being felt, are excluded. Such an approach means all available clues about the pathogenesis are not considered in diagnoses, and so a practitioner may underestimate or overestimate the pathology against incorrectly 'recognised' pulse qualities rather than using all the information that is available. The obvious problem with this is that the lost pulse information may signal the difference between treatment that aims to tonify against one that aims to disperse.

4.1.1 Practical implications of confusion in CM pedagogy

The ultimate outcome of this confusion is great variance in terminology between CM texts affecting the practical application of pulse diagnosis. This includes the application of pulse diagnosis in:

- Treatment planning within clinical practice
- Educational purposes and pulse learning
- Research investigations involving traditional methods of diagnosis.

4.1.1.1 Pulse pedagogy and treatment planning

The absence of standardised pulse terminology has implications for the use of pulse diagnosis in clinical practice, where the role of pulse is thought to have various applications in diagnosis, in treatment formulation and as an immediate indicator of the effectiveness of the treatment (Birch & Felt 1999). When used for these purposes, it is vital that the pulse information is reliable, ensuring that the patient receives the correct diagnosis and so appropriate treatment. This is particularly important when using herbal medicine, as an incorrect diagnosis and hence an incorrect herbal prescription may result in a worsening of the condition. Similarly in acupuncture, there are some systems that rely on pulse assessment as the primary means of diagnosis and so treatment is dependent on a reliable and accurate assessment.

4.1.1.2 Pulse pedagogy and learning

In Asia and elsewhere Birch and Felt (1999) note that there has been a shift away from clinically based pulse teaching to a model that emphasises intellectual or theoretically based knowledge. As a result, intensive clinically based training in pulse diagnosis has fallen out of common use. The theoretical approach is commonly applied in other areas of CM education, and this pedagogical approach is usually based on the premise of a standardised and workable theoretical data set such as that used in Eight Principles differential diagnosis (Ba Gang) or Five Phases (Wu Xing). Such a standardised theoretical approach is often in contrast to the theoretical information on pulse diagnosis, with its characteristic ambiguous descriptive terms which lack clarity.

Consequently, Birch & Felt (1999: p. 235) proposed that the pulse literature was intended as a supportive adjunct to practice-based teaching, and so explains its apparent failings when used as the only form of teaching. Accordingly, they claimed, it was never meant to be the primary means of imparting knowledge in this area. Birch & Felt based their claims on historical texts that documented the traditional teaching methods of pulse diagnosis. The repetitive practice of pulse palpation under a teacher's guidance in clinic was once the mainstay of education in this area.

Yet even this explanation of the failings of the pulse pedagogy warrants questioning. For example, even as far back as the second century CE, where traditional master–apprentice teaching methods for learning pulse diagnosis were used, Wang Shu-he (author of the *Mai Jing*) wrote of the difficulty in distinguishing between pulse qualities, even when having memorised the definitions. He used an example in which the Bowstring, Tight, Floating and Scallion Stalk pulses could be seen to share some common characteristics. This, he observed, made these pulses easy to mistake for one another, even with the use of a standard pulse terminology:

> The mechanisms of the pulse are fine and subtle, and the pulse images are difficult to differentiate. The bowstring and the tight, the floating and the scallion-stalk confusingly resemble one another. They may be readily distinct at heart (that is, their verbal definition may have been memorized), but it is difficult for the fingers to distinguish them. If a deep pulse is taken as a hidden one, the formula and treatment will never be in the right line. If a moderate pulse is taken as a slow one, crisis may crop up instantly. In addition, there are cases where several different kinds of pulse images appear all at the once or several different categories of disease may exhibit the same type of pulse
> *(Wang, Yang (trans) 1997: p. xi).*

Other CM authors argue that pulse taking should not be difficult to learn (Porkert 1995, Flaws 1997), stressing the importance of the theories and of learning the standard textbook definition of each pulse quality (King 2001: p. 37). However, it can be strongly argued that it is precisely the lack of clarity of the standard definitions that cause problems. Wiseman and Ye (1999) note a lack of precision and non-standardised definitions arise when authors and practitioners have failed to identify exactly what they mean when stating or describing pulse characteristics (Wiseman & Ye 1999).

4.1.1.3 Pulse pedagogy and research

In research, ideally, an appropriate study method requires detailed documentation of all facets of the design process, detailing how information was collected, interpreted and decisions made using CM methods of diagnosis, leading to the development of a treatment protocol. Therefore a clear and unambiguous terminology is required here as well. In addition, the careful detailing of both treatment and diagnostic processes should be included in clinical trials (Birch 1997), not only to enable replication of the studies but also to provide clinically relevant information for the CM profession.

A failure to standardise pulse terminology and descriptions hinders the evaluation of traditional-based systems of CM, where the role of pulse is given equal weighting with other assessment approaches. For example, a holistic perspective and a method of treatment tailored to the individual are integral components of the traditional approach to CM. This involves the systematic gathering and collating of patient data to construct a diagnosis and subsequent treatment protocol. With a treatment based directly on the diagnostic assessment, it is vital that this initial process is both objective and reliable. As Flaws notes: 'In TCM, a correct pattern discrimination is vitally important. It is the guide and foundation to successful, individualised treatment' (Flaws 1997: p. 3).

4.2 Pulse diagnosis, subjectivity and the need for reliable assessment methods

A subjective procedure is one in which an observation or outcome arises from the individual; it is dependent on the individual's own interpretation and therefore cannot be objectively measured or confirmed. The pulse diagnosis method, by definition, is such a procedure. Subjective procedures are prone to ambiguity, and this is clearly reflected in the pulse literature where there may be two quite contradictory descriptions for the same pulse quality. Subjective procedures are also prone to variability in their application; different practitioners may interpret the same patient's pulse in different ways. Alternatively, the same practitioner may interpret the same patient's pulses differently on subsequent examinations at the same sitting, as was reported by Craddock (1997).

In part, it is thought that such variability is due to the pulse's sensitivity to external temporary influences such as physical activity and emotions (Maciocia 2004). In this respect, rather than the reliability of the method being at fault, it is suggested that the patient's variability is responsible for pulse reading discrepancies (King 2001: p. 37). However, this is somewhat tenuous, particularly in the absence of any standardised terminology or pulse taking procedure, as differences in a patient's pulse characteristics may be due to inconsistent pulse technique or the pulse taker's own subjective interpretation of the pulse changes.

Because of the perceived subjectivity not only of pulse diagnosis but also of other aspects of the CM diagnostic procedure, there has been debate about whether the treatment and choice of acupuncture points should be based on conventional medical diagnostic procedures rather than CM theories (Bensoussan 1991, Hammerschlag 1998, Smith 1998, Ulett 1992 cited in King 2001: p. 38). This has particular relevance for CM research involving clinical efficacy, where diagnostic procedures need to be shown to be objective, reliable and reproducible, and also have validity.

37

Table 4.3 ● Comparison of pulse quality definitions of the Slow pulse

Author and source	Definition	Page no.
Deng (1999)	A slow pulse . . . refers to three beats per breath, or one less than normal	117
Guanzhou Chinese Medicine College (1991)	Generally regular rhythm 40–60 beats per minute	
Kaptchuk (2000)	Fewer than four beats per respiration	197
Porkert (1995)	. . . less than four beats per breath (on the adult)	38
Wiseman & Ellis (1996)	Three or less beats per respiration	119

(As an aside, the term 'objective' refers to information that is uncoloured by the practitioner's perceptions and interpretation. In the context of pulse diagnosis, the parameters of pulse rate and rhythm are two common CM pulse characteristics that can be objectively verified and the measurements validated by others. Interestingly, this is also reflected in the literature, in which the pulse descriptions for pulses defined by rate or rhythm have a higher consensus among different authors (Table 4.3). Yet many other variables remain subjective, reinforcing the need for unambiguous terminology and concrete operational definitions for applying the pulse taking procedure.)

4.3 Pulse in changing contexts

The available pulse literature identifies a range of factors as contributing to the variability of the pulse and so needing to be factored into assessment processes when interpreting pulse findings. However, the associated effects on the pulse are often based on assumptions. This is because there have been so few studies investigating the clinical relevancy of even the most basic assumptions underlying radial pulse diagnosis. These assumptions include the relationships between pulse and age, gender, season and body types. For example, it is assumed that the left side pulse in men is stronger than the right side pulse, while in women the reverse is the case. This is stated in the CM classics *Nan Jing*, *Mai Jing* and *Bin Hue Mai Xue*, in addition to similar claims by modern authors such as Hammer (2001: p. 95) and Rogers (2000: p. 88). The claims regarding this and other relationships first appeared over 2000 years ago in a society that was fundamentally very different in terms of culture, society, geography and economics from contemporary modern society. As Hammer (1993: p. 125) noted: 'Much of what has come down to us as Scripture does not stand the test of time.'

The veracity of long-held CM assumptions may change over time for many reasons. For example, temporal changes in diet, lifestyle, environmental pollution

and the changed pace of modern life may impact on the general health of a population, generating different health problems. Similarly, technological advances in biomedical practices and medication have seen the eradication of some diseases and the control of others. Conditions once considered incurable or terminal are now treatable or manageable, and so it can be strongly argued that the related pulses are no longer seen in individuals presenting in primary CM practice in the developed countries. Conversely, conditions once rarely seen in east Asia are occurring with greater frequency in modern society. For example, in Western countries the rise of cardiovascular diseases such as arteriosclerosis and hypertension has been linked to genetic, lifestyle and environmental factors, and these diseases are now occurring more often in Asian populations.

Any of these factors may indeed impact in some way on the pulse characteristics of the general population. Some clinical support for this was provided by the report of the existence of a new pulse quality, tentatively termed the *Fluctuating pulse* (Zhou & Rogers 1997). Rather than an oversight of the ancient CM practitioners and scholars, they suggested that the appearance of this additional quality was: 'A pulse quality that developed in modern times in response to a changed, and changing, environment' (p. 91).

Obviously, the recognition of new pulse qualities may equally mean that some of the traditional pulse qualities may no longer manifest as frequently in the population as may have happened in centuries past. While applying the knowledge and skills contained in older CM texts, modern practitioners should also continue to broaden their knowledge base to encompass changing environment and demographic factors.

4.4 The normal pulse

If pulse qualities are evolving, then the CM image of a normal pulse (usually described as moderate in speed, located neither superficially nor deeply, with an even and regular rhythm) may no longer be valid for contemporary Western urban society, or indeed, contemporary urban Chinese or Japanese society. The notion of what constitutes a normal pulse is further complicated by the assumption that the pulse is prone to seasonal changes, resulting in particular changes that are considered to be normal for the season. Other influences on the pulse include age, gender and time of day. An extensive English-language literature review has not revealed any large-sample demographic study to assess the types of pulse occurring in the general population or their cyclical change through the seasons.

Confusion concerning the features of a normal pulse is not limited to CM practice. In their text on arterial pulses O'Rourke et al (1992: p. 47) point out that it is difficult to define the normal pulse since: 'The arterial pulse shows a range of patterns under normal conditions. Different patterns are seen . . . in the same artery at different ages, in the same artery under different physiological conditions.'

This view is similar to that of the CM theory regarding pulse, where it is claimed that a range of pulse qualities constituting the normal pulse may be seen, according to the influence of age, gender, body type or season. Although the classical literature notes the effects of these variables on the pulse, in a modern context there are no data demonstrating these effects or evidence of exactly how they manifest in a clinical setting.

4.5 Reliability and validity of the pulse diagnosis process

Discrepancy between what is written in the classics regarding pulse and what may be occurring in contemporary industrialised populations raises further issues of the validity of the available body of pulse knowledge. Together with inconsistencies of pedagogy and palpatory technique, this brings us to ask a further critical question: Is pulse diagnosis a sound diagnostic tool, and can it be relied on to produce consistent results?

How one chooses to answer this question probably depends on one's ideological perspective on the practice of pulse diagnosis. From an evidenced-based perspective, the answer is ambivalent as so few studies have been undertaken to confirm or disprove the palpatory technique and its associated assumptions. For example, there are insufficient empirical data either supporting or refuting the notion that changes in the organ system are reflected at the associated radial arterial pulse positions, and too few studies to determine whether practitioners can reliably and consistently discern these changes (Walsh et al 2001: p. 25).

While accepting there is not a large body of firm evidence, there are ways of ensuring that the reliability of pulse taking is maximised, which is the point of this book. This entails ensuring that all abstractions con-

cerning measurement of the pulse are made concrete and the pulse measurement procedure must be shown to be reliable. Stern & Kalof (1996) note that this should involve the development of appropriate operational definitions to determine which variables are being measured and how they will be measured. For pulse diagnosis, it is essential to use concrete operational definitions to ensure that the correct finger positions are located and that consistent methods of palpation are adopted for identifying variations in the pulse wave. If pulse assessment is undertaken the same way every time, then any perceived changes are likely to be the result of illness rather than being variations introduced through inconsistent application of palpatory technique by the practitioner.

Reliability also refers to relating any identified changes in pulse characteristics to pathology through a consistent means of interpretation. This largely depends on the use of the body of literature, the pedagogy, used for categorising any such pulse changes felt. In this sense, reliability can apply not only to the consistent use of a technique by the practitioner but also to the intrinsic validity of the technique. Reliability is, in effect, a product of the literature, theories and systematic clinical use of pulse diagnosis in practice.

4.5.1 Inter-rater reliability

In its basic form pulse taking is a measurement tool for assessing changes in pulse characteristics. A measurement procedure is considered reliable if it produces the same (or similar) scores when separately used on the same set of individuals under the same conditions (Gravetter & Wallnau 1996). This is termed *inter-rater reliability*. From a clinical perspective, inter-rater (or inter-observer) reliability testing is the process used to substantiate the extent to which practitioners are in agreement with each other regarding patient assessment using a specific measurement tool, in this case pulse diagnosis. The measurement tool is considered to be reliable if it can be shown to reproduce similar results when used by two or more independent assessors to evaluate the same group of patients (King 2001: p. 39). A high level of agreement between the assessors means a high level of inter-rater reliability (Polgar & Thomas 1995).

4.5.1.1 Pulse inter-rater reliability research

Relatively little attention has been paid to testing the validity of the basic theory underlying CM diagnostic procedure. Clinical research into acupuncture and CM focuses primarily on determining the mode of action of acupuncture (involving identification of neurological and biochemical pathways), and herbs (receptor interactions and physiological effects on function) (Lewith & Vincent 1998). Relatively few studies have been carried out to evaluate the reliability of CM diagnostic processes. The existing studies concerning pulse diagnosis have generally reported low levels of inter-rater reliability in relation to the agreement about pulse and the perceived differences in pulse characteristics.

Practitioner inter-rater reliability studies (King 2001: pp. 40–41)

A common finding in the limited research carried out to evaluate the reliability of CM pulse diagnosis is the inverse relationship between the degree of complexity of pulse qualities and levels of inter-rater reliability. A study by Craddock (1997), investigating the reliability of the CM pulse diagnostic process, found that the levels of inter-rater and intra-rater reliability decreased with the increasing complexity of pulse qualities being measured. Since this pilot study included only four practitioners and eight subjects, generalisations of findings require caution. In this study, raters were blinded to subjects, which removed any visual bias from the assessment process. This helped to ensure that the diagnosis was pulse dependent only and not influenced by the physique and appearance of the subject having their pulse assessed (as this is also considered to be part of the CM diagnostic process). The results of a study by Kass (1990) also suggested that levels of inter-rater reliability decreased as more subtle levels of pulse discrimination were required. However, in this study inter-rater reliability was determined using both manual palpation and an electronic pulse detection device, so it is difficult to compare these results with those solely using manual palpation.

The effect of non-standardised pulse terminology and methodology is also reflected in the results of Cole's British study (1977) of the use of pulse diagnosis in Britain. This research also reported generally low levels of inter-rater agreement between CM practitioners. In addition, a tendency for individual practitioners to favour particular pulse patterns when recording pulse information was also identified: in examining the same group of subjects one practitioner recorded a higher number of 'normal' pulses while another practitioner, recorded approximately equal numbers of 'normal' and 'unbalanced' pulses. Cole surmised that this could have been due to both the practitioners' preconceived notions about what to expect in the pulse (possibly influenced by other diagnostic criteria available) and to their individual subjective interpretation of the presentation of the pulse characteristics, but unless specific pulse terminology and detailed methodology was provided, it could be equally interpreted as the result of differing measurement techniques and pulse terminology used to evaluate the pulse.

In a study using 5 practitioners and 26 subjects, Birch & Ida (1998, personal communication) found a range of inter-rater reliability agreement in the pulse assessment component of research undertaken to examine diagnostic assessment methods. However, all practitioners had the same access to each subject's medical history and the raters were able to see the subjects whose pulses they were palpating, which may have had some influence on their evaluation of pulse assessment. The pulse qualities of depth, strength and rate were rated on a 1–5 scale. Using Spearman rank correlation, results ranged from zero ($r = -0.004$) or no agreement to near-perfect correlation ($r = 0.93$) or agreement, with most results lying between 0.38 and 0.45.

Because the diversity of the pulse diagnosis systems used in the above studies, it is difficult to compare the findings. However, the generally low levels of inter-rater reliability may be perceived to reflect a systemic weakness: poorly defined pulse definitions and pulse palpation methodology. It is assumed that all practitioners in the same study were purportedly using the same pulse taking system and definitions of pulse qualities. However, unless the exact pulse taking method was prescribed and the pulse qualities clearly defined, the assessors may well have used their own interpretations of the pulse qualities and their own methods of pulse palpation. This is likely, given the wide range of definitions for each of the pulse qualities found in the pulse literature. This also applies to the pulse taking techniques, most notably differences in finding the levels of pulse depth or the traditional pulse positions. These studies reinforce the need for standardisation of both terminology and method when conducting research into aspects of pulse diagnosis.

The relationship between unambiguous, concrete definitions and reliability was clearly demonstrated in a study by King et al (2002), in which levels of inter-rater agreement were statistically significantly better than chance alone. In this study, the descriptive terminology often used to describe the specific CM pulse qualities was not used. Instead, the pulse was broken down into simple components, termed parameters, that related to the actual tactile sensations perceived under the fingers during palpation, but which, when reconstructed, also form the traditional pulse qualities. By operationally defining each parameter, the reliability of the pulse measurement system was demonstrated by two independent assessors. A high level of inter-rater reliability was also demonstrated in a replication phase of the study.

Subsequent studies have shown this parameter method is reliable for pulse characteristic evaluation when used in the context of CM, limiting the source of variability between assessors (King et al 2002, King et al 2006, Walsh 2003, Walsh & Cobbin 2001). In this way, developing a pulse pedagogy that is unambiguous and clearly defined assists in achieving reliability of pulse measurement.

Student inter-rater reliability studies

Relevant inter-rater reliability research on pulse has generally focused on practitioners. There has been little investigation of a student's ability to learn pulse diagnosis and implement pulse theory in the discrimination of radial pulse characteristics. This is surprising, since it is as a student that potential practitioners must learn correct technique and appropriate pulse taking procedures and reliable pulse diagnosis (Walsh et al 2001).

The inconsistent interpretation of pulse types by students, and even practitioners, may be attributed primarily to pulse descriptions that are open to subjective interpretation. Finch & Crunkilton (1993) describe this as 'constraints of content' (p. 164); stating that it is content, rather than the inability of the students or the practitioners to integrate information, that inhibits the learning process. This view was supported by a study to assess the inter-rater agreement levels among CM students (Walsh et al 2001), where student participants failed to maintain the number of pulse characteristics for which statistically significant agreement levels were achieved from the initial baseline measures over the following 12 month period. Using a single-blind study design and large sample size, students were tested on three occasions, at the beginning of pulse diagnosis classes (C1), at the completion of the 14 week pulse classes (C2) and one year later (N = 35, 29, 20). Surprisingly, the last collection showed the lowest level of inter-rater agreement among the students. In addition, of the three collections, the second collection alone showed a level of agreement greater than that expected by chance. Walsh found that overall levels of agreement about some basic pulse characteristics (such as depth, speed and length) differed very little from those obtained by chance alone. The study's findings showed a decrease in the number of pulse characteristics for which inter-rater agreement levels were achieved over time with exposure of the cohort to further curriculum studies (C3) as compared to frequency levels achieved at C2. Significantly, in C1 and C2, the participants used pulse descriptions from a single source in their CM course: the class notes. A further 12 months' exposure to a set curriculum and extracurricular reading of the CM literature may have contributed to an increased variance in the students' ability to reach consensus in discriminating differences in the pulse at C3. It was surmised that, rather than stemming from an inability to learn pulse diagnosis, low levels of agreement reflected the conflicting and subjective information about pulse diagnosis in the available CM literature.

4.5.2 Addressing reliability issues

If the practitioner interprets the pulse sensation using a specific set of rules that allows others to understand why and by what means the pulse sensation was interpreted, this begins to establish reliability. This should be the role of pulse terminology: to provide a framework for identifying which procedures were used, how these were applied in palpating the pulse and why a decision regarding the pulse in terms of health or pathology was made. This requires a standardised system of pulse terminology that is still relevant to contemporary clinical practice of pulse diagnosis, but is not subject to the limitations of the traditional literature.

Wiseman & Ye (1999) emphasise the necessity for a standard terminology for unequivocal communication in Chinese medicine. However, this may result in over-classifying pulse terminology to the point where it no longer has any clinical relevance to the practitioner or to aspects of the pulse wave being palpated. As O'Rourke et al (1992) quoted Broadbent who was referring to Galen's pulse descriptions, 'it is easy to confuse the essential features of the important variations in the pulse by overwhelming them in minute distinctions of no practical significance' (p. 5). It is necessary then, when developing appropriate terminology, to ensure that it remains clinically relevant, so not adding more confusion to the process.

In developing an unambiguous terminology for use with pulse palpation, it is first necessary to determine the essential parameters or the characteristics that are involved in the physical manifestation of the radial pulse. This approach is equally applicable to all pulse assumption systems used in CM; whether founded on lineage teachings, on instructions recorded in the classics or on those found in more contemporary constructs such as Five Phase acupuncture.

Such an approach to developing unambiguous terminology is not a recent concept. Wang Shu-he recognised this in the *Mai Jing* by applying a name to a group of descriptive terms in identifying the pulse qualities he used. In more recent times Wiseman & Ye (1999: p. 56) discuss the analysis of pulse terminology written by Zhou Xue Hai in 1896, in which he determined that there were four main pulse characteristic parameters:

- position (wèi) at which the pulse could be felt (Cun, Guan or Chi, that is length)
- pace (shò) of the pulse (relating to both rate and rhythm)
- form (xíng) of the pulse (level of depth and width)
- dynamic (shì), i.e. the strength of the pulse on arrival and departure.

In this way, some specific CM pulse qualities could be defined by a single parameter, whereas others are defined by two or more parameters. This method of pulse assessment has been partially touched on by contemporary authors such as Lu (1996) and Townsend & De Donna (1990), and a range of other contemporary texts from various sources. The terminology applied to describing pulses and identification of pulse types used throughout this book employs a similar approach to that detailed by Zhou Xue Hai. We have termed this the *pulse parameter method*.

From an extensive examination of pulse terminology, it was determined that it is the varying combination of the presence or absence of changes in these parameters that forms the basis of the specific CM pulse qualities. For example, the Sinking pulse (Chén mài) is noted for being felt most forcefully at the deep level of depth (regardless of the overall pulse force) and its lack of presence at the superficial level of depth.

The specific CM pulse qualities can be further categorised into simple and complex CM pulse qualities, according to the number of pulse parameters involved in their presentation. The Intermittent pulse (Dài mài) is categorised as a simple CM pulse quality, as rhythm is the only parameter involved. Conversely the Scallion Stalk (hollow) (kōu mài) pulse is classed as complex because of the involvement of changes in a number of parameters including pulse force, depth, arterial wall tension and width. These parameters and associated CM pulse qualities are discussed in further detail in Chapters 6 and 7.

4.6 Radial pulse palpation method

As well as differences in the 'standard' pedagogy in the literature, there are also differences in palpatory technique and a lack of detailed instruction on how to palpate the pulse. This means that idiosyncratic techniques have evolved for locating the levels of depth of the pulse, each with its own methods.

The CM literature concerning pulse diagnostic methodology is fraught with inconsistencies concerning the numerous techniques for pulse taking. Differences occur within and between pulse diagnosis systems and can be related to the specific assumption systems underlying them, influencing the interpretation of the findings in a diagnostic context. For example, there are varying methods for locating the different levels of the pulse among CM texts. Townsend & De Donna (1990) proposed that the superficial pulse could be found by increasing light pressure until a definite pulse could be felt. Other texts suggested placing the fingertips lightly on the skin surface without applying pressure (Deng 1999 Li (Huynh trans) 1991, Wiseman & Ellis 1996). The methods of examining the deep level of the pulse were also varied, with simplistic instructions such as 'felt by pressing firmly' (Wiseman & Ellis, 1996) or 'the physician presses quite hard' (Kaptchuk 2000). Townsend & De Donna (1990) suggested compressing the pulse until it vanished and then decreasing the pressure slightly until the pulse returned, while another author suggested pressing down to the area between the tendon and bone (King 2001).

Generally, CM texts tend not to fully define all aspects of the pulse taking procedure. Instead emphasis is placed on the clinical indications of the different CM pulse qualities and associated disease patterns, while neglecting the very methods used to identify them. This is reflected in the ambiguous and often contradictory pulse definitions. Confusion often occurs over terms used to name specific CM pulse qualities and others that are used as descriptive terms. For example, the Firm pulse (Láo mài) is described in one text (Lu 1996) as being deep, forceful, large, wiry and long and the indications of its solitary presence in each of the individual positions is described. Yet in the same text, the Long pulse (Cháng mài) is defined as being longer than the normal length of Cun, Guan and Chi, therefore raising the question of how a pulse that is 'long' could possibly be present only in a single pulse position.

The subjective methods of the CM classical literature and the use of analogies to define the amount of pressure exerted to find specific levels also have little relevance to modern-day experience, and only confuse the application of techniques further. For example, in the Fifth Difficult Issue of the *Nan Jing*, the pressure needed to distinguish between the five different levels of depth is described in terms of the weight of a number of beans. In commentaries on the Fifth Difficult Issue discussing how to palpate the different levels of the pulse, there is a comment about the difficulty of understanding the 'bean method' (Unschuld (trans) 1986: p. 114), another referenced using pressure to the bone, so it is apparent that there have always been difficulties associated with the various methods of palpation when using descriptive terminology.

4.6.1 Pulse method reliability

Although an unambiguous and concrete terminology is essential for radial pulse diagnosis, it is now apparent that it is equally important to have a consistent method with which to palpate the pulse. A consistent method refers to:

- How and when to apply the pulse taking method: the order of gathering information from the pulse.
- The different techniques (depth, length, strength of application) and required body part (pulse position)
- A consistent application of the techniques in the same way every time.

A consistent method of application is vital, as many of the specific CM pulse types are dependent on the measurement of pulse parameters in specific positions. For example the Long pulse is defined as the presence of pulsations at the three traditional pulse positions Cun, Guan and Chi and beyond these positions, distally and/or proximally. Therefore, it is crucial that the practitioner understands precisely how to locate these positions, in order to be able to identify the CM pulse quality correctly if it is present. This has particular importance in specific methods of radial pulse diagnosis such as the Five Phase method, where the pulses in each of the three traditional pulse positions at the superficial and deep level are rated in terms of overall force: either as deficient, excessive or 'normal' (appropriate strength). This is significant because the resulting treatment protocol is primarily based on this diagnostic pulse pattern. Other examples of such systems requiring precise palpatory methods include the Japanese keiraku chiryo system which interprets the organ (Zang Fu) pulse positions into four primary diagnostic categories of organ pairings (Birch 1998: p. 45) and the San Jiao or Three Heater method for looking at a comparative strength differences. Consequently, if the traditional pulse positions are not located in a similar fashion or if there are differences in the methods used to palpate the pulse at different levels of depth, there will be no reliability. The development of a correct and consistent pulse method is detailed in Chapter 5.

References

Agdal R 2005 Diverse and changing perceptions of the body: communicating illness, health, and risk in an age of medical pluralism. Journal of Alternative and Complementary Medicine 11(S1):S67–S75

BAC 2000 The British Acupuncture Council guidelines for acupuncture education. British Acupuncture Council, London

Bensoussan A 1991 The vital meridian: a modern exploration of acupuncture. Churchill Livingstone, Melbourne

Birch, S J 1997 Testing the claims of traditionally based acupuncture. Complementary Therapies in Medicine 5:147–151

Birch S 1998 Diversity and acupuncture: acupuncture is not a coherent or historically stable tradition. In: Vickers A (ed) Examining complementary medicine: the sceptical holist. Stanley Thornes, Cheltenham, pp 45–62

Birch S, Felt R 1999 Understanding acupuncture. Harcourt Brace, London

BMA 2000 Acupuncture: efficacy, safety and practice. British Medical Association report. Harwood Academic Publishers, London

Cheung C, Belluomini J (trans) 1982 An overview of pulse types used in traditional Chinese medical differential diagnosis. Journal of the American College of Traditional Chinese Medicine 1(1):15–36

Cole P C 1977 Pulse diagnosis and the practice of acupuncture in Britain [PhD]. University of Sussex, Sussex

Craddock D 1997 Is traditional Chinese medical pulse reading a consistent practice: a comparative pilot study of four practitioners [BAppSc]. University of Technology Sydney, Sydney

Deng T 1999 Practical diagnosis in traditional Chinese medicine. Churchill Livingstone, Edinburgh

Finch C, Crunkilton J 1993 Curriculum development in vocational and technical education: planning, content, and implementation. Allyn & Bacon, Boston

Flaws B 1997 The secret of Chinese pulse diagnosis, 2nd edn. Blue Poppy Press, Boulder, CO

Gravetter F, Wallnau L 1996 Statistics for the behavioural sciences, 4th edn. West Publishing Company, St Paul

Guanzhou Chinese Medicine College 1991 Inspection of the tongue and pulse taking. Guanzhou Chinese Medicine College, Guanzhou

Hammer L 1993 Contemporary pulse diagnosis: introduction to an evolving method for learning an ancient art – part 1. American Journal of Acupuncture 21(2):123–139

Hammer L 2001 Chinese pulse diagnosis: a contemporary approach. Eastland Press, Seattle

Hammerschlag R 1998 Methodological and ethical issues in clinical trials of acupuncture. Journal of Alternative and Complementary Medicine 4(2):159–171

Kaptchuk T 2000 Chinese medicine: web that has no weaver. Revised edn. Rider Books, London

Kass R 1990 Traditional Chinese medicine and pulse diagnosis in San Francisco health planning: implications for a Pacific rim city. Online. Available: http://www.acupuncture.com/library/research

King E 2001 Do the radial qualities of traditional Chinese medicine provide a reliable diagnostic tool?: an examination of pulse relationships stated in modern and classical Chinese texts [MSc]. University of Technology, Sydney

King E, Cobbin D, Walsh S et al 2002 The reliable measurement of radial pulse characteristics. Acupuncture in Medicine 20(4):150–159

King E, Walsh S, Cobbin D 2006 The testing of classical pulse concepts in Chinese medicine: Left- and right-hand pulse strength discrepancy between males and females and its clinical implications. Journal of Alternative and Complementary Medicine 12(5):445–450

Lewith G T, Vincent C A 1998 The clinical evaluation of acupuncture. In: Fllshle J & White A (eds) Medical acupuncture: a western scientific approach. Churchill Livingstone, Edinburgh, Ch 13, pp 205–224

Li S Z, Huynh H K (trans) 1981 Pulse diagnosis. Paradigm, Brookline, MA

Li S Z, Flaws B (trans) 1998 The lakeside master's study of the pulse. Blue Poppy Press, Boulder, CO

Lu Y 1996 Pulse diagnosis. Shandong Science and Technology Press, Jinan

Maciocia G 2004 Diagnosis in Chinese medicine: a comprehensive guide. Churchill Livingstone, Edinburgh

Manaka Y, Itaya K, Birch S 1995 Chasing the dragon's tail. Paradigm, Brookline, MA

Morant G, (Grinnell L, Leveque M , Jeanmougin C, trans) 1994 Chinese acupuncture. Paradigm, Brookline. MA

NASC 2001 National Academic Standards Committee for Traditional Chinese Medicine. The Australian guidelines for traditional Chinese medicine education. Australian Acupuncture and Chinese Medicine Association, Brisbane

O'Connor J, Bensky D (trans and eds) 1981 Acupuncture: a comprehensive text. Eastland Press, Seattle

O'Rourke M, Kelly R, Avolio A 1992 The arterial pulse. Lea & Febiger, Pennsylvania

Polgar S, Thomas S 1995 Introduction to research in the health sciences, 3rd edn. Oxford University Press, New York

Porkert M 1995 Classical acupuncture: the standard textbook. Phainon, Dinkelscherben

Rogers C 2000 The five keys: an introduction to the study of traditional Chinese medicine, 3rd edn revised. Acupuncture Colleges Publishing, Sydney

Smith A 1998 Five Phase diagnosis: the art of science or the science of art. Pacific Journal of Oriental Medicine 5:20–26

Stern P, Kalof L 1996 Evaluating social science research, 2nd edn. Oxford University Press, Oxford

Townsend G, De Donna Y 1990 Pulses and impulses: a practitioner's guide to a unique new pulse diagnosis technique. Thorsons, Wellingborough

Ulett G 1992 Beyond yin and yang: how acupuncture really works. Warren H Green, St Louis

Veith I 1972 The Yellow Emperor's classic of internal medicine. University of California Press, Berkeley

Walsh S, Cobbin D, Bateman K et al 2001 Feeling the pulse: trial to assess agreement level among TCM students when identifying basic pulse characteristics. European Journal of Oriental Medicine 3(5):25–31

Walsh S 2003 The radial pulse: correlation of traditional Chinese medicine pulse characteristics with objective tonometric measures [PhD]. University of Technology Sydney, Sydney

Walsh S, Cobbin D 2001 The suitability of the parameter pulse method in teaching undergraduate students: a longitudinal study comparing two methods of pulse diagnosis in the teaching environment. In: Cochran W (ed) The professionalisation of traditional Chinese medicine. Proceedings of the 6th Australasian Acupuncture and Chinese Herbal Medicine Conference 9 Sept. p. 6

Wang S H, Yang S (trans) 1997 The pulse classic: a translation of the Mai Jing. Blue Poppy Press, Boulder, CO

WHO 1999 Guidelines on basic training and safety in acupuncture. World Health Organisation, Geneva

Wiseman N, Ellis A 1996 Fundamentals of Chinese medicine. Revised edn. Paradigm, Brookline, MA

Wiseman N, Ye F 1999 Translation of Chinese medical pulse terms: taking account of the historical dimension. Clinical Acupuncture and Oriental Medicine 1:55–60

Zhou C, Rogers C 1997 The fluctuating pulse: description of a recently identified pulse. In: Cochran W (ed). Towards unity: integrating theory and practice. Proceedings of the Third Australasian Acupuncture and Chinese Herbal Medicine Conference, 13 July. p. 15

Getting started:
pulse techniques, procedures and the development of a methodical approach to pulse assessment

5

Chapter contents

5.1 Positioning the patient 46
5.2 Locating the radial artery 47
5.3 Locating the pulse positions for assessment 49
5.4 Practitioner positioning 51
5.5 Assessing the parameters 51
5.6 Locating the pulse depth 53
5.7 The normal pulse 56
5.8 Assessing health by the pulse 57
5.9 Channel, organ and levels of depth 58
5.10 Comparison of the overall force of the left and right radial pulse 58
5.11 Pulse method 59
5.12 Other considerations when assessing the pulse and interpreting the findings 61
5.13 Summary 68

Although an objective terminology is essential for radial pulse diagnosis, it is equally imperative to have reliable procedures and a consistent method when palpating the pulse. Pulse procedures refers to the processes preceding pulse assessment as well as the actual techniques used during this process. These procedures encompass:

- Positioning of the patient and practitioner
- Procedure for locating the three pulse positions
- Techniques for locating and assessing the different levels of depth
- Assessment of the arterial structure and pulse wave contour.

The ordering of these techniques and procedures is described as the pulse method. As we established in Chapter 4, pulse method refers to:

- How and when to apply the pulse taking
- The order of gathering information from the pulse using the different techniques (depth, length, strength of application) and required body part (pulse position)
- The consistent application of the pulse method and techniques used in the same way every time.

Identification of many of the specific CM pulse qualities depends on the measurement of pulse parameters in specific positions, so a consistent method is of vital importance. The objective for developing and using a consistent method of pulse palpation is to limit the variance of pulse findings attributable to technique. Once such variances are controlled, then any findings with palpation can be confidently attributed to the occurrence of actual pulse differences.

This chapter focuses extensively on the first stage of the pulse diagnosis process – the application of correct technique and procedures. A further stage of the pulse diagnosis process, interpreting pulse assessment findings diagnostically, is dealt with extensively in Chapters 6 and 7. We also investigate the organization of the techniques and procedures and their order of application, and discuss the benefits of developing a pulse method that is systematic in its application.

5.1 Positioning the patient

Before the pulse is assessed, the patient needs to be positioned appropriately. Appropriate patient positioning allows the practitioner maximal access to the radial artery for assessment purposes while preventing any postural changes that may affect blood flow. For example, if the patient slouches, their respiration will be poor and this will cause a corresponding decrease in pulse strength. Postural slouching and arterial compression from poor arrangement of the upper limbs impede blood flow from the central arteries into the peripheral arteries, limiting the propulsion effect that the pressure wave has on moving blood. In this situation any assessment of the pulse will be inaccurate and unreliable.

The pulse is most commonly taken when the patient is seated, but assessment can also occur when the patient is lying supine (Box 5.1). Irrespective of the positioning approach used, the arm is always placed at the level of the patient's heart. Holding the arm lower or higher than the heart level affects the pulse pressure, causing changes in the pulse wave. Ensuring that the arm is level will minimise these postural related pressure differences. Pulse examination is undertaken on both the left and right arms (Fig. 5.4).

If sitting, the patient's legs should be uncrossed with feet placed flat on the floor. Their posture should be relaxed but upright so that the thorax region is not constricted during respiration, allowing the lungs to expand and contract freely. The wrist should be extended straight with the palm facing upwards (Fig. 5.1). Similarly, when lying supine, the patient should have their legs uncrossed, wrist extended with the palm facing upwards (Fig. 5.2).

A folded towel or small cushion can be used to support the wrist if necessary in either the supine or sitting positions. This ensures that the radial artery is easily accessible and that the blood flow is unimpeded. Additionally, such support limits any movement in the wrist that maybe introduced by the practitioner when applying finger pressure to assess the pulse at different levels of depth.

5.1.1 Speaking

Ideally there should be no speaking between the practitioner and patient during the pulse assessment process. When the patient speaks this will change their respiration, position of the diaphragm and oxygen requirements, also changing the pulse contour and pulse rate.

When the practitioner speaks during the pulse assessment, this often is a sign that they are not focused on the assessment process. Occasionally, speaking is required and is usually done in response to further elucidation of any pulse findings. For example, the presence of missed beats requires further questioning to determine whether the patient was aware of this. This should be kept to relevant questions if concurrently assessing the pulse.

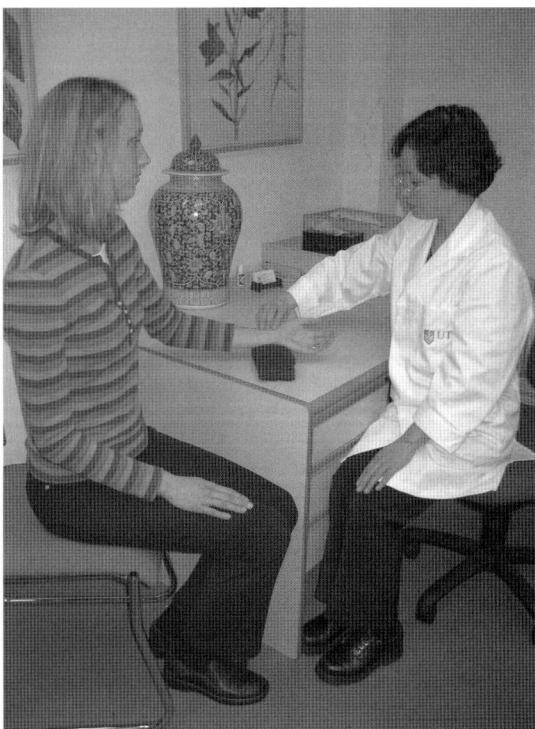

Figure 5.1
Positioning of the practitioner taking the pulse when the patient is sitting. The patient's legs uncrossed, feet flat on floor, with palms upwards. The patient should be in a comfortable upright position and their wrists supported.

Box 5.1

Positioning the patient for assessing the pulse

- Arm level with the heart
- Patient's legs uncrossed
- Patient should be sitting upright or lying supine
- Support the wrist when extended with a towel or cushion

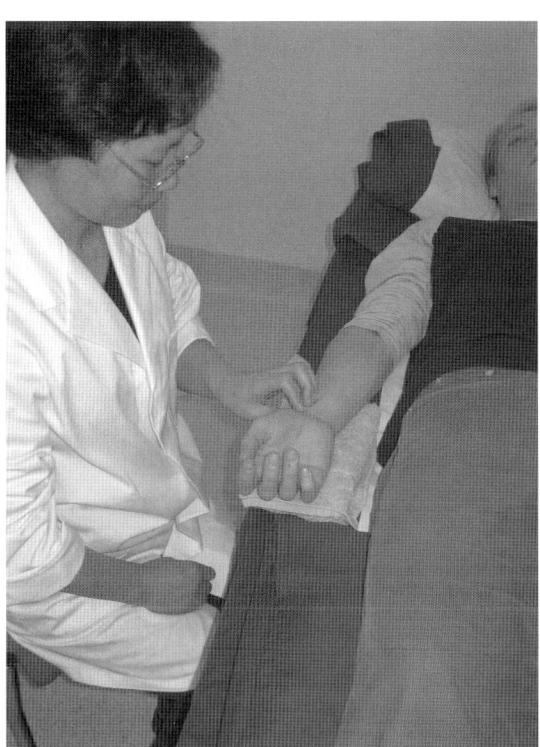

Figure 5.2
Positioning of the practitioner taking the pulse when the patient is supine. Note that the patient's arm is by their side and the wrist is supported for maximal access to the artery.

A

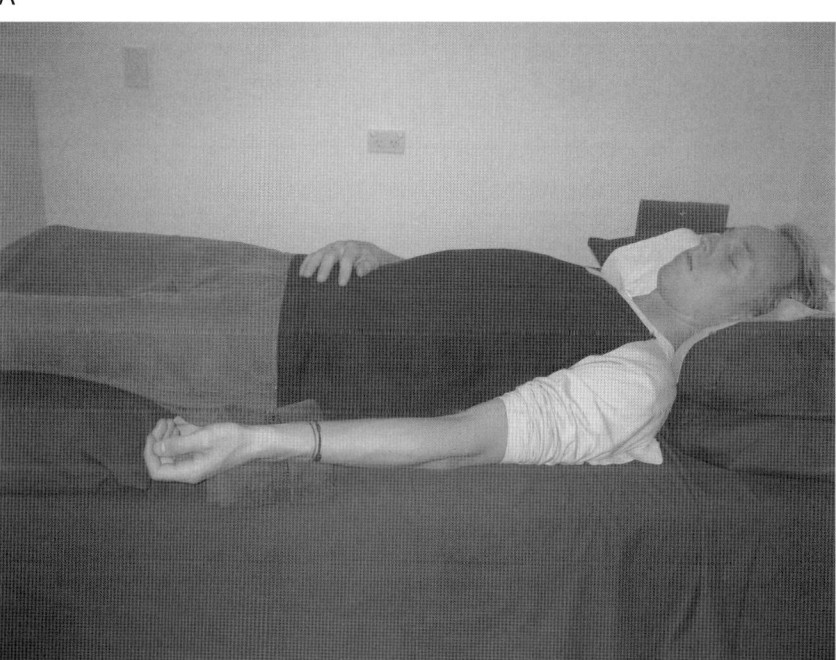

B

5.2 Locating the radial artery

Once the patient and wrist region are appropriately positioned, the next step is to locate the artery, and in particular, the radial pulse sites used for pulse examination. As described in Chapter 2, the radial artery is located on the lateral portion of the anterior forearm. It extends from the elbow, where the brachial artery bifurcates, to the wrist crease, at which point the radial divides further into other arterial segments. (When seen from the perspective of channel physiology, the radial artery follows the course of the

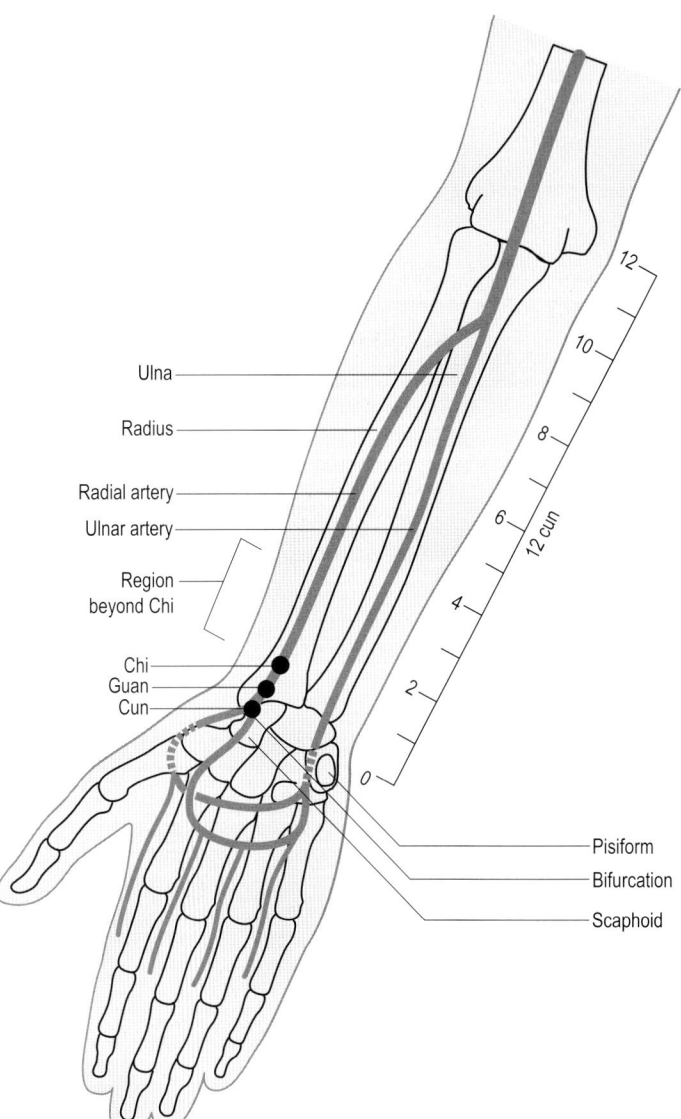

Ulna

Radius

Radial artery
Ulnar artery

Region
beyond Chi

Chi
Guan
Cun

12

10

8

6

12 cun

4

2

0

Pisiform

Bifurcation

Scaphoid

Figure 5.3
Styloid process, the radial artery and
location of the three pulse positions Cun,
Guan and Chi and other related anatomical
structures. The Cun (inch) measurements
indicate the portion of the artery used for
pulse assessment.

Lung channel.) The CM pulse sites used for pulse assessment are located in the wrist portion of the artery only. At this region, the radial artery is usually quite easily palpated because of its close proximity to the skin surface and its position over a hard surface – in this case the radial bone. The radial bone provides a firm support to the radial artery when external pressure is applied. If there were no support then it would be difficult to clearly distinguish the pulse parameters or apply different levels of pressure without the artery moving.

The portion of the radial pulse used for assessment is located proximal to the wrist crease directly above the pulsation of the radial artery adjacent to the styloid process of the radius. This is known as the Cun Kou pulse, and from the time of the *Nan Jing* it was considered to be the convergence point of movement through all the conduit vessels. The Second Difficult Issue in the *Nan Jing* discusses the length of the Cun Kou position, describing it as 1.9 Cun in length. Proportionally, this is about one sixth of the area between the transverse elbow crease and the wrist crease, assuming the length of the forearm is 12 Cun (or anatomical units) (see Fig. 5.3). In metric measurement this is approximately 3– 5 cm. However, exact measurements are not necessarily applied because locating the pulse positions primarily depends on the location of the styloid process and the relative size of the patient.

A clear and discernable rhythmic movement should be apparent at this region when palpated. If there is no pulse detectable then this can indicate:

- Incorrect anatomical region
- Incorrect finger placement
- Correct location and finger placement but the radial artery is not located at the wrist. This is termed a *deviated artery*.

5.2.1 Deviated artery: abnormalities of the radial artery

In a small percentage of people the radial artery is anatomically deviated from the anterior to the lateral portion of the arm as it nears the wrist. In these individuals the artery winds laterally around the styloid process and travels on the posterior side of the wrist (in the anatomical position) as if following the path of the Large Intestine channel through the anatomical snuff-box rather than the path of the Lung channel. This is termed a *Fan Guan Mai* or simply a 'pulse on the back of the wrist' pulse by Wiseman & Ye (1998: p. 473, p. 470).

5.2.2 When to look for a deviated radial artery

If the pulse appears to be absent or extremely faint, look for the presence of a pulsation on the posterior or lateral part of the wrist, in the vicinity of the radial styloid process. If there is a significant pulsation, this indicates a deviated radial artery. In this case, the radial artery runs very superficially and both the artery and pulsations can be easily observed. When the artery is located at this region, the pulse cannot be used for palpation purposes except for assessing rate and rhythm.

A deviated arterial artery is not considered pathological from either a CM or a biomedical perspective. Such deviations represent normal individual variation. However, if the pulsation is not felt in the Cun Kou area or an alternative position, then this may be perceived as pathological. The Cun Kou area should be re-examined, with particular attention to the deep level of depth.

5.2.3 Other abnormalities

Other 'abnormalities' that can similarly affect the presentation of the arterial pulsation include:

- Ganglions
- Bone spurs and growths
- Surgical procedures for carpal tunnel syndrome rearranging soft tissue structures
- Other surgical procedures for arthritis in which carpal bones can be removed
- Scarring, especially keloid tissue
- Inflammatory conditions of the tendons.

5.3 Locating the pulse positions for assessment

Once the Cun Kou region of the artery proximal to the wrist is located, the pulse positions used for pulse assessment must be identified. There are three of these positions, and they are found by dividing the Cun Kou region into three portions using the styloid process of the radius as a guide. The three positions are:

- Cun (inch): Located proximal (or closest) to the wrist crease
- Guan (bar): Located medial to the styloid process of the radius
- Chi (cubit): Most distal (furthermost) position from wrist crease.

Because the three pulse positions are determined proportionally according to an individual's size, this means that the same procedure needs to be followed every time to ensure exact location of these positions within the same physique and between different physiques (Box 5.2). Of the three positions Cun, Guan and Chi, it is the central position Guan which is associated with a specific surface anatomical landmark; the styloid process. For this reason, the Guan position should always be located first as the locations of the Cun and Chi positions depend on the initial location of Guan.

5.3.1 Locating Guan

The Guan position is found first as it is easily located adjacent to the styloid process of the radius. The styloid process is a flaring of the radial bone, and can be

---

Box 5.2

Locating the three positions

- Index finger is placed at the Cun position
- Middle finger is placed at the Guan position
- Ringer finger is placed at the Chi position
- Thumb is placed on the underside of the wrist

identified as a bony protuberance on the lateral side of the wrist, proximal to the wrist crease (in the anatomical position). To locate the styloid process it is best to palpate the bone as it is not always easy to identify this landmark by observation alone. By gently running the index finger over the region a distinct 'bump' can be felt where the styloid process flares away from the shaft of the radius. The styloid process can also be clearer to palpate with radial/ulnar deviation, causing the soft tissue to stretch and expose the bone. Once it is located, the practitioner moves directly medial towards the soft skin of the anterior wrist above the radial artery. The arterial pulsations are often felt most distinctly in this position, and the outer border of the styloid process may be felt at the margin of the finger when positioned on the artery. This is the Guan position. When the middle finger is placed on the Guan position, the other two fingers should fall naturally into their positions: the index finger on Cun, located adjacent to the scaphoid bone, and the ring finger on Chi, proximal to Guan.

The actual finger placement is proportional to the size of the wrist: on a tall person the wrist is larger, and so the three positions and fingers are spaced further apart. Conversely, on a shorter person the wrist is proportionally smaller and so the three fingers are positioned closer together. However, for all patients the positioning of the fingers on the pulse should always be undertaken in reference to the styloid process and the location of the Guan position. Using either the Cun or the Chi position for this purpose will lead to incorrect placement of the fingers. (This doesn't work with children.)

With the practitioner's thumb resting lightly on the back of the patient's wrist the fingers should be arranged so that the tips are level with one another. It is the tips of the fingers which should be used for palpation, exerting equal pressure to feel the three pulse positions simultaneously. The fingers can be used:

- Simultaneously to palpate all three pulse positions on one arm
- For comparative purposes, assessing the overall pulse in one side with the other
- Individually to assess pulse positions at different levels of depth.

5.3.2 Placement of the thumb

In the process of placing the fingers on the appropriate pulse positions and undertaking assessment, the thumb is of particular importance. The thumb is used to stabilise the wrist against movement that may occur when different pressures are applied by the fingers to the pulse. If the patient's wrist moves during palpation this will render the reliability of the findings questionable.

For example, if a particular amount of strength is used to move the fingers into the deep level of depth, but the wrist is unsupported, then the wrist may move so that rather than palpating the deep level the practitioner may assess only the middle level of depth without realising this is the case. For this reason, the thumb is placed on the posterior wrist region to provide support to the wrist and leverage for the fingers when palpating the pulse.

5.3.3 The anatomy of the radius and support of the radial artery

Because of the shape of the radial bone and the depression formed between it and the styloid process, the support provided by the styloid to the radial artery at the wrist varies. For example, at the Guan position the pulse wave and arterial structure are both felt more distinctly than at the Cun or Chi position alone. Because of the support offered by the styloid bone at the Guan position, the artery sits relatively superficial. Less skin, and thinner epidermal/fasciae layers, mean a 'clearer' pulse image when palpating and facilitates better detection of arterial parameters such as tension.

At the Chi position the radial bone sinks away from the surface with the artery similarly becoming deeper. In order to detect pulses clearly it is often necessary to provide support under the artery. Having the artery supported means it can be compressed and so the pulse is detectable for diagnostic purposes. If no support is provided then the artery and pulses remain indistinct. For this reason palpation of the Chi positions often results in a pulse that is felt deeper or less strongly when compared to the pulse at the Guan positions. It is only after pressure is applied and the artery is supported by the bone that the pulse is felt distinctly. Sometimes the direction of finger pressure needs to be adjusted to ensure that the artery is being compressed into a firm surface, such as the tendons located medially to the radial artery. (This may account for the traditional description of the pulse at this position, the Kidney pulse, being located like a 'pebble at the bottom of a stream' or described as 'insects crawling around the bone'.)

The Cun pulse positions are in a depression between two bony structures. These structures are the styloid process and the scaphoid bone. For this reason, the pulse and artery are less supported at the Cun position than at the Guan position, but are felt more distinctly than the Chi positions because of the stabilisation offered to the artery by these bones. However, as at the Chi position, the lack of direct underlying support under the cun positions often means the pulse and artery are not felt as distinctly at the Guan position, but are not as deeply located as the Chi position.

5.4 Practitioner positioning

When taking the pulse the practitioner should sit opposite or next to the patient. Using the tips of the fingers (Box 5.3), the practitioner's left hand is used to feel the pulses of the patient's right hand and the practitioner's right hand is used to feel the pulses on the patient's left (Box 5.4). Similarly, if the practitioner were to palpate their own pulses on the right wrist, the practitioner's left hand wraps under the wrist with the index, middle and ring fingers sequentially falling on the three pulse positions Cun, Guan and Chi. This is reversed if feeling the left hand pulses. This ensures that the same fingers are always used to palate the same pulse positions (Fig. 5.4). For example, the right index finger is always placed on the left Cun position, irrespective of whether the practitioner is palpating someone else's pulse or their own. This will assist in ensuring that a level of sensitivity and a reference range of pulses are built up for that particular finger and this in turn assists with reliable identification and assessment of any changes in the pulse parameters at the related pulse site.

5.5 Assessing the parameters

Once the pulse positions are located, the fingers are moved in different directions and depths to assess the pulse wave and the anatomy of the arterial wall at each of the positions. In particular, discrete increments of pressure are applied by the fingers to feel the three levels of pulse depth. The fingers are also moved from side to side to assess the width and tension of the arterial wall, and longitudinally to assess pulse length. Of the three movements, depth assessment is particularly important in CM, as each pulse site can be further divided into different levels of depth with each level theoretically reflecting a different region of the body.

Assessment of pulse depth is discussed in greater detail below, and this requires a specific technique to locate the levels of depth. Lateral and longitude assessment of the pulse are respectively discussed in Chapter 6 in the section on assessing the pulse parameter length and in Chapter 7 in relation to assessment of the pulse parameter arterial wall tension.

5.5.1 Relevance of the different pulse positions

In CM, each of the three pulse positions is used to assess the overall pulse, as is done in biomedical practice, but each of the three positions is also viewed as reflecting a specific function or region of the body. Because of this, the pulse at each position is sometimes viewed as three distinctly different pulses, in spite of the three pulse positions being located on the same arterial segment and with the same blood flowing through them. The Cun positions are often ascribed to the upper region of the torso, the thoracic cavity, and changes in the pulse specifically at these two positions (the left and right Cun) indicate dysfunction of this region. Similarly, the Guan and Chi positions are ascribed respectively to the abdominal and pelvic cavities and the pulses are said to infer the function of these regions. The thoracic, abdominal and pelvic cavities are termed the upper, middle and lower Heaters (or Jiao) respectively. The pulse positions Cun, Guan and Chi also are simultaneously assigned to different channels, organs or regions of the body depending on the system used for interpreting the pulse information. In this sense then, the left Cun position for example is associated with the Heart and Small Intestine channel, the anatomical region of the chest, as well as reflecting the upper Jiao when paired with the right Cun position (Fig. 5.5). Besides associating each position to specific organ and channel entities, the three pulse positions are used for assessing the overall pulse qualities. These qualities include specific changes in the pulse wave and arterial structure that often occur across the three positions and are used to infer the nature of an illness and the effect it is having on the body.

51

Box 5.3

Fingertips and fingernails

- The fingertips are the most sensitive regions of the finger. Individuals who play the guitar will find that the skin thickens at the tips of the fingers and for this reason, sensitivity to the pulse is often substantially lessened, if not absent. In such instances the finger pads rather than the tips should be used for assessing the pulse.
- The length of the fingernails can also prevent the use of the fingertips for pulse assessment. In such circumstances, the finger pads can be used or the nails regularly trimmed.

Box 5.4

- The fingers of the right hand are used to palpate the left wrist pulse.
- The fingers of the left hand are used to palpate the right wrist pulse.

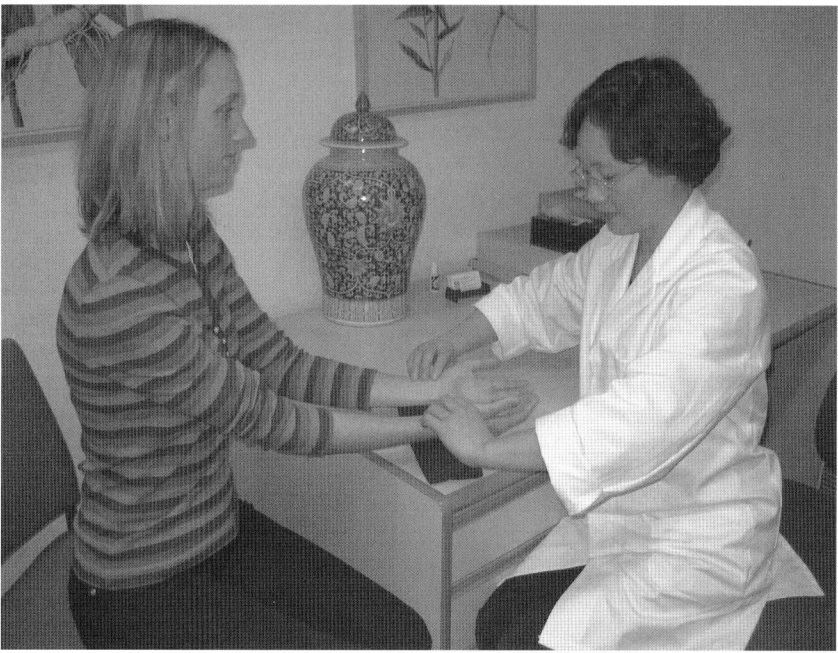

A

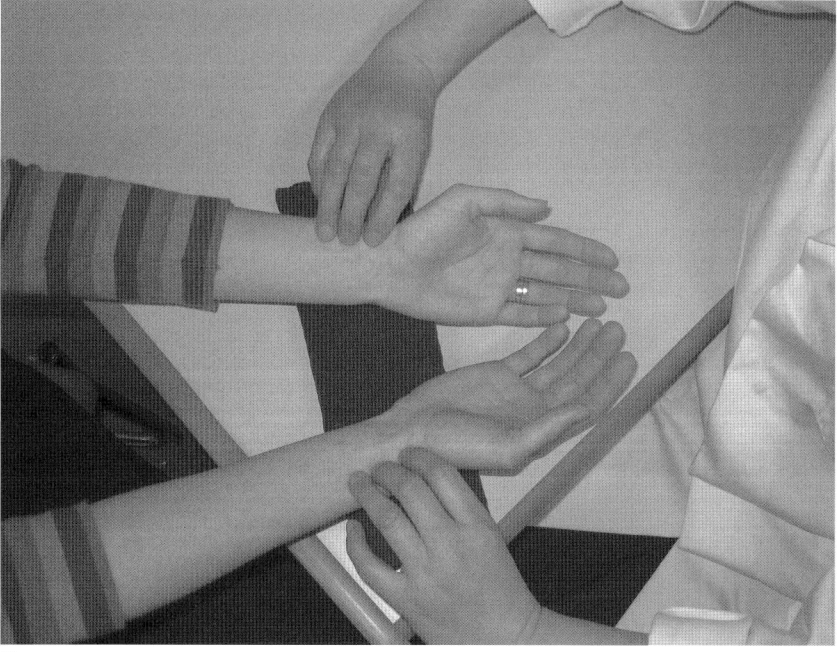

B

Figure 5.4
Bilateral hand palpation. The practitioner's left hand is palpating the right pulse and the right hand is palpating the left hand the pulse.

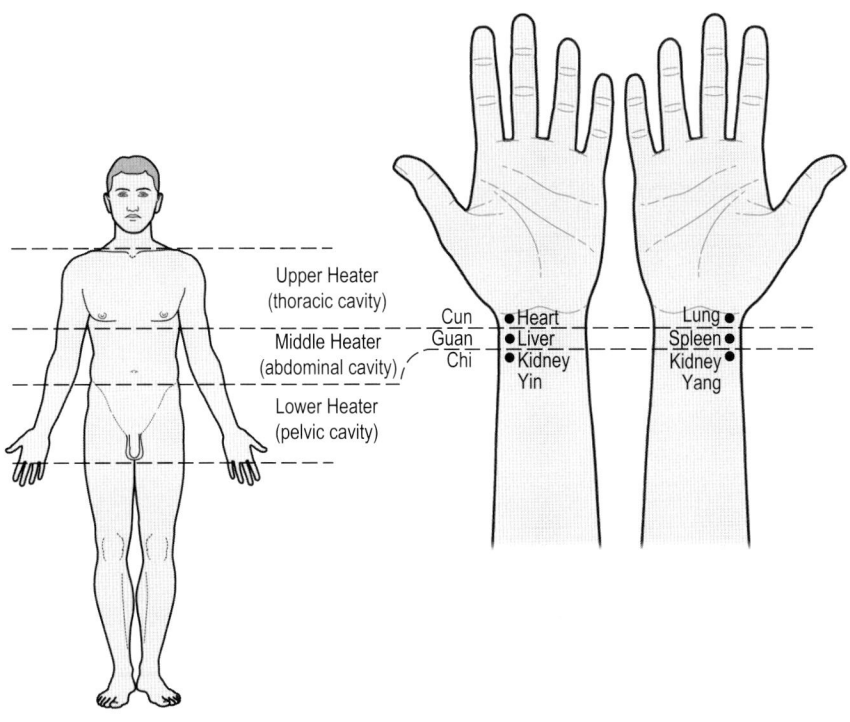

Upper Heater
(thoracic cavity)

Middle Heater
(abdominal cavity)

Lower Heater
(pelvic cavity)

Cun	● Heart	Lung ●
Guan	● Liver	Spleen ●
Chi	● Kidney	Kidney ●
	Yin	Yang

Figure 5.5
Association of the three pulse positions to the three regions of the body and their relationship to the organs.

5.6 Locating the pulse depth

A consistent technique for correct location of the levels of depth is just as important in pulse diagnosis as correct anatomical location of the Cun, Guan and Chi pulse positions. Each pulse/position site can be further divided into two levels (superficial and deep) of depth or three (superficial, middle and deep), depending on the theoretical CM model used. For example, in Five Phase pulse diagnosis, only the superficial and deep levels of depth are assessed (Fig. 5.6). In determining overall pulse qualities as presented in the *Mai Jing* and *Bin Hue Mai Xue*, three levels of depth are often required for pulse assessment. There are even systems of pulse assessment based on the writings of the *Nan Jing* that palpate up to five levels of depth, and other systems state up to eight levels of depth (Hammer 2001), but these systems are not widely used. There are three commonly used levels of depth: superficial, middle and deep.

The parameter of pulse depth may be interpreted in two ways. Firstly, it refers to the level of depth where the radial arterial pulsation is found to be the strongest, regardless of the overall intensity of the pulsation. That is, we need to determine the relative strength of each level of depth. An integral part of determining pulse depth involves examination of the effect on radial pulsation of differing amounts of pressure exerted on the radial artery.

Secondly, pulse depth can refer to the level of depth at which the radial artery is physically located. This may be the result of anatomical structural variations within the subcutaneous layer of tissue overlying the radial artery, or the anatomical variations in the musculature and tendinous insertions around the forearm and wrist area. Diagnostically, the level of depth may be affected by pathological processes occurring within the body, resulting in either a pulse that can be felt strongest at the superficial or deep level of depth, or perhaps equally strong at all three levels of depth. Other factors affecting where the pulse can be felt include the strength of cardiac contraction.

5.6.1 Locating the three levels of depth

The three levels of depth should always be examined during pulse taking to determine the level at which the pulsations are strongest overall. This process is repeated as many times as necessary to correctly identify the strongest level. This is achieved by using consistent pressure across all three fingers to palpate to each of the three levels of depth; the superficial level of depth initially, followed by the deep and then middle levels of depth. Pulses at the three depths are found as follows.

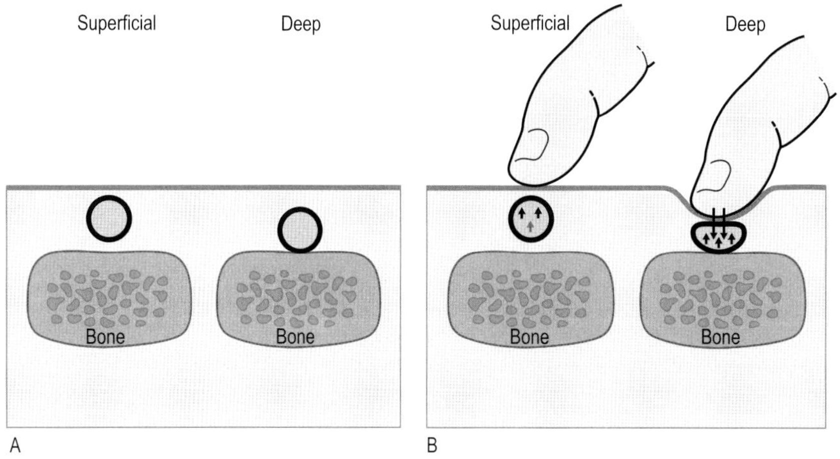

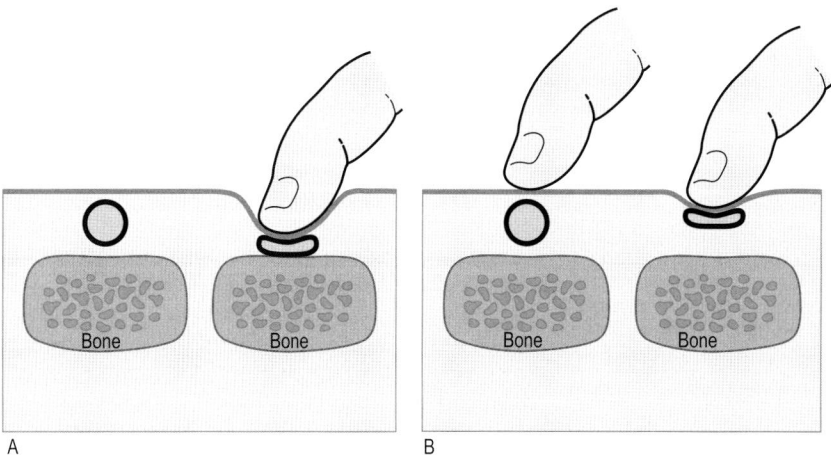

Figure 5.6
Radial artery, the pulse and assessment of pulse depth. The pulse depth relates to either the physical presence of the artery situated superficially or deep (A) or can be classified by the degree of finger pressure required to feel the strongest pulsation between the three levels of depth (B). Two examples are shown. One where the pulse is strongest at the superficial level of depth the other where the pulse is felt strongest at the deep level of depth.

Figure 5.7
Compression of the artery by finger pressure to assess the ease of pulse occlusion. In (A) compression of the artery occurs only when heavy pressure is applied by the finger, where the bone provides a stabllising support against which to occlude the artery. In (B) the artery is easily compressed at a more superficial level because of the lack of arterial pressure due to vacuity (deficiency) patterns of Qi or Blood.

- Superficial: This is found by resting the fingertips lightly on the skin surface. No pressure should be applied except that of the resting pressure of the fingers on the skin surface. (The superficial level of depth is *not* the depth at which the pulse is first felt.) The superficial level is defined as being located directly below the skin level. It is common not to feel any pulse at this level of depth; this is diagnostically just as important as having felt a pulse at the superficial level.

- Deep: This level of depth is found by occluding the radial artery (pressing the artery firmly against the radial bone) and then releasing the pressure gently until the pulse can be felt again. (The *Mai Jing* states 'press to the bone and then release the pressure' to feel this level of depth; alternatively, the pressure required is greater than the weight of 12 soybeans (Wang, Yang trans 1997).) This approach creates an initial rush in the blood flow when pressure is released slightly after occluding the pulse. A few seconds should be allowed to enable the pulse to equalise before assessment. It is important to take care not to release so much pressure as to move the fingers into the middle level of depth (Fig. 5.7).

Note: With some pulses it may seem extremely difficult to occlude the artery, with the pulse still felt beyond Chi. When this occurs, it is not a failure to occlude the pulse but rather it is the continuing presence of pulse waves moving from the heart to the periphery and hitting into the side of the palpating finger. When pulses are detected on the side of the finger during pulse occlusion, this is usually a sign of strength in the pulse. Whether the pulse strength reflects health or illness requires further assessment. When enough pressure is applied to stop movement of the pulse *under* the fingers then the pulse is considered to be occluded whether or not the pulse continues to be felt at the side of the ring finger.

- Middle: This level of depth is found by applying a moderate pressure to the radial artery (not sufficient to occlude it), somewhere between superficial and deep. It is detected by exerting more pressure than required to palpate the superficial level but not enough to occlude the pulse. The middle level is located after initially locating the superficial and deep levels, which are found first in order to ascertain the amount of pressure required to palpate to the middle level. This level is an estimate of the halfway point between the two pulse depth extremes.

The order of finding the levels of depth is important to ensure that assessment is occurring at the correct level of depth. It is relatively easy to observe whether assessment is occurring at the superficial level of depth but difficult to locate the middle level of depth, located at the 'halfway mark', without first knowing the degree of strength required to find the deep level. As the pulse taker moves from the superficial level to deeper within the pulse, believing that they are at the deep level of depth, they may in fact only be in the middle level of depth. This can occur because no baseline has been established to give a context to both the middle and deeper levels of depth.

5.6.2 Defining a pulse by the level of depth

Different pulses are often described as being felt strongest at a particular level of depth. When a pulse is described as being located at the deep level of depth this can mean one of two things:

- The pulse is felt strongest at this level of depth; it may still be felt with less finger pressure at the other levels of depth, superficial and middle, it is just less strong
- The pulse cannot be felt at middle or superficial and only felt at the deep level of depth.

In these scenarios, the level of depth of a pulse is the level at which the pulse is felt strongest. Several pulse qualities are defined or identified in this manner. For example, the Floating pulse is defined by the fact that it is felt strongest at the superficial level of depth and sequentially less at the other levels of depth when finger pressure is increased. In this way the Floating pulse is determined not only by the presence at the superficial level of depth but also by its diminishing strength at deeper levels. With other pulse qualities, too, it is both the presence of strength at one level of depth and the absence of strength or a detectable pulse at another level of depth that is used for identifying that particular pulse. Another example is the Scallion Stalk (Hollow) pulse which is also felt strongest at the superficial level of depth and is absent at the middle and deep level of depth when further finger pressure is applied. (Note, however, that for the Scallion Stalk pulse other parameters in addition to depth assessment are of equal importance in defining the pulse.) The level of depth where the pulse is felt strongest is also often the level of depth where the arterial wall and pulse contour are clearly felt as well.

5.6.3 Diagnostic meaning of the levels of depth

5.6.3.1 Superficial and deep level of depth

In a CM context a pulse felt strongest at the superficial level of depth is broadly categorised Yang and a pulse felt strongest at the deep level of depth is categorised Yin. When the fingers move from the superficial to the deep level of depth, so the pulse progressively moves from reflecting Yang to reflecting Yin. This is reversed when palpating from the deep to the superficial levels of depth, when the pulse progressively reflects Yang.

If the pulse is viewed from an anatomical or pressure wave perspective, then the superficial pulse indicates an artery located near the skin surface or a pulse with sufficient force for the flow wave to expand the blood vessel. A pulse felt strongest at the deep level of depth can also indicate either an artery obscured by the skin and overlying tissue, or an artery with insufficient support, or simply a pulse that is strongest at the deep level. This may reflect a poor pulse force, which does not allow the flow wave to expand the vessel; and this may be due to a poor heart function or dilution of pulse strength through other factors such as arterial dilatation (see Chapter 2). The vessel wall can also constrict or be compressed by the surrounding connective tissue, restricting clear expansion of the pulse wave. From

Box 5.5

- Superficial level of depth reflects Yang: exterior
- Deep level of depth reflects Yin: interior
- Middle level of depth reflects the balanced interplay between Qi (function) and Blood (form)

Box 5.6

Other circumstantial information gained from the process of pulse palpation

- Finger nails: Is there any cracking or deformity in the fingernails? Observe the colour of the nails and nail bed. A pale colour indicates poor circulation and can be related to blood vacuity. A bluish colour can indicate hypoxia and relates to poor lung and cardiac function. White indicates complete vasoconstriction.
- Skin: Feel the temperature and texture of the skin and flesh overlying the artery. Is the skin warm, cold or clammy? Is the skin texture rough, indicating dryness, or soft, indicating fluid retention?
- Wrist size: Observe the size of the wrist to make a judgement on whether the arterial width is appropriate. Is the artery proportional to individual's body size?
- Veins: Observe the colour and shape of the veins. Can they be easily observed? Are they distended (indicates stagnation or increased arterial pressure)? Are they blue, green or red in colour?
- Radial artery: Is the artery easily observable? Are there visible pulsations? A visible artery can indicate an increase in arterial tension while visible pulsations indicate pulse force or a superficially located pulse.

these examples, it can be seen that probably a number of different mechanisms are involved in the formation of a deep pulse. However, irrespective of why a deep pulse occurs, a pulse felt strongest at the deep level of depth is broadly categorised as Yin. The Eight Principles (*Ba Gang*) approach to pulse assessment in particular categorises pulse in this way, categorising a pulse as either Yin or Yang.

5.6.3.2 Meaning of the middle level of depth

Located between the deep and superficial levels of depth, the middle level of depth can be viewed from a CM perspective as the point of interchange between Yin and Yang, the fluxing between the two 'poles' of form (deep level) and function (superficial level) (Box 5.5). When the pulse is felt strongest at the middle level of depth this is viewed as a sign of balance between Yang or function (Qi) and the interplay with Yin or form (Blood). The middle level of depth is where the pulse should be felt strongest on most individuals. When the pulse is felt strongest only at the superficial or only at the deep levels of depth then this more than likely reflects ill health, dysfunction or maybe a prognostic sign inferring ill health. In this scenario, a pulse occurring strongest at the superficial level of depth reflects Yang-type illnesses or conditions that have caused Yang to become hyperactive. This is seen in cases of febrile conditions producing delirium, or in conditions with dream-filled restless sleep. Similarly, a pulse occurring strongest at the deep level of depth reflects Yin-type illnesses or conditions that have constrained or depleted the Yang, causing the pulse to contract into the deeper regions of the artery. Yin conditions often involve organ dysfunction.

In their simplest form, the overall CM pulse qualities in the literature are used in this context, identifying the nature and location of an illness, whether Yin or Yang. In this way, the superficial level of depth reflects the Yang, the middle level of depth the action of Qi with Blood, and the deep level of depth the organs/Yin.

5.6.3.3 Combining depth assessment with the other parameters

Through additional procedures and techniques for assessing the pulse wave and arterial wall, the practitioner combines the information derived from depth assessment for better understanding of the pulse (Box 5.6). The cumulative end to this process is combining the assessment of the different pulse aspects or parameters of the pulse wave and arterial structure in the identification of the traditional overall CM pulse qualities. However, not all individuals will present with a distinctly identifiable CM pulse quality as described in the CM literature. In these situations assessment of the parameters individually can be critical to using the pulse to inform diagnosis and treatment. These CM pulse qualities and the associated parameters that define them are discussed in detail in Chapters 6 and 7.

5.7 The normal pulse

The normal pulse is a template used to identify variations in the pulse from an expected health range. Given that the pulse is a manifestation of the interaction of several different parameters, it is logical to also consider the normal pulse as a range of values within which the pulse can present and still be considered a reflection of health. For example, the normal pulse rate ranges from 60 to 90 bpm.

Yet the normal presentation for one pulse parameter does not necessarily exclude the potential that another pulse parameter is simultaneously presenting abnormally. For example, a pulse rate of 70 bpm is considered healthy, within the normal range, but when accompanied by increased arterial tension, where the arterial wall becomes hard, then the pulse is not normal. When determining whether the pulse is normal or not, all aspects of the pulse therefore need to be considered.

There are a range of additional variables specific to the individual that also need to be given consideration when determining if the pulse is normal or not. They include body size, physique, exercise levels, age, gender and seasonal variables. In this sense, the normal pulse refers to an individual's usual pulse.

5.8 Assessing health by the pulse

5.8.1 Shen, Stomach Qi and Root

In a CM context, a pulse is described by some contemporary authors as having three attributes or factors (Maciocia 2004, Townsend & De Donna 1990). These are Shen, Stomach Qi and Root.

- Shen: This refers to the relative strength of the pulse, which has a constant rate and regular rhythm. The Shen is used in this sense to refer to physical heart function: the parameters associated with the strength of pulsation and regularity of heart contraction. It represents the functioning of Qi of the Heart. Assessment of this attribute or factor should occur at any level of depth and any position. What constitutes healthy and unhealthy presentation of the parameters for this pulse attribute is discussed in Chapters 6 and 7 in the discussion on pulse rate, pulse rhythm and pulse force.
- Stomach Qi: This refers to the rate of rise and decline in the blood flow wave as it passes under the fingers, where the contour of the pulse reflects Stomach Qi. The attribute or factor refers to adequate levels of Qi and blood and their interaction. There is an obvious relationship to dietary factors and adequate intake of appropriate food to produce blood and Qi. Ni's (1995) translation of the *Nei Jing* states that the Yang pulses reflect the health of the Stomach Qi. Pulses lacking strength, arterial expansion and are short are therefore classified as Yin or as pulses which lack Stomach Qi (p. 30). This relates to the blood quantity filling the artery and sufficient Qi to motivate blood expansively.
- Root: This is used to refer to the Kidneys (assessed at the Chi pulse positions) or assessment of the Kidneys at the deep level of depth across all three positions. (The association of the Kidneys with the deep level of depth is discussed at length in the *Mai Jing*.) The concept is used to refer to a pulse with foundation. That is, there should be at least some presence of the pulse in the deeper levels of the

artery. This is not always the case with certain illnesses, but in health, presence of Root means the Yin is anchoring the Yang. In this way, a pulse overly strong at the superficial level of depth indicates the lack of Yin anchoring the Yang.

Of the three concepts, the Root is of most importance. The Shen level may be transient and more affected by moment-to-moment changes than the other two levels. Poor sleep will result in decreased strength at the Shen level, yet the Root should remain unaffected. The Root reflects the foundation of health in the body. As long as the Root is present then prognosis is good, as it is when the pulse has a regular rhythm and a constant strength.

When the pulse rhythm, strength or contour begins to fluctuate, whether from moment to moment, or within the same individual over a longer period of time, then the outlook is indicative of potential and/or actual dysfunction.

5.8.2 Parameters and a healthy pulse

Assessment of a healthy pulse from a parameter perspective is assessed on four aspects. These are:

- Timing of the pulse
  - Rate: 60–90 bpm
  - Rhythm: Regular
- Presence of the pulse
  - Depth: Felt at all three levels of depth but relatively strongest in the middle or deep level of depth
  - Length: Felt at the three pulse positions Cun, Guan and Chi, and/or beyond Chi
- Arterial structure
  - Width: Appropriate to the individual's physique and the circulation reaching the periphery to warm the skin, toes and fingers
  - Arterial tension: There should be some tensile strength in the arterial wall, but it should be capable of being externally indented when moderate finger pressure is applied, or internally expanded by the arterial pulse wave
  - Pulse occlusion: With increasing finger pressure the pulse should be felt at least at two levels of depth before being occluded. Pulsation on the body side of the ring finger is likely to be present when occluded
- Pulse waveform
  - Force: Pulse hits the fingers with strength with a distinct rise and fall in the pulse amplitude – pulse rises against the fingers
  - Contour and flow wave: Smooth uninterrupted flow.

5.9 Channel, organ and levels of depth

The idea that the superficial level of depth reflects Yang and the deep level of depth reflects Yin is used to associate a particular channel and organ to each of the pulses found at these two levels across the three positions. In particular, the three positions of each wrist at the superficial level of depth are said to reflect the functional strength of the Yang channels and organs. In the deep level of depth, at the corresponding positions, the pulses are considered to reflect the functional strength of the Yin channels and organs. This gives a total of 12 pulse positions: 6 located superficially and 6 deep.

There are various arrangements of the organs or channels at the wrist pulse positions that have been described in the CM literature in the past. Variations in arrangement of the organs and channels are discussed extensively in many texts and are not repeated here. However, listed below are two most commonly used arrangements which are relevant to contemporary clinical practice. Each of these arrangements is described in the *Nan Jing* and *Bin Hue Mai Xue*. The first relates to the arrangement of channels, the other to the organs. The channel arrangement at the wrist pulse positions is often used in acupuncture, while the organ arrangement at the wrist positions is often described for use in herbal medicine. There is also a third arrangement that blends aspects of the acupuncture channel and herbal organ arrangements together. These distinctions can be further described as follows:

- Acupuncture channel arrangement: So called because of the association of the small intenstine (SI) and large intenstine (LI) pulses at the superficial level of depth at the left and right Cun positions. In this arrangement the SI partners the Heart (HR) channel and the LI partners the Lung (LU) channel. The Yin and Yang pairing of the fire and metal elements is complete, as represented in the LI/LU and SI/HR channels being located together on the upper limbs. Acupuncture affects the channels and so the arrangement reflects the channel location in the body (Table 5.1).

- Herbal organ anatomical arrangement: This places the SI and LI respectively at the superficial regions of the left and right Chi positions. This is done as the SI and LI organs are located in the lower regions of the body and so the pulse arrangement of the organs at these positions reflects this arrangement. This model is often explained by the focus in herbal medicine on organic disease. Herbs traditionally interact with the organs (Table 5.2).

Secondary English sources of the classics further distinguish the Kidney pulses in the *Bin Hue Mai Xue* model, with the Kidney pulse on the Left side reflecting Kidney Yin and the Kidney pulse on the right side reflecting Kidney Yang. The division of the Kidney pulse in this way appears to be a contemporary adaptation. For example, Birch (1992) in his literature review on radial pulse positions notes the division of the pulse into Kidney Yin and Kidney Yang as not occurring in the classical pulse literature he reviewed, whereas secondary English translations often denote this division.

Table 5.1 ● The pulse positions and their relationship to the 12 main acupuncture channels as noted in the *Nan Jing*

Left side	Superficial	Deep		Deep	Superficial	Right side
	Small intestine	Heart	Cun	Lung	Large intestine	
	Gallbladder	Liver	Guan	Spleen	Stomach	
	Bladder	Kidney	Chi	Pericardium	Triple Heater	
	Yang	**Yin**		**Yin**	**Yang**	

Table 5.2 ● The pulse positions and the relationship to the organs as listed in the *Bin Hue Mai Xue*

Left side	Superficial	Deep		Deep	Superficial	Right side
	Chest	Heart	Cun	Lung	Chest	
	Gallbladder	Liver	Guan	Spleen	Stomach	
	Small intestine	Kidney (Yin)	Chi	Kidney (Yang)	Large intestine	
	Yang	**Yin**		**Yin**	**Yang**	

There are more ways of associating the different levels of depth than these mentioned above. Further information can be found in the *Nan Jing*, *Mai Jing* and various other contemporary texts on the topic.

5.10 Comparison of the overall force of the left and right radial pulse

In addition to the techniques for locating the pulse positions and different pulse depths, pulse assessment and some associated theoretical pulse assumption systems require examination of the *relative differences* in pulse strength, irrespective of the actual degree of strength or overall force in the pulse. Whether a pulse is forceful or forceless is irrelevant when assessing relative strength differences, as assessing relative differences in strength is achieved by:

- Comparing one position to another position (within and between different sides)
- Comparing one level of depth to another (also within and between different sides)
- Comparing the overall pulse on the left with the right side pulse
- Comparing the pulse of one individual to another.

5.10.1 Comparing left and right pulses

Comparisons are made by simultaneously palpating the left and right radial pulses. In making a comparison, all three positions on each wrist are palpated using an even pressure. All three of the levels of depth need to be evaluated consecutively. For example, at the superficial level of depth the practitioner assesses the overall strength of the pulse when palpating the Cun, Guan and Chi positions simultaneously. This procedure is repeated at the middle and deep levels of depth. The overall strength at all three levels of depth is then averaged to arrive at the strength for the left and right side pulse. To exclude a dominant hand bias due to better discrimination skills depending on whether the practitioner is left or right hand dominant, the subject should be asked whether the pressure exerted by the assessor on each side's pulse is felt as equal. If necessary, the finger pressure is adjusted and then the pulse on each side should be examined at each of the levels, simultaneously. In this approach, pulse assessment primarily focuses on the parameter of force. Chapter 9 discusses a number of assumption systems where pulse diagnosis focuses primarily on assessing relative differences in strength.

5.11 Pulse method

A pulse method is a systematised approach that puts together the pulse procedures into an organised examination process. This includes:

- Deciding whether pulse diagnosis is an appropriate technique to use
- When to take the patient's pulse in the consultation
- Order of gathering information from the pulse
- Interpreting the information within a diagnostic context.

5.11.1 Is pulse taking appropriate?

Like all examination techniques used in the diagnostic process, pulse taking is not always required, nor necessarily an appropriate assessment method to use in all situations. Take the case of an acute sprained ankle. Pulse assessment of the radial arterial pulse is not likely to contribute any significantly useful information when determining the extent and level of damage sustained to the ankle, or meaningfully inform treatment protocols for the acute presentation of this condition. In contrast, pulse diagnosis is considered necessary for assessing the functional state of the channels and related organs in Five Phase or constitutional acupuncture.

Pulse diagnosis is viewed in the literature at one extreme as a technique that can be used for diagnosing any condition and used in all situations, through to the other extreme where it is useful only for assessing heart function. The decision to incorporate pulse into diagnosis into the examination process therefore rests largely with the consulting practitioner and relates to their personal views and perception of health, their education, practise of CM and experience.

Situations derived from the various views of authors where pulse diagnosis is considered an appropriate assessment technique to use generally include:

- Disorders affecting the organs and their related functions
- Dysfunction in the movement, production or storage of Qi, Blood, Essence and Fluids
- Problems associated with the emotions
- Psychological based illnesses including some forms of addictive behaviour and substance abuse
- Management of long-term illness and dysfunction.

5.11.2 When to take the pulse during diagnosis

Pulse diagnosis sits within the four examination approaches of CM. These include questioning, observation, listening/smelling and palpation, including pulse diagnosis. In CM, there is no strict order of obtaining this information. In spite of this, there are divergent opinions on the appropriate time during consultation to feel the radial pulse. One view is that pulse should be undertaken at the beginning of consultation, while the other viewpoint states the reverse, claiming it should be undertaken at the conclusion of consultation after the other examinations have been completed. Each viewpoint has a valid rationale and this is often based on the perceived value that pulse assessment contributes to the examination process.

- At the beginning of the consultation: Assessment of the pulse at the beginning of consultation allows the practitioner to get a general overview of what is happening in the body, without being influenced by too much additional information. Obviously once the patient is seen, visual diagnostic information is already being processed; the way they move, talk, breathe, the colour and condition of the facial features and skin, the hair, expression, eyes and general demeanour of the patient. This, in conjunction with the information obtained from pulse diagnosis, will also help to direct the practitioner along the diagnostic process.

  When using pulse assessment at the beginning of consultation the practitioner needs to guard against assessing increased pulse rates due to any exertion undertaken by the patient before the consultation. If pulse is taken at the beginning of consultation, it is advisable that the patient be left to rest before pulse assessment commences.

- At the end of consultation: The end of the examination process is often when radial pulse diagnosis takes place, often as a confirmatory process, to further corroborate what the other signs and symptoms have already revealed. However, taking pulse at this stage can present problems: there is the danger of trying to fit the assessed pulse pattern into the diagnosis determined by the other diagnostic processes such as questioning, looking and listening. At this stage of consultation, it can be argued that it is easy to ignore certain characteristics that do not fit in with diagnosis, or to perceive changes that do not really exist. This may especially occur when a specific CM quality is not clearly present in a definitive form. (By using the pulse parameter system, we can take into account the various degrees of all changes that are occurring within the pulse.)

Despite the two contradictory views there are some general guidelines regarding the appropriate time to take the pulse.

- When the patient has rested and introductions have been made (make sure the heart rate is not effected by extensive conversation, exertion, exercise or prior movement).
- Use pulse diagnosis at the beginning of the assessment process rather than at the end to ensure that the reading is not being biased by other information.
- If pulse diagnosis is used as an adjunctive or confirmatory diagnostic tool, then pulse at the conclusion of questioning may be appropriate, bearing in mind that pulse assessment at this stage may be influenced or biased by prior findings through other means of assessment.
- It is important to remember that the patient may provide responses to questions that are contradictory, or they may be elusive. In this case, the pulse may give a better indication as to what is occurring than the patient's answers. Questioning can be guided by the pulse findings, and at least used to gain a better perspective in broad terms about what may be occurring.
- Consuming food will disturb the pulse. Assessment should therefore occur at the end of the consultation if the patient has eaten beforehand.

5.11.3 The order of gathering pulse information

Once it is established that pulse assessment is appropriate and when to take the pulse, the practitioner then needs to use a methodical approach in gathering the information by pulse assessment.

This will assist with:

- Analysing the pulse for purposes of systemic comparisons
- Establishing a routine which will lend itself to heightened focus when assessing pulse
- Ensuring that all aspects of the pulse are assessed and none are missed.

It should be clearly noted that there are a number of different methods described in the literature, and different practitioners will inevitably favour one approach over another. Some practitioners also develop their own methods to gather information about the different parameters of the pulse. There is no right or wrong approach to gathering the information. However, the practitioner should always aim to develop a consistent method for pulse assessment.

To illustrate by what is meant by a consistent method, we have provided an example below. This method involves two stages, each of which can be further divided into steps. The first stage focuses on the pulse taker's general impressions of the pulse without actually 'measuring' or apportioning a 'value' to the different parameters. Apportioning a value is the second stage, and requires a rigorous and exact assessment of each of the parameters.

Stage 1: initial impressions

Step 1: Locate the pulse positions and place the fingers on these

Step 2: Feel the overall pulse with all fingers on the three pulse positions Cun, Guan and Chi

Step 3: Feel the overall pulse at the other levels of depth.

Stage 1 is about overall impressions of the pulse, so it isn't strictly necessary to locate the three levels of depth exactly. Rather, simply move the fingers towards the bone, occlude the pulse and gently raise the fingers back towards the superficial level of depth.

When arriving at an overall impression of the pulse it is useful to consider the following questions:

- Is the pulse easy to find?
- Is the pulse felt clearly?
- Are there any distinct or unusual presentations of the pulse and related parameters? That is, is the pulse noticeably superficial, or is there noticeable tension in the arterial wall?
- Is the pulse strong, weak or of normal strength?
- Does the pulse have a contour or does the arterial wall dominate?
- Does the pulse rebound against the finger when pressure is released?
- Do your first impressions correlate with the individual's physical build and apparent state?
- Does the pulse feel fast or slow? (Note that this initial stage of assessment is about your first impressions of the pulse and it is not necessary to actually take the actual measure of pulse rate at this stage).

When first feeling the pulse it is important not to be swayed by your first impressions into making a premature diagnosis. When feeling the pulse, what often occurs is that a particular change in one of the pulse parameters is quickly apparent when illness is present. For example, there may be an increase in arterial tension, or the pulse is noticeably strongest at the superficial level of depth, or pulse force is greatly reduced or pulse rate increased. In this instance caution must be used not to classify the pulse into a CM pulse quality based on the most apparent change in the one parameter alone. For example, it would be easy to call any pulse that has an increase in arterial tension a Stringlike (Wiry) pulse. This would be incorrect, as there are several distinctive pulse qualities that all manifest with an increased in arterial tension and the Stringlike (Wiry) pulse is simply one of these. Also, the Stringlike (Wiry) pulse is associated with changes in other pulse parameters and not simply based on arterial tension alone. If a pulse is forcibly classified into one of the overall qualities, then important information is lost that can mean the difference in making a correct diagnosis and formulating appropriate treatment.

Stage 2: specific pulse assessment; the parameters

Next, it is necessary to palpate and make an assessment of the presentation of each specific parameter. Start with a measured assessment of pulse rate, using a watch, and then determine whether the rhythm is regular. Rate and rhythm are the easiest of the parameters to assess. This makes them useful for focusing the mind for assessment of the other parameters. Next assess the other parameters in the following order:

- Depth: At which level of depth is the pulse felt strongest?
- Length: Is the pulse long or short?
- Width: Is the pulse thin or not thin?
- Force: What is the overall force of the pulse? How does the strength vary between positions and at different levels of depth?
- Pulse occlusion: Is the artery easy or hard to occlude?
- Arterial wall tension: Is this increased, normal or absent?
- Contour and flow wave: Are there any changes in the contour and texture of the flow wave?

By following a set of procedures and methods in this way, the practitioner is able to build a diagnosis based on the pulse by adding the assessment of one pulse parameter to another. As a picture of the parameters builds up, it may become apparent that the parameters are presenting in such a way that they form one of the traditional CM pulse qualities described in the literature. However, if the pulse parameters do not combine to form an easily identified pulse quality, this need not be a cause for concern. Often, the pulse doesn't present as described in the literature, so assessing the individual aspects or parameters of the pulse, such as depth, width and length, is still just as informative. Table 5.3 is a summary of the parameters listed in Stage 2 and gives a diagnostic context of the parameter and related changes within a CM framework when using the parameters in this way.

Information pertaining to the specific assessment of the pulse parameters in Stage 2 above is given in

61

Table 5.3 ● Summary of the pulse parameters, variations in their presentation and the relationship to CM theory

	Description	CM theory	How the pulse is affected
Depth	Level of depth at which the pulse can be felt the strongest	May indicate: 1. Where disease is located. The superficial level generally refers to external, while deep refers to internal 2. Yang Qi's ability to move outwards 3. The strength of Yin Qi and its ability to anchor Yang Qi	A pulse felt strongest at the deep level and unable to be felt superficially can indicate: 1. Deficiency of Qi and Blood 2. Obstruction of Qi and Blood A pulse felt strongest at the superficial level of depth can indicate: 1. External attack 2. Floating of Yang Qi due to deficiency of Yin (Yang loses the anchoring effect of Yin)
Width	Diameter of the artery The area that the arterial wall displaces laterally on the palpating finger	Can indicate a number of factors: The volume of Yin fluids and Blood Relates to the arterial tension Affected by Damp	Increased width: Hyperactivity of Yang: Yang excess disturbing Qi and Blood, causing them to expand and fill the artery Floating of Yang due to deficiency of Yin not restraining Yang, whose nature is to move outward and upward Lack of volume to fill artery pulse feels 'hollow', easily occluded Decreased width: Deficiency of Yin fluids or Blood Damp can compress the arteries
Rate	Number of beats per minute	Functional activity of Yang Qi	Increased rate: hyperactivity of Yang or relative hyperactivity of Yang due to deficiency of Yin Decreased: deficiency of Yang or excess Cold
Rhythm	Interval between beats: should be regular	Indicates the state of Heart Qi and functional activity of the organs	Irregular rhythm may occur at irregular or regular intervals. The more often they occur, the more severe the condition
Length	Presence or absence of pulsations at Cun, Guan, Chi, beyond Cun and beyond Chi	Indicates: Amount of Qi and Blood Presence of heat Obstruction of Qi and Blood	Hyperactivity of Yang: Yang excess disturbing Qi and Blood, causing them to expand and fill the artery
Arterial tension	The tone of the arterial wall, giving it definition. Related to the elasticity of the arterial wall. Contributes to the feeling of 'hardness' of the artery wall when palpated	Reflects the activity of Yang Qi May reflect the presence of pathogenic Cold	Hyperactivity of Yang Qi can lead to increased tension in artery wall Decreased activity of Yang Qi can lead to decreased tone of arterial wall, leading to less definition Stagnation of Qi, whether due to vacuity or repletion may cause increased tension Pathogenic Cold may cause contraction of the arterial wall leading to increased tension

Table 5.3 ● Summary of the pulse parameters, variations in their presentation and the relationship to CM theory—cont'd

	Description	CM theory	How the pulse is affected
Force	The intensity with which the pulse strikes the palpating finger	Reflects the functional activity of Yang Qi Reflects volume of Blood/Yin fluids May reflect presence of a pathogenic factor May reflect strong Zheng Qi (antipathogenic Qi)	If Yang Qi is deficient, the pulse will be forceless, due to lack of motive force to propel blood. Deficiency of Blood/Yin fluids: less fluid being propelled and filling out the artery, therefore forceless If the pulse is forceful, this may indicate: Strong functioning of Yang Qi, or May indicate obstruction of Qi and/or blood Presence of pathogenic factor that has entered the body
Pulse occlusion	Refers to the amount of pressure needed to occlude the radial pulse	Influenced by the pulse force, volume, width and arterial tension	If the blood volume is decreased the pulse may feel 'empty'. If there is sufficient Qi and blood, then pulse may require force to occlude If Yang Qi is hyperactive causing stagnation, increased tension in the pulse can make it difficult to occlude. A lack of Yang Qi to provide the arterial wall with tone may lead to easy occlusion
Flow wave	Refers to the longitudinal movement of blood through the artery	Reflects the quality and volume of blood Also related to amount of Yang Qi, providing pulse with impetus to move	Hyperactive Yang Qi due to stagnation of Qi can cause blood flow to be restrained Deficiency of Blood/Yin fluids can cause blood flow to become turbulent If Yang Qi is deficient then blood flow is less forceful, may be slower
Pulse contour	Refers to the texture of the blood flow and shape of the pulse	Related to Yang Qi controlling the tone of the arterial wall Also related to volume of blood	An increase of fluid within the system leads to an increase in force and rounded contour If blood is deficient, the pulse force will vary in intensity, unable to fill the vessels If Yang Qi is hyperactive and the arterial walls are less flexible then arterial walls don't expand and contract as readily Damp in the tissues may compress the arteries, leading to a narrowing of the arteries (less able to expand normally)

Chapters 6 and 7, along with a system of diagnostic interpretation of assessment findings, including the related traditional CM pulse qualities. This chapter has focused on the technique required to locate the positions and levels of depth for assessing the parameters. Other techniques for assessing length, width, pulse occlusion, strength and contour are included with the appropriate parameters to which they relate in Chapter 6 and 7 as well.

5.12 Other considerations when assessing the pulse and interpreting the findings

In addition to the difficulties of applying different pulse assumption systems and pulse descriptions from the literature, the complexity of the CM radial pulse diagnostic process is heightened by other factors that must be taken into account when evaluating the pulse according to the patient's individual characteristics and environment (Maciocia 1989). These include influences such as seasonal effects, gender, age, level of fitness, occupation and body type (Deng 1999, Maciocia 1989, O'Connor & Bensky 1981).

It has been assumed that these variables impact on the physiological presentation of the pulse, and therefore obviously have important implications for the interpretation of an individual's pulse qualities. As a result, it is necessary to consider these factors when examining the pulse, to determine whether the pulse quality is appropriate for the individual rather than being caused by a pathological disturbance. For example, the Slow pulse in CM theory is usually associated with a Cold condition. However, if the patient is accustomed to regular exercise (such as an athlete) then a Slow pulse may be quite normal. What might appear to be a pathological pulse, when taken in the proper context and in the absence of any other abnormal signs and symptoms, could be considered to be normal for the individual in question.

The following discussion on factors affecting the radial pulse is reproduced and modified with permission from King (2001).

5.12.1 Radial pulse assumptions in classical and modern CM literature

Contemporary CM texts have a tendency to accept the classical pulse information, often incorporating the term 'traditionally' to qualify their material. Frequently there is little reference to the actual sources from which this information was obtained. This creates problems in terms of placing the information in a historical perspective and identifying the theoretical framework being utilised. In addition, this makes it difficult to determine whether (and if so, where) the modern authors have expanded on the information, adding their own commentary. In some instances, CM texts mention that the pulse varies with age, gender and body weight, but neglect to elaborate on how these factors affect the pulse characteristics.

Despite the effects that such factors are believed to have on the pulse, such claims remain untested and continue to appear unchallenged in many contemporary CM texts. As such, we have presented these factors as a summative collection of information from the relevant literature.

5.12.2 Seasonal effects

The philosophical theory of Yin and Yang, on which Chinese medical theory is based, is thought to have evolved as a result of observing cycles occurring in nature. This theory, which proposed that all phenomena exist as a result of the variable interaction of opposite but complementary qualities, could be seen in the cyclical nature of day and night, the tides and seasonal changes.

The human body was seen as a reflection of the universe, a microcosm within the macrocosm, and therefore subject to the cyclical effects of nature. Health was dependent on living 'in accord with nature' (Ni 1995: p. 53). This interaction of human beings with their surroundings meant that changes in the environment were believed to be capable of affecting the individual. The effect of the environment on the body is discussed at great length in the *Nei Jing*. Different climatic circumstances resulted in different type of diseases. The seasons influenced the type of illnesses that occurred, where they occurred within the body and the way that treatment was conducted.

> The weather . . . affects every living creature in the natural world and forms the foundation for birth, growth, maturation, and death
> (Ni 1995: p. 19).

> The cycles of heaven and earth reflect in the constant changes in nature. Take the example of seasonal weather changes . . . Every organism in nature adapts and changes along with the seasonal cycles of germination in the spring, growth and development in the summer, maturity and harvest of the autumn, and storing or hibernating in the winter. The human pulse also corresponds to these changes
> (Ni 1995: p. 64).

In particular, the effect of the four seasons on the pulse has been noted a number of times, with descriptions of the qualities that the pulse reflected in each season.

> In the spring, the pulse will mirror nature and become slightly wiry or round; in the summer, it will enlarge and become flooding; in the fall, the pulse will float to the surface; in the winter, it will sink to the interior.
> (Ni 1995: p. 65)

> The relationship between the eight winds and four seasons, the flow between one season and another, will all determine the normal pulses in the body.
> (Ni 1995: p. 57)

As a consequence, when diagnosing it was necessary to take the normal seasonal variations of the pulse into consideration.

The influence of the seasons on the pulse is a concept that pervades the history of CM literature. Chapter 15 of the *Nan Jing* is devoted to the discussion of the appropriate quality for the pulse in each season. If the pulse did not reflect this quality, this indicated illness and an explanation of the type of pathological pulse and its implications is included. Likewise, the *Mai Jing* discusses the effect of season on the radial pulse in relation to the normal quality of each season.

In both the classical and modern texts, there is some agreement concerning the presence of seasonal variations in pulse. These changes generally relate to the depth and quality of the pulse. For example:

> These [seasons] influence the pulse, it being deeper in Wintertime and more superficial in Summertime
> *(Maciocia 1989: p. 166).*

> The human body is subject to influence by climatic changes over the four seasons . . . These changes are reflected on the pulse. During spring the tension of the pulse gradually increases and becomes wiry. During summer . . . the pulse overflows (like a hook). During autumn . . . the pulse becomes empty, floating, soft and fine (like a hair). During winter . . . the pulse becomes deep and strong
> *(Li, Huynh trans 1985: p. 8).*

> In the spring . . . the tension of the pulse is enhanced and the wiry pulse appears; in the summer . . . the pulse will be fully filled and thus a full pulse presents; in the autumn . . . a pulse that is felt soft, light and floating, like a feather of a bird, occurs; in the winter . . . Yang Qi of the human body also hides in the depth or the interior of the body, causing the pulse to be deep and very forceful. No matter how the pulse changes, as long as the changes correspond to the seasons and are felt forceful and unhurried, it is a normal pulse
> *(Lu 1996: p. 96).*

> In moderate climates, the regular change of the seasons and their typical weather produces slight inflections of the pulse on healthy individuals which may be described in spring as an inflection in the direction of a stringy pulse, in summer . . . a flooding pulse, in autumn . . . a superficial pulse and in winter . . . submerged pulses . . . Yet none of these inflections, taken in isolatedly, may be interpreted as a symptom of disease
> *(Porkert 1983: p. 245).*

In *The Practical Jin's Pulse Diagnosis*, a modern Chinese pulse text utilising a pulse diagnostic system based on a combination of CM and biomedical knowledge, the influence of seasonal change is still acknowledged. Changes in the pulse are attributed to physiological changes in the body coping with the extreme changes of temperature through the four seasons. For example, the pulse is 'deep and solid' in winter and 'full . . . strong when it rises and weak when it sinks' in summer, as a result of the body's attempt to regulate its temperature (Wei, Lu (trans) 1997: p. 108). Elsewhere in the text, changes in the rate of the pulse are noted in winter (slow) and summer (rapid), while the spring pulse is said to be slightly wiry.

> The wiry pulse, which is strong, thick, hard and wiry, is often felt in the spring; the full pulse, which is felt strong when it rises and weak when it sinks, is usually seen in summer . . . in autumn . . . the pulse is often felt full and feather-like in shape; and in winter, the pulse is usually deep and solid . . .
> *(Wei, Lu (trans) 1997: p. 108).*

> Rapid . . . in summer . . . slow . . . in winter'
> *(Wei, Lu (trans) 1997: p. 63).*

5.12.2 Gender

The notion of a gender-based difference in pulse strength has persisted from early CM teachings. Statements regarding the comparative strength of men and women's pulses can be found in many classical and modern CM texts. This includes various differences in the strength of the left and right hands, in the relative strength of the Cun, Guan and Chi positions and an overall difference in strength (and sometimes pulse quality) between genders.

The difference in strength according to gender appears to have its basis in Yin–Yang theory. According to this theory, the left side of the body is considered Yang and the right side Yin. Males should have more Yang energy, therefore males should have a stronger left side. Women, being associated with Yin, should have a stronger right side. This follows for the difference in the relative strength of the positions. In Yin Yang theory the upper position, equated with Cun, is Yang and the lower position, equated with Chi, is Yin. Therefore, in men the Cun position should be slightly stronger than Chi and vice versa for women.

The *Nei Jing*, one of the oldest extant Chinese medical classics, devotes a number of chapters to the methodology, pathology and significance of the palpation of arteries around the body. Differences in the pulse are noted in relation to pregnancy.

> When examining the pulses, if one finds the Yin pulses are distinctly different from the Yang pulses, this indicates pregnancy
> *(Ni: 1995: p. 33).*

If in women the hand shaoyin or the heart pulse is prominent, pregnancy is indicated *(Ni: 1995: p. 74).*

The Nineteenth Difficult Issue in the *Nan Jing* introduces the concept of gender difference regarding movement of energy in the vessels throughout the body. Gender was to be taken into account when feeling the pulse to determine whether the pulse was normal. It was considered normal for a male pulse to be 'stronger above the gate' (corresponding to the Cun position) and in a female for the pulse to be stronger 'below the gate' (corresponding to the Chi position). Using this system, doctors could identify the gender of their patient by pulse alone. Patterns that would be considered normal in one gender would be, if found in the other, pathological.

> In males [a strong movement in] the vessels appears above the gate; in females [a strong movement in the] vessels appears below the gate.
> *(Unschuld 1986: p. 259)*

> When males display a female pulse it is a sign of deficiency disorder within; when females display a male pulse it is a sign of a disorder of excess in the extremities
> *(Furth 1999: p. 50).*

Differences in the overall force and qualitative aspects of the pulse are noted in relation to gender. The *Mai Jing* describes the differences in quality and strength between female and male:

> The pulses in females are inclined to be more soggy and weaker than in males . . . For males, the left (pulse) being larger is favourable, while for females the right being larger is favourable'
> *(Wang, Yang (trans) 1997: p. 10).*

Li Shi Zhen's *Pulse Diagnosis* states:

> The left is Yang and the right is Yin. Men have more Yang Qi . . . their left hand is stronger. Women have more Yin blood . . . their right hand pulse is stronger.
> *(Li, Huynh (trans) 1985: p. 4).*

However, although this was disputed by Flaws (1995), a modern TCM author, in his book *The Secret of Chinese Pulse Diagnosis*, he neglects to elaborate further his own findings.

> '[Bin Hu says] . . . it is normal for men's pulses to be larger on the left and women's to be larger on the right. I have not found this to be the case in my clinical practice
> *(Flaws 1995: p. 49).*

This opinion was revised in a later edition of the same book:

> Personally, I would say women's pulses are smaller on the left, at least in the bar and cubit positions, due to their monthly loss of blood
> *(Flaws 1997: p. 59).*

In another translation of Li Shi Zhen's classic, *The Lakeside Master's Study of the Pulse* (Li, Flaws (trans) 1998) the relative strength of the Cun and Chi according to gender is discussed.

> As long as the pulse remains normal in number of beats (and/or size and shape) throughout the four seasons, it is normal for a woman's pulse to be sunken in the inch and a man's pulse to be sunken in the cubit
> *(Li, Flaws (trans) 1998: p. 70 footnote).*

A modern author in support of this view, stated that:

> In men, the Front [Cun] position should be very slightly stronger, while in women the Rear [Chi] position should be so. This also follows the Yin-Yang symbolism according to which upper is Yang (hence male) and lower is Yin (hence female)
> *(Maciocia 1989: p. 166).*

Alternatively, a 'somewhat hook-like pulse' is considered to be normal for everyone, with the pulse starting off deep in the Chi position and then rising to become relatively floating in the Cun position (Flaws 1997: p. 61). This would appear to correlate with the physiological positioning of the radial artery which is situated deeper at the Chi position and then becomes more superficially located due to support of the radial bone at Guan (refer to section 5.6.1).

Gender specificity in relation to pulse strength differences between right and left appears to be abandoned in some modern Chinese texts, with references instead to overall differences in strength. In particular, women's pulses are generally said to be weaker and faster than men's pulses:

> In adult females, the pulse is usually softer and weaker than the males, because they have more fat covering the vessels and their constitution is relatively weaker than males.
> *(Lu 1996: p. 37).*

> In general, the pulse of men will be somewhat large and women will be relatively weak, slightly fine and somewhat fast.
> *(Deng 1999: p. 92).*

> Women usually have thready, weak and a little rapid pulse.
> *(Wei, Lu (trans) 1997: p.109).*

A woman's pulse is usually softer and slightly faster than a man's
(Kaptchuk 2000: p. 196).

Contemporary Western CM texts tend to reiterate the traditional theory regarding left/right differences. O'Connor & Bensky (1981) state that women's right sides are usually stronger than their left, while the opposite occurs in men. In addition, such pulse information is believed by some to be able to predict the sex of an unborn child, so that if the pregnant woman's right side is stronger then the child is female and if the left is stronger, it is male.

In their examination of the use of the pulse across cultures, Amber & Babey-Brooke (1993) state that the CM pulse taking procedure differed according to sex; men have their left side examined first and women the right side. This is explained by traditional theory that the left side corresponds to Yang (associated with males) and the right side corresponds to Yin (associated with females). Using this theory further, the left indicates disease in males while the right side indicates disease in females. It is also noted that:

> (the) left side is positive and the right side is negative in the male; the right side positive and the left side negative in the female
> *(Amber & Babey-Brooke 1993: p. 148).*

In the absence of further clarification, it is assumed that the authors are referring to comparative strength.

5.12.3 Pregnancy and the pulse

A number of changes occur in the haemodynamic system during pregnancy, including the following:

- An increase in the amount of circulating blood, mostly in the form of plasma. Blood volume can increase from 30% to 50% and starts around 12 weeks of gestation, peaking at 28–34 weeks (Estes 2006). Other sources note that plasma volume starts from about 6 weeks gestation (Blackburn 2003 cited in Coad & Dunstall 2005).
- Cardiac output is greatly increased but arterial blood pressure remains the same, mostly due to stroke volume.
- Heart rate increases by 10–15 bpm. Basal metabolic rate usually increases by 15–25% due to increased oxygen consumption and to foetal metabolic demands (Estes 2006).
- Peripheral resistance to blood flow is reduced and blood flow to extremities (hands and feet) is increased due to peripheral vasodilatation resulting in warm hands and feet (Stables & Rankin 2005).
- Oestrogen levels in blood plasma rise.

- This is a general relaxation of peripheral vascular tone in early pregnancy: it decreases by 5 weeks, lowest level by 16–34 weeks (Stables & Rankin 2005).

5.12.3.1 Pregnancy and the effect on the radial artery pulsation

Many of these cardiovascular changes may account for the perceived changes to the contour of the radial artery pulsation during pregnancy. For example, the Slippery pulse is indicative of increased Yang (Heat) and this is reflected in the increased metabolic rate, which results in an increased pulse rate. The Slippery pulse also reflects the increase in body fluid that occurs as a normal part of pregnancy, resulting in an increase in blood volume of up to 30–50%. The combination of these factors, plus the decreased peripheral resistance, lead to a greatly increased cardiac output.

5.12.4 Age

Differences stated in relation to age mainly concern children and adults (young and old) in terms of pulse rate and strength, with younger people generally considered to have more forceful pulses than older people (Fig. 5.8). This reflects the belief that Qi and Blood decline with age and this is reflected in the pulse. An increased heart rate in children is noted in a number of TCM texts. In children the pulse rate is significantly faster; it decreases through childhood into adulthood. A newborn baby is likely to have an average heart rate of 140 bpm (Estes 2006: p. 253). One author (Wei, Lu (trans) 1997) noted that in adults, the pulse is slower in younger people and faster in older people:

> Children's pulses tend to be faster than those of adults
> *(Townsend & De Donna 1990: p. 70).*

> In general, younger people have stronger pulses than older people
> *(Townsend & De Donna 1990: p. 71).*

> The Qi and blood of elderly people are vacuous and weak, and the pulse is vacuous and without force. The Qi and blood of young, strong people are effulgent and exuberant, and the pulse arrives replete and with force
> *(Deng 1999: p. 92).*

> (The pulse) is usually . . . rapid and hard in the aged, slow and forceful in the young . . .
> *(Wei, Lu (trans) 1997: p. 63).*

> Young people with a strong constitution usually have a strong pulse beat, while the aged usually have a weak and hard pulse because

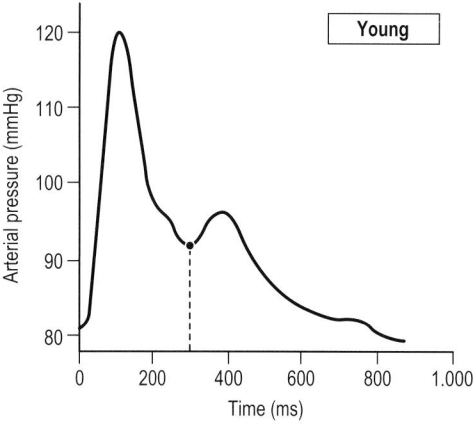

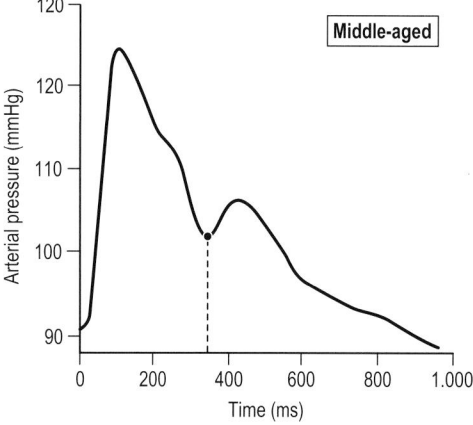

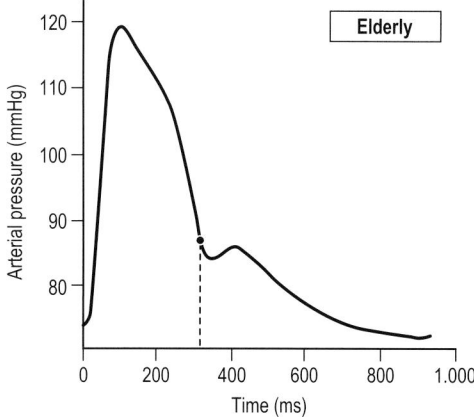

Figure 5.8
Variation in pulse wave form with age. Age-related differences are attributable to stiffening of the arterial walls, causing the reflective wave to move from the diastole to systole. This causes a higher mean sustained pressure in systole in older people. (After Figure 3.2.4 in AtCor Medical 2006, A clinical guide: pulse wave analysis, with permission of AtCor Medical Pty.)

they are weak in constitution and their elasticity of the vessels is lowered
(Lu 1996: p. 37).

5.12.5 Body type

In general, there is little information about body type and its influence on the pulse. Most texts refer to the physiological presentation of the radial artery in terms of its depth and the amount of overlying tissue. A heavier person may have a deep pulse and a slim person may have a relatively superficial pulse. This is not necessarily considered to be pathological. Similarly, someone who is tall has a wider artery, while someone who is short in height has a thin artery. If nothing else, this simply relates to proportional difference in physiques. There are some also references to body type and pulse rate in the literature, with heavier people assumed to have a slower pulse.

Some of the references in the literature to body size and influence on the pulse are as follows:

Heavily built people tend to have slower pulses than slighter people
(Townsend & De Donna 1990: p. 70).

A heavy person's pulse tends to be slow and deep, while a thin person's is more superficial
(Kaptchuk 2000: p. 196).

A thin body with thin muscles will have a somewhat floating pulse; a fat body with thick layers will have a somewhat deep pulse. These cannot be taken as pathological
(Deng 1999: p. 92).

A thin person with fine muscles mostly presents relatively superficial pulse; and a fat person with thick fat in the epithelium, most presents deep pulse, or the pulse in the lower level
(Wei 1997: p. 106).

Fat people mostly have a deep pulse. Skinny people have comparatively large pulses
(Flaws 1997: p. 60).

Obese people tend to have fine and deep pulses, while thin people have large pulses
(Wiseman & Ellis 1996: p. 118)

5.13 Summary

Although assumptions concerning the pulse and the effect of factors such as seasonal changes, gender, age and body type are usually included in modern CM pulse literature, this often appears cursory, with little elaboration on why or how these variables influences pulse characteristics. While physiologically based differences may help to possibly explain, to some degree, the influence of body type, age and gender on the pulse, the effect of the seasons appears to be slightly more esoteric.

The seasonal effects on the pulse are described in great detail in the classical literature such as the *Nei Jing* and *Mai Jing*, but have largely tended to fall out of favour in modern texts. This may reflect the theoretical rather than clinical relevance of the information. It should also be remembered that CM theory developed in a country with a wide geographical diversity, where the seasonal differences are sharply pronounced and temperature ranges extreme. This may indeed explain why certain disease patterns are more prevalent in certain regions of the country and at certain times of the year. Such effects on the body would therefore be expected to impact on the pulse. However, this may not translate into countries experiencing milder climatic changes.

One aspect of the seasonal relationship with pulse that may have some relevance to clinical practice is the body's response to changes in temperature. It is well documented in biomedicine that in response to increased body temperature, there is vasodilatation of the blood vessels close to the surface of the skin to help release heat into the surrounding environment. Conversely, with decreased body temperature there is vasoconstriction, so that the blood vessel walls contract inward to conserve body heat. This may partially explain the CM assumption that the pulse is more superficial in summer and deeper in winter. Clinically, a deep pulse presenting in a patient in very hot weather may therefore be an indication of dysfunction, reflecting an inability of the body to regulate itself.

The information pertaining to the pulse and the effect of season, gender, age and body type has existed from early CM literature, yet there has been very little investigation into the validity of these relationships in a modern context. There is a paucity of demographic information available to document the effect of any of these factors on the pulse generally and it is therefore difficult to definitively say how these will impact on the pulse presentation in a clinical setting. Preliminary demographic investigations into the pulse and some of these variables, using a reliable pulse taking methodology and pulse terminology (shown to have high levels of inter-rater reliability), have revealed some interesting gender differences in a healthy group of subjects (King 2001). Male pulses were generally rated as more forceful than female, with the pulse also rated as more easily occluded in females than males. Differences in the length of the pulse were also apparent, with males classified with long pulses (90%) more often than females (56%). There was no support for the perceived CM gender-based difference in pulse strength between left and right sides, with a significant majority of subjects found to have a stronger pulse on the right side regardless of gender (73% of females and 69% of males) (King 2001: p. 85). It was surmised that this may have been due, in part, to the fact that most subjects were right handed and therefore blood flow to the dominant hand may be influenced by increased muscle mass; further research using a larger cohort of left-handed subjects is necessary to examine this theory. However, CM theory states that the relative increase in strength on one side compared to the other is influenced only by gender, not necessarily by handedness.

This study also provided some limited support for the existence of three individual pulse positions at the wrist area, with differences in strength perceived between Cun, Guan and Chi. It was found that the Chi position was found to be the weakest position overall in both males and females, while Cun or Guan were most frequently rated as the strongest (King 2001: p. 138). There was also support for the existence of three levels of depth, with the pulse rated as strongest at the middle or deep levels of depth in the majority of subjects. This would be expected in a healthy cohort and gives some credence to the CM theory of the healthy pulse having Root, that is, a presence at a deeper level of depth.

Body type and the relationship to pulse depth were also examined in the study. Generally, it was found that the pulse was less frequently found at the superficial level of depth in heavier people (body mass index (BMI) >25), while in slimmer people the pulse was found to be present more frequently at both the superficial and deep levels of depth.

Body type was also an important feature in the findings of an individual's pulse being categorised as forceful or not forceful as reported by Walsh (2003). Generally, although it was not statistically significant, there was an overall trend towards the pulse being reported as less forceful as body weight increased (ANOVA, $p = 0.06$). However, when gender was considered in analysis using correlation coefficients, women with a greater body weight were more often reported to have 'not forceful' pulses in correlation assessments of tonometry and manual palpation. Further, when objective tonometry measurements of the time taken for the heart to contract were considered as well, there was a significant relationship between weight, gender and increase in systolic heart contraction variables, with an accumulative 81% explanation of the nature of the relationship for an assessor's selection of the pulse as 'forceful' or 'not forceful'. Women were reported to have less forceful pulses than men.

The concept of a seasonal effect on the pulse and level of depth was given limited support by the finding that generally the pulse was rated strongest at a relatively deeper level of depth in winter than summer, in the same group of subjects (King 2001: p. 143). However, the sample size was relatively small in this case, so replication of these findings in a larger sample size is necessary.

The scope for research into the most basic underpinnings of CM pulse theory is great. Many of the fundamental concepts for the various systems of pulse interpretation such as Five Phase and San Jiao are based on the assumption that three pulse positions exist at the wrist region, yet very little research has been undertaken to investigate the validity of this concept. This also holds true for the theoretical existence of different levels of pulse depth, which is particularly relevant for Five Phase pulse diagnosis and the traditional CM pulse qualities. Further demographic information needs to be collected about the features of the 'normal' pulse before the possible effects of factors such as body type, gender and seasonal effects can be investigated. Therefore, although they are interesting, the assumptions about these factors should be used with a degree of caution. It is more clinically valuable to examine a patient's pulse in terms of the changes in individual pulse parameters and evaluate how these contribute to the pattern manifesting with the other presenting signs and symptoms.

References

Amber R, Babey-Brooke A 1993 The pulse in Occident and Orient. Santa Barbara Press, New York

Birch S 1992 Naming the Unnameable: A historical study of radial pulse six position diagnosis. TAS 12:2–13

Coad J, Dunstall M 2005 Anatomy and physiology for midwives, 2nd edn. Elsevier, Edinburgh

Deng T 1999 Practical diagnosis in traditional Chinese medicine. Churchill Livingstone, Edinburgh

Estes M E 2006 Health assessment and physical examination, 3rd edn. Thomson Delmar Learning, Australia

Flaws B 1995 The secret of Chinese pulse diagnosis. Blue Poppy Press, Boulder, CO

Flaws B 1997 The secret of Chinese pulse diagnosis, 2nd edn. Blue Poppy Press, Boulder, CO

Furth C 1999 A flourishing yin: gender in China's medical history, 960–1665. University of California Press, Berkeley

Hammer L 2001 Chinese pulse diagnosis: a contemporary approach. Eastland Press, Seattle

Kaptchuk T 2000 Chinese medicine: web that has no weaver, revised edn. Rider, London

King E 2001 Do the radial qualities of traditional Chinese medicine provide a reliable diagnostic tool?: an examination of pulse relationships stated in modern and classical Chinese texts [MSc]. University of Technology, Sydney

Li S Z, Flaws B (translator) 1998 The lakeside master's study of the pulse. Blue Poppy Press, Boulder, CO

Li S Z, Huynh H K (translator) 1981 Pulse diagnosis. Paradigm, Brookline, MA

Lu Y 1996 Pulse diagnosis. Shandong Science and Technology Press, Jinan

Maciocia G 1989 The foundations of Chinese medicine. Churchill Livingstone, Edinburgh

Maciocia G 2004 Diagnosis in Chinese medicine: a comprehensive guide. Churchill Livingstone, Edinburgh

McCance K L, Huether S E 2006 Pathophysiology: the biologic basis for disease in adults and children, 5th ed. Elsevier/Mosby, St Louis

Ni M S (translator) 1995 The Yellow Emperor's classic of medicine: (huang di nei jing su wen ling shu). Shambhala, Boston

O'Connor J, Bensky D (translators and editors) 1981 Acupuncture: a comprehensive text. Eastland Press, Seattle

Porkert M 1983 The essentials of Chinese diagnostics. Acta Medicinae Sinensis Chinese Medicine Publications, Zurich

Stables D, Rankin J (editors) 2005 Physiology in childbearing with anatomy and related biosciences. Elsevier, Edinburgh

Townsend G, De Donna Y 1990 Pulses and impulses: a practitioner's guide to a unique new pulse diagnosis technique. Thorsons, Wellingborough

Unschuld P, (translator) 1986 Nan-ching: the classic of difficult issues. University of California Press, Berkeley

Walsh S 2003 The radial pulse: correlation of traditional Chinese medicine pulse characteristics with objective tonometric measures [PhD]. University of Technology, Sydney

Wang S H, Yang S (translator) 1997 The pulse classic: a translation of the Mai Jing. Blue Poppy Press, Boulder, CO

Wei J, Lu Y (translator) 1997 The practical Jin's pulse diagnosis. Shandong Science and Technology Press, Shandong

Wiseman N, Ellis A (translators and editors) 1996 Fundamentals of Chinese medicine, revised edn. Paradigm, Brookline, MA

Wiseman N, Ye F 1998 A practical dictionary of Chinese medicine, 2nd edn. Paradigm, Brookline, MA

Simple CM pulse qualities and associated pulse parameters

6

Chapter contents

6.1 Introduction 72
6.2 The simple pulse parameters 73
6.3 Rate 73
6.4 CM pulses defined by rate 78
6.5 Rhythm 83
6.6 CM pulses defined by rhythm 88
6.7 Depth 91
6.8 CM pulse qualities defined by level of depth 94
6.9 Length (longitude) 100
6.10 CM pulse defined by length 101
6.11 Width (latitude) 103
6.12 CM pulse qualities defined by arterial width 110
6.13 Summary 112

Pulse diagnosis is often complicated in the clinical context because pulse manifestations as they present in the radial artery do not present as nice discrete 'images' as posited in the literature. Indeed, expectations of always feeling a classical pulse quality are misplaced and will lead to difficulties and frustration on the part of the pulse taker. Rather, it should be expected that the pulse may ordinarily present as no recognisable traditional pulse quality. This is to be expected, as each person will not always respond the same way to the same illness: a person's constitution and the relative strength of their Qi and blood means the body responds differently. Other factors such as lifestyle (work, exercise, dietary) and life history only add further variability.

There may be instances when the pulse taker assesses the pulse when the immune system is just responding to a pathogenic agent so the pulse is felt while it is moving from the individual's normal or healthy pulse to the pulse that reflects the nature of the pathogenic illness and the body's response to that illness. In this situation, the pulse is not yet fully formed and may also not fit nicely into the distinctive CM pulse qualities described in the literature. Alternatively, the body's response to the illness is such that the pulse quickly forms a recognisable quality and it is over time as the body's energies are depleted or the pathogen mutates that the pulse quality may assume a less recognisable form.

In this sense, the pulse can be thought of in terms of a continuum (Fig. 6.1). The idea of the pulse as a continuum is purposely used to denote that the pulse is not a static sign, nor is the body a static organism. In this sense, there are no 'absolutes' as to how the pulse should be, it always just *is*. It is reflective of the relative degree of the body's ability to maintain normal healthy function or homeostasis in response to the constant demands of living. In terms of illness or dysfunction, the idea of the continuum refers to the changing flux of the pulse between two points of reference. At one reference point are those pulses reflecting health, usually assumed to be the individual's usual pulse state; at the other point of reference are those pulses that reflect illness or

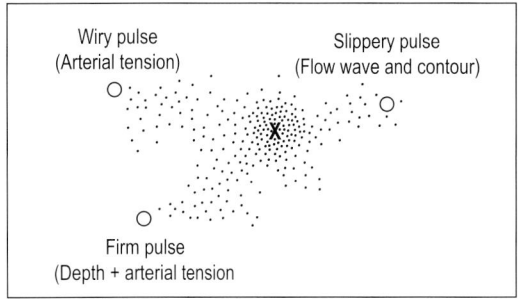

Figure 6.1
Schematic of the pulse in a continuum. The pulse formation illustrated has aspects of the Firm pulse, Slippery pulse and Floating pulse and so does not discretely fit into any of these pulse categories as they are defined within the literature.

dysfunction – the potential end manifestation of the pulse flux if no treatment intervention is provided to counter the pathogen/dysfunction.

Sometimes the pulse palpated is in flux on a continuum between two pulse types that both reflect illness or dysfunction; there may be a worsening or improvement in an illness, but not necessarily resolution of the illness. Chronic inflammatory conditions such as arthritis are examples of diseases in which there are acute periods of inflammation interspaced with periods of generalised symptoms. In this respect, certain pulse qualities develop slowly, progressing through stages in response to physiologic changes associated with disease progression or resolution. Such a process is comparable to that described by Katz (2000) in relation to the problems of defining heart failure.

> . . . this condition is not a disease but instead represents the final common pathway by which a number of disorders damage the heart so as to cause disability and premature death. These disorders include coronary disease, hypertension, valvular disorders, and a diverse group of heart muscle diseases referred to as cardiomyopathies. Furthermore, because this syndrome establishes a number of vicious cycles, heart failure begets more heart failure. (p. 7)

The description is particularly pertinent to pulse diagnosis. In this respect, pulses reflecting chronic illness and dysfunction arising from the consumption of vital substances occur over time. Some of the traditional pulse qualities are reflective of this chronological progression of illness and will only occur as an end result of a long disease process. Other pulses occur only in an acute situation. Some other pulse qualities occur only when fundamental substances of Qi, Blood and

Fluids are abundant; when these are depleted, then those pulse qualities will not occur.

Potentially there is an immense range of combinations of the pulse parameters; it is the interaction of these and their various manifestations that produces unique pulses that do not fit easily into the discrete pulse images presented in the literature. In such instances, recording and noting the pulse in terms of its constituent parameters allows important diagnostic information to be available for use, rather than lost within an incorrect application of a pulse quality name.

6.1 Introduction

The term *pulse parameters* refers to the fundamental variable characteristics that contribute to the formation of the radial arterial pulse. The 27 traditional CM pulse qualities form when there are specific changes in these parameters. A traditional pulse quality can form when there is a change in a single parameter only; other traditional pulse qualities form when there are changes in several parameters. In the pulse parameter system of radial pulse diagnosis, we have identified 9 pulse parameters that determine the 27 CM pulse qualities:

- Rate
- Rhythm
- Arterial width
- Depth
- Length
- Arterial tension
- Ease of occlusion
- Force
- Pulse contour.

6.1.1 Parameters and the arrangement of the CM pulse qualities

In Chapter 6 and 7 we present each of the 27 specific CM pulse qualities in conjunction with their relevant defining parameter(s). A pulse's defining parameter refers to the variable change in the presentation of the pulse that is *most* apparent. For example, the Rapid pulse is defined by an increase in the frequency of pulsations. Consequently, the Rapid pulse's defining parameter is pulse rate.

Where distinct changes in two or more parameters are involved in the formation of the CM pulse quality, we have categorised the CM pulse quality by using the parameter that plays the most important role in its formation. For example, the Skipping pulse features interruptions to the pulse's regular rhythm and is accompanied by an increase in pulse rate. Yet it is the rhythm changes that are its most defining parameter and it is consequently categorised under the rhythm parameter.

However, this categorising of the pulse qualities is by no means the only way to classify them. Some of the more complex CM pulse qualities presented in Chapter 7 could be classified under more than one parameter. Categorising a pulse based on parameters is flexible.

Depending on the number of parameters involved in a pulse's formation, the traditional CM pulse qualities can be additionally categorised as simple or complex. *Simple* refers to pulse qualities that are defined by a change in one parameter only, like the Rapid pulse. *Complex* refers to pulse qualities that are defined by a change in two or more parameters, such as the Firm pulse. The terms 'simple' and 'complex' can equally apply to the pulse parameters themselves. For example, pulse rate is a simple pulse parameter as it is characterised only by the pulse frequency. In contrast, pulse force is a complex pulse parameter because it depends on a range of variables such as the strength of cardiac contraction, blood volume and the tensile compliance of the arterial wall. It is how these variables combine that determine the force of the pulse.

In addition to presenting the traditional 27 pulse qualities with their relevant defining parameters, we also present the pulses according to the complexity of their defining parameter. Each of the parameters are defined, assessment techniques are detailed and the related CM pulse qualities noted along with their clinical significance. Simple pulse parameters and the related CM pulse qualities are presented in this chapter. Complex pulse parameters and related CM pulse qualities are presented in Chapter 7.

6.2 The simple pulse parameters

The simple pulse parameters covered in this chapter are:

- Rate
- Rhythm
- Depth
- Length
- Width.

Related changes in these five parameters are associated with 12 of the 27 traditional CM pulse qualities. The CM pulse qualities associated with the simple pulse parameters are:

- The Slow, Rapid and Moderate pulses (defined by rate)
- The Skipping, Bound and Intermittent pulses (defined by rhythm and accompanied by changes in rate)

- The Sinking, Floating and Hidden pulses (defined by level of depth)
- The Long and Short pulses (defined by length)
- The Fine pulse (defined by its width).

These pulses can be classified as simple pulse qualities because they are generally defined by a change in a single parameter. Exceptions are the Bound pulse and Skipping pulse, which form as a result of changes in two parameters, rhythm and rate. However, the Bound pulse and Skipping pulse are still considered 'simple' pulse qualities as they are defined by two of the most objectively evaluated parameters.

These five parameters are also defined as simple because they are relatively easy to assess in a clinical context. Indeed, these five parameters are deemed the least subjective of the nine parameters, involving the evaluation of distinctive physiological characteristics of the artery and the pulse wave. For example, manual palpation of the radial arterial diameter is assessed for the parameter of width. Pulse length is assessed by the presence or absence of pulsations at Cun, Guan and Chi pulse positions and beyond these positions. The parameter of depth entails an appraisal of the levels of depth where pulsations are relatively strongest. The rate and rhythm of the pulse can be calculated with standardised formulae of beats per minute in the case of rate, and comparison of the length of intervals between beats for rhythm. Pulse rate and rhythm can also be accurately assessed using electronic devices such as electrocardiography, and arterial width can be measured using Doppler ultrasound.

In a biomedical context, the three parameters of rate, rhythm and width are used primarily to provide information about the functional performance of the cardiovascular system, particularly the heart. The parameters of depth and length are not extensively used in the biomedical diagnostic sense, but are used as an indicator of the circulatory system's integrity. This is best seen in acute traumatic injury of the limbs in which circulation may be compromised through swelling and fractures causing arterial occlusion, and also occurs in chronic conditions in which arteries narrow and blood flow is impeded. Palpating the length of the artery is useful in identifying the point of arterial occlusion, and pulse depth is used to assess the strength of blood flow and pressure in the vessel.

6.3 Rate

Three traditional CM pulse qualities are associated with the pulse rate parameter:

- Slow pulse (section 6.4.1)
- Rapid pulse (section 6.4.2)
- Moderate pulse (section 6.4.3).

The parameter of pulse rate additionally encompasses a fourth pulse quality in addition to the three CM pulse qualities listed under this rubric: the 'normal' pulse rate. This is really not a pulse quality but rather a baseline standard for identifying abnormal pulse rate changes; whether the pulse rate is occurring faster or slower than would normally be expected.

There are clear guidelines in the literature that detail when to interpret pulse rate measures outside the normal stated pulse rate range as healthy. This often depends on a range of variables including gender, age and exercise. Therefore, in clinical practise it is important to record the pulse rate every time you palpate an individual's pulse, to establish a normal baseline measure for their particular pulse rate.

6.3.1 Pulse rate and its measurement

The pulse wave that we ultimately feel in the radial artery originates in the heart, due to the rhythmic contraction (systole) and relaxation (diastole) of the heart's left ventricle as it pumps blood throughout the body. Each systole and the following diastole is known as one *cardiac cycle*. Therefore, pulse rate is an expression of the heart rate, describing the number of times the cardiac cycle occurs each minute.

Assessment of pulse rate involves noting the presence of pulsations and the frequency with which these occur in one minute. Although pulse rate is expressed in beats per minute, it isn't always necessary to assess the pulse frequency for a full minute. For example, one method for assessing pulse rate involves counting the number of beats for 15 seconds then multiplying this value by 4, or counting the number of beats for 30 seconds, then multiplying this value by 2, to obtain a measure of pulse rate in beats per minute (bpm).

The assessment method used for obtaining a measure of pulse rate should be repeated at least twice and the findings averaged. This is useful in two ways. Firstly, it assists in determining the accuracy of the value obtained for the pulse rate. Secondly, by obtaining a second measure of pulse rate, any transient changes affecting heart rate are more readily identified by noting any large variations between the two measured values. This also increases the reliability of pulse rate assessment. (See Box 6.1 for further considerations when interpreting pulse rate diagnostically.)

6.3.1.1 Pulse rate versus heart rate

The terms pulse rate and heart rate are often used interchangeably to mean the same thing. This is based on the assumption that since heart contraction produces the pulse wave, all pulse movements felt at the radial artery should correspond to the same number of heart

---

Box 6.1

Questions to consider when assessing pulse rate

- Is this a first-time patient?
- Has the patient been hurrying to the appointment?
- Are they nervous or stressed?
- Does the patient exercise regularly? What type of exercise do they do?
- Have they exercised recently before their appointment?
- Have they taken any medications/supplements?
- Has the patient consumed tea or coffee recently? Are there any other dietary sources of caffeine, for example carbonated or energy drinks, herbal supplements?
- Is the pulse wave rising slow, normal or fast?
- Is there aversion to heat or cold?
- Is a fever present?
- What is the weather like?

---

contractions. However, there are certain biomedical conditions affecting the heart and arterial structures in which two distinct pulse waves can be felt for every heart contraction. Sometimes the heart contraction can be weak and the pulse wave cannot be felt in the radial artery. In other cases the pulse is being occluded, as in thoracic outlet syndrome. It should be noted then that in certain circumstances, the pulse rate and the heart rate do not correspond.

6.3.2 Normal pulse rate

The average resting pulse rate in a healthy adult is about 70–80 bpm, but this 'normal' range is usually extended to 60–90 bpm. Normal pulse rate will also vary depending on the level of physical activity. In a healthy adult, it can decrease to 40 bpm during sleep. At the other extreme, pulse rates of up to 180 bpm may occur during intense exercise (Epstein et al 1992: p. 7.9).

6.3.3 Variables affecting pulse rate

Of all the pulse parameters, pulse rate is the most variable. It is easily affected by several factors, including:

- Gender
- Age
- Exercise
- Medications
- Body temperature
- Emotions.

The 'normal' heart rate and hence pulse rate in a healthy individual may consequently differ from the traditionally defined normal pulse rate range of 60–90 bpm. For example, although there are specific guidelines for identifying rapid or slow pulses, it should be remembered that for someone with a customarily slow pulse (that is, <60 bpm), a rapid pulse for this person might still fall into the normal range of rate (60–90 bpm). This might be seen in individuals who undertake aerobic exercise, in whom a pulse rate of less than 60 bpm is normal. When this individual falls ill, then the pulse rate may increase to 75–80 bpm, a normal pulse rate by definition, but abnormally high for that individual. In this sense, determining the normal pulse rate for an individual should be done with respect to the relevant factors affecting that individual.

6.3.3.1 Gender and pulse rate

Estes (2006: p. 253) asserts that women have a slightly faster resting pulse rate than men:

- Women: 72–80 bpm (average 75)
- Men: 64–72 bpm (average 68)

Gender-related pulse rate differences are thought to result from the relative size of the heart. Men have relatively larger hearts than women resulting in a greater proportion of blood being pumped through the arterial system with each cardiac contraction. In women, if the heart is relatively smaller, to maintain the same blood volume movement as men the heart rate needs to increase. (This gender difference is a generalisation, as commonly both men and women will have normal resting heart rates greater than or less than the ranges listed.)

6.3.3.2 Age and heart rate

There is an inverse relationship between heart rate and age; heart rate decreases slightly with increasing age. This is a result of decreasing responsiveness of the β-adrenergic receptors in the cardiac cells to chemical stimulus, combined with decreasing sinoatrial node automaticity (McCance & Huether 2006) (see the description of the intrinsic conduction system in section 6.4.5).

From a CM perspective this correlates to Yang Qi decreasing with age. Children and infants, considered to have more Yang Qi intrinsically, have a significantly higher heart rate, with newborns likely to have a heart rate of 140 bpm. Resting heart rate for a fetus can be as high as 140–160 bpm (Marieb 2001: p. 708). Table 6.1 lists a range of normal heart rate ranges for different age groups.

The relationship between age and heart rate is clinically reflected in the diagnostic interpretation of the resting heart rate. For example, a slow heart rate occurring in a younger person, when not associated with any form of aerobic training, is seen as a poor sign of

Table 6.1 ● Normal heart rate measures according to age

Age (years)	Range (bpm)	Average (bpm)
Newborn	100–170	140
1	80–160	120
3	80–120	110
6	70–115	100
10	70–110	90
14	60–110	85–90
Adult	60–100	72
Adult men	64–72	68
Adult women	72–80	75

Source: Estes (2006: p. 253).

health. In older people, Perk et al (2003) found a strong correlation between heart rate and all-cause mortality in elderly women in a study examining the relationship between heart rate and mortality in the elderly (average age of subjects was 70 years). Although there was a similar trend for elderly men, this was not statistically significant. Perk et al (2003) found that women with a heart rate greater than 77 bpm had three times the mortality rate of those whose heart rates were less than 77 bpm ($r = 0.25$, $P = 0.0003$). This means that a relatively fast resting heart rate (that is, on the higher side of the normal range) in an older person is a mortality risk sign and can be viewed as a sign of poor health (Perk et al 2003). In a CM context, this probably reflects vacuity of the heart associated with depletion of essential substances, notably Qi.

6.3.3.3 Exercise and heart rate

Like any other muscle in the body, the more exercise the heart receives the better toned it becomes and therefore the more efficient in moving blood. This is particularly noticeable in individuals who undertake endurance training and consequently have a slower than normal resting heart rate (50–60 bpm) with elite athletes resting heart capable of falling below 50 bpm (McCance & Huether 2006: p. 1048). A slower heart rate in this situation results from:

- Increased vagal stimulation (which slows the heart) and decreased sympathetic stimulation
- Increase venous return of blood to the heart due to lowered peripheral resistance leading to increased stroke volume.

Stroke volume (SV) is the amount of blood pumped out by a ventricle with each heartbeat. As the heart rate (HR) slows down, this allows longer ventricular filling, which in turn increases stroke volume. The relationship between SV and HR is termed cardiac output (CO), defined as the amount of blood that is pumped out by each ventricle in one minute and dependent on the heart rate and stroke volume:

$$CO \text{ (ml/min)} = HR \text{ (bpm)} \times SV \text{ (ml/beat)}$$

Therefore, increased SV helps to compensate for a slower rate to maintain CO.

When cardiac fitness is poor, the heart functions less efficiently and so SV is diminished, with less blood being ejected from the heart with each cardiac contraction. In this situation, the HR increases to maintain CO. In individuals who exercise little, or whose cardiac muscle tone is poor, their normal resting heart rate is consequently raised.

6.3.3.4 Medication, herbal supplements and heart rate

There are many medications and herbal supplements that affect heart rate, and appropriate texts should be referenced for further information. Many of the routinely used over-the-counter medications such as cold and flu medications contain compounds such as pseudoephedrine (a decongestant) that may cause heart and pulse rate to increase. Common asthma-relieving medications such as salbutamol, found in bronchodilators, are β-adrenergic agonists which may cause an increased heart rate or tachycardia in some patients. Many herbal medicines and supplements such as guarana (*Paullinia cupana*), aconite (Fu zi, *Aconitum carmichaeli*) and ephedra (Ma Huang, *Ephedra sinica*) have stimulant effects on the heart and pulse rate. Nicotine also has a stimulatory effect on pulse rate (while cannabis has a primary effect on the pulse contour). Digitalis and other drugs such as beta-blockers, which block the β-adrenoreceptors and prevent stimulating chemicals from attaching, may slow down the heart rate.

6.3.3.5 Body temperature and heart rate

An increase in body temperature results in increased heart rate because of a rise in the metabolic rate of cardiac cells. This is commonly seen with fever. Conversely, a decrease in body temperature can slow down heart rate and contractility. Individuals exposed to cold and suffering hypothermia routinely present with slowed heart rates. In a CM context, cold is seen as retarding the body's Yang Qi and so the pulse slows.

Generally, environmental conditions associated with the seasons similarly affect the pulse. In summer, the pulse is felt strong, relatively superficial and slightly fast, and this is seen as a 'normal' response to the environment rather than a pulse representing pathology. Cold weather or seasonal conditions can cause the arterial tension to increase, and pulse width may decrease in an attempt to maintain body warmth. The classical CM literature also described the pulse as being deeper in winter.

6.3.3.6 Emotions such as fear, excitement, anxiety or stress

Extremes of emotion may cause changes in heart rate. Anxiety may cause tachycardia, commonly experienced as a 'panic attack'. Depression may affect the Shen, thereby affecting the heart's control of blood and the vessels. Stress stimulates the sympathetic nervous system increasing production of epinephrine (adrenaline) and elevating body heat as a consequence of increased metabolic activity (Estes 2006: p. 255). As noted previously, increase in body temperature can increase heart rate.

6.3.3.7 Pregnancy and heart rate

Early in the first trimester of pregnancy a number of hemodynamic changes take place in order to meet the demands of the growing foetus. Increased cardiac output is due to an increase in both heart rate and stroke volume. The increase in heart rate occurs as early as 4 weeks after conception and increases on average by about 15 bpm (Stables & Rankin 2005: p. 233).

6.3.3.8 Other causes affecting heart rate

There are a number of factors additionally associated with changes in the pulse rate parameter and which are always seen as a pathological response. These include (but are not limited to):

- Decreased potassium (hypokalemia), which delays ventricular repolarisation and may have varying effects on rate; bradycardia – a slow pulse, atrioventricular block or paroxysmal atrial tachycardia (McCance & Huether 2006: p. 105).
- Inhibition of the vagus nerve can cause tachycardia (McCance & Huether 2006: p. 1049).
- Shock and hypovolemia (low blood pressure) due to blood loss, plasma loss or interstitial fluid loss. Initial compensatory mechanisms include increases in heart rate and systemic vascular resistance to elevate cardiac output, by release of catecholamines by the adrenals (McCance & Huether 2006: p. 1628).
- Thyroid hormones cause changes in heart rate. Hyperactivity or hypoactivity of the thyroid affects metabolism and core body temperature (McCance & Huether 2006: pp. 692–5).

6.3.4 Regulation of heart rate: CM perspective

The rate of the pulse provides a general indication of the functional activity of Yang Qi in the body (Box 6.2). Yang Qi is seen as a motive force, giving rise to and ensuring the regularity of the movement of both Qi and blood:

Box 6.2

Traditional CM method of pulse rate assessment

The objective evaluation of heart rate with a timepiece such as a watch was not available at the time the CM classics were written. Instead, a method was devised for the purpose of evaluating whether the pulse rate was faster or slower than it should be. This method was based on the number of beats per complete respiration cycle of the patient (one inhalation and one exhalation) or the respiratory rate of the practitioner, depending on the CM literature reviewed. The following quote from the *Su Wen Nei Jing* describes this approach:

In man,
during one exhalation, the vessels exhibit two movements.
During one inhalation, the vessels exhibit two movements too.
Exhalation and inhalation constitute one standard breathing period.
If the vessels exhibit five movements,
this is an intercalation [of a fifth movement] because of a deep breathing.
That is called a 'normal person'.
Su Wen
(Unschuld 2003: p. 257)

From the pulse literature, the normal pulse rate per complete respiration cycle breath should be 4–5 pulse beats (see Table 6.2 for age-related respiratory rates). A later expansion of the *Su Wen* passage by a commentator suggested that a patient's condition should be assessed by making a comparison with the pulse frequency of someone who is not ill, such as the healthy physician.

Disadvantages of the traditional method of pulse assessment

The obvious disadvantages of the respiratory method include:

- The assumption that the practitioner is in good health and therefore has a 'normal' rate of respiration to provide a reliable baseline comparison. This is not always the case.
- Lack of agreement between literature sources relating to the use of the respiratory rate of the practitioner or the patient as the baseline comparison.
- If using the patient's respiratory rate, it may be difficult to observe the complete respiratory cycle, as it is not always easy to see inspiration and expiration clearly, particularly if the patient's breathing is shallow or irregular.

That which is quiet is Yin; that which moves is Yang
That which is retarded is Yin; that which is accelerated is Yang.
Su Wen 7
(Unschuld 2003: pp. 88).

The pulse rate is affected when the Yang Qi is affected. In this context, changes in pulse rate occur when Yang Qi is affected by:

- External factors causing heart rate to increase or decrease depending on whether the cause is of a hot or cold nature. External factors include dietary and pathogenic causes.
- Internal factors causing heart rate to become hyperactive (often due to Yin vacuity so the Yang is no longer controlled) or hypoactive (through Yang Qi vacuity, in which the Yang Qi is no longer sufficient to move the heart and blood) at its customary rate.

Additional changes in the pulse parameters of force (generally increased in replete patterns and decreased in a vacuous patterns) and depth are used to further differentiate the pulse rate changes and the causes. Information obtained from assessment of the pulse rate parameter is always used with information obtained from the assessment of other pulse parameters. Pulse rate assessment alone does not supply sufficient information to identify the location (internal or external) or the nature (vacuity or replete) of disease/dysfunction.

6.3.5 Regulation of heart rate: biomedical perspective

From a biomedical perspective, there are three regulatory mechanisms which control heart rate (the following information is from McCance & Huether 2006):

- Intrinsic conduction system: The fundamental rhythm of the heart is set by the sinoatrial (SA) node, a small area of cells that function as a pacemaker due to their spontaneous electrical nature. They continuously depolarise and initiate action potentials that spread to the rest of the heart, via a conduction system, causing it to contract. The conduction system includes the atrioventricular (AV) node, the AV bundle (bundle of His), the right and left bundle branches and the Purkinje fibres (conduction myofibres).
- Autonomic nervous system (ANS): The ANS (parasympathetic and sympathetic divisions) helps to modify the heart rate according to the needs of the body. The sympathetic nervous system is activated in times of stress, excitement and exercise, the 'fright, flight or fight' response. It increases heart rate by stimulating the release of

77

norepinephrine (noradrenaline), making the pacemaker fire more quickly.

The parasympathetic nervous system (PNS), via the vagus nerves (vagal tone), slows down heart rate by the release of acetylcholine. At rest the heart is predominantly under control of the parasympathetic nervous system. In fact, it slows down the heart rate set by the SA node so that the normal resting heart rate is about 75 bpm. Baroreceptors (located in the aortic arch and carotid arteries) that respond to changes in blood pressure can also produce reflex changes in heart rate.

- Chemical factors: Hormones such as epinephrine (adrenaline) and norepinephrine (noradrenaline), from the adrenal medulla, increase both heart rate and contractility. Thyroid hormones have a similar effect. Growth hormone and pancreatic hormones may also affect heart rate (McCance & Huether 2006). Changes in concentrations of potassium (K^+), calcium (Ca^{2+}) and sodium (Na^+) ions affect heart rate through affecting the depolarisation threshold of nerves and muscle contractility. (Refer to appropriate physiology texts for further information.)

6.4 CM pulses defined by rate

6.4.1 Slow pulse (Chí mài) 迟脉

6.4.1.1 Requisite parameters

The Slow pulse is a simple pulse quality defined solely by the pulse rate.

It is characterised by a decrease in pulse rate to below the normal range of 60–90 bpm.

6.4.1.2 Clinical definition

The Slow pulse has a rate that is less than or equal to 60 bpm.

6.4.1.3 Classical Description from *Mai Jing*

> The Slow pulse is a pulse that beats three times for one respiration, very slow in coming and going
> (Wang, Yang (trans) 1997: p. 5)

'Three beats for one respiration' refers to the number of pulsations per one inhalation and one exhalation or one respiratory cycle (Table 6.2).

6.4.1.4 CM indications for the Slow pulse

The Slow pulse can be considered a sign of either good health or pathology.

Slow pulse indicating health

The Slow pulse may be a 'healthy' pulse, often observed in athletes, denoting cardiac fitness. In elite individuals, the resting normal heart rate may be below 50 bpm. From a CM perspective, this is seen as clear and unobstructed flow of Qi and blood. A healthy slow pulse would form when Heart Qi is strong and Blood is abundant.

A healthy slow pulse can be differentiated from an unhealthy slow pulse by two factors (Fig. 6.2, Table 6.3):

- Length of interval between beats
- Duration of systole, also known as ejection duration.

Table 6.2 ● Resting respiratory rate: breaths per minute versus age

Age (years)	Range	Average	Equivalent bpm using CM theory of 4 beats/breath
Newborn	30–50	40	160
1	20–40	30	120
3	20–30	25	100
6	16–22	19	76
10	16–20	18	72
14	14–20	17	68
Adult	12–20	18	72
Bradypnea[a]	<12/minute		<48–60
Tachypnea[b]	>20/minute		>80–100

[a] Caused by barbiturates, alcohol, narcotics, head injury depressing respiratory centre.
[b] Caused by hypoxia, metabolic acidosis, stress, anxiety – respiratory rate is elevated due to the release of catecholamines.
Modified from Estes (2006: pp. 250–251).

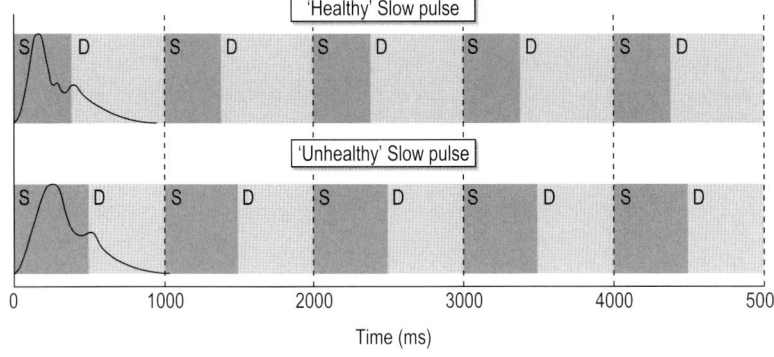

Figure 6.2
Variation between the systolic (S) and diastolic (D) components of the pulse wave between the formation of a healthy slow pulse and an un-healthy slow pulse.

Table 6.3 ● Summary comparison of CM patterns presenting with decreased pulse rates (<60 bpm) and their differentiation

	Pulse presentation	**Signs and Symptoms**	**Physiological response**
Yang vacuity	Slow and forceless	Desire for warmth, no thirst, bright-pale face, cold limbs	Long systole, small pulse amplitude
Pathogenic cold	Slow and forceful	Pain, thirst for warm drinks, pale face, cold limbs	Normal systole, increased amplitude, increased arterial tension
Pathogenic heat	Slow and forceful	Heat signs such as fever, abdominal pain	Normal systole, increased amplitude
Health	Slow and forceful	No cold or heat signs. No aversion to cold or heat	Short systole, long diastole

This will be explained further in the section on biomedical perspective (6.4.1.5).

There is also a third differential factor, but this is more subjective or sensory dependent. Constant (1999: p. 32) describes this as the sense of a 'tap' against the fingers. When the heart contracts strongly and quickly, the pulse wave also expands quickly to its peak and this is felt as a 'tap' against the fingers. When the heart contraction is slower, the pulse may rise or lift against the finger but there is no tap.

Slow pulse indicating pathology
According to CM theory, 'When Qi moves, blood moves' (Flaws 1994: p. 58). Therefore decreased movement of Qi leads to decreased flow rate of blood. This occurs in two ways:

• The presence of strong pathogenic Cold may result in a decrease in pulse rate. 'Cold leads to the contraction of Qi' (Flaws 1994: p. 59) and this retards the movement of Qi and blood.

• A vacuity of Yang Qi may result in a pulse rate slower than normal, as there is insufficient Yang Qi to propel the blood normally.

As a pathological pulse type, the Slow pulse may indicate three possible patterns:

Invasion of external pathogenic cold (Slow and forceful)
Cold has a contracting nature, causing contraction of both blood vessels and muscles and resulting in constrained flow of Qi and blood. It acts as a counter to the Yang's warming and expansive nature and constrains the movement of Qi, contributing to a slowing of the heart rate. The presence of an external pathogenic factor will be felt as an increase in the force of the pulsation. (See the Floating pulse and the Tight pulse for specifics on the pulse in the presence of an external pathogenic agent (EPA) of Cold).

Vacuity of Yang Qi (Slow and forceless)
Yang Qi provides the motive force to move blood. 'When Qi moves, blood moves' (Flaws 1994: p. 58). Consequently, deficient Yang Qi will lead to impaired flow of blood. The *Nei Jing* notes in Chapter 18 that, compared to that of a 'normal' pulse, a pulse that beats only twice per complete respiration signifies a deficiency of Qi.

> When man exhales once and his vessels exhibit one movement and when he inhales once and his vessels exhibit one movement, that is called 'short of Qi'.
> *(Unschuld 2003: p. 258).*

79

Yang Qi provides the momentum to the heart to initiate systolic contraction and propel blood through the arteries. Therefore deficient Yang also reduces strength of heart contraction, thereby affecting both the amount of circulating blood that enters the circulatory system and the impetus with which the blood moves. This will result in a pulsation that is lacking in force.

Pathogenic heat

Lu (1996) describes an occurrence of the Slow pulse in the presence of pathogenic Heat in the intestines causing obstruction. Heat causes fluids to congeal, so obstruction of Yang Qi leads to a Slow pulse, but the pulse is forceful and accompanied by signs and symptoms associated with heat rather than cold signs.

6.4.1.5 Biomedical perspective

Termed *bradycardia*, the pathological Slow pulse is defined as having a heart rate slower than 60 bpm which is accompanied by a systole that is slower (or longer) than normal. This can be due to a number of factors including low body temperature, medication such as digitalis, hypothyroidism, heart problems and electrolyte imbalances (Ca^{2+}, Na^+, K^+). Carotid sinus syndrome can result in bradycardia due to hypersensitivity of the carotid artery walls to pressure. Mild external pressure triggers a strong baroreceptor reflex which results in vagal stimulation that has a parasympathetic effect, thus slowing the heart rate (Guyton & Hall 2006: p. 148).

Pathologically, an extremely slow pulse may be due to heart block, where there is impairment of the normal electrical conduction pathway through the heart that causes normal cardiac contraction. (In CM this is viewed as Heart Yuan Qi vacuity.) There are different degrees of heart block, linked to the level of impairment of the heart's conduction system. Signs range from delayed heart contraction through to compromised circulation and eventual heart failure. Treatment protocols also vary, ranging from medications to physical insertion of an artificial pacemaker to replace the heart's own natural pacemaker (SA node: see section 6.3.5).

6.4.2 Rapid pulse (Shuò mài)
数脉

6.4.2.1 Requisite parameters

The Rapid pulse is a simple pulse quality defined only by changes in the pulse rate parameter. There is an increase in pulse rate above that of the normal heart rate range, 60–90 bpm.

6.4.2.2 Clinical definition

The rate of the Rapid pulse is greater than or equal to 90 bpm.

Note that the rate of 90 bpm for classifying a rapid pulse is different from the biomedical definition of a rapid pulse or tachycardia, commonly listed as 100 bpm. See 6.4.2.5 Biomedical Perspective, below, for further information. Also see Box 6.3, Racing pulse.

6.4.2.3 Classical description from the *Mai Jing* and *Nei Jing*

> The rapid pulse is a pulse coming and going abruptly and urgently [beating 6–7 times in one respiration in another version; named an advancing (pulse) in yet another]
> *(Mai Jing; (Wang, Yang (trans) 1997: p. 3).*

> Rapid is defined as more than five beats per breath of the doctor
> *(Nei Jing; Ni (trans) 1995: p. 31).*

6.4.2.4 CM indications for the Rapid pulse

The Rapid pulse may indicate health or pathology depending on the age of the individual.

Health

In children, a rapid pulse is considered 'auspicious' or favourable (Li, Flaws (trans) 1998: p. 75), as children's pulses are usually more rapid than those of adults. This is attributable to their Yang nature and so a rapid pulse is an appropriate pulse to manifest. The *Mai Jing* notes specifically that 'In children between four and five years, the pulse is fast, beating 8 times per respiration' (Wang, Yang (trans) 1997: p. 10). The normal pulse rate for adults is described as 4–5 beats per respiration, which means that the normal children's pulse rate is twice that of adults when using the old respiration method.

Pathology

In an adult, the Rapid pulse always indicates pathology involving heat or hyperactivity of Yang. Any hyperactivity of Yang Qi may augment pulse movement of Qi and blood, resulting in an increased heart rate. This may indicate the presence of pathogenic Heat or Fire, as seen in febrile diseases. Alternatively, a rapid pulse may also result from an inability of Yin to control Yang, allowing Yang to move without its usual constraints:

> When the Yin fails to contain the Yang, the flow in the channels will become rapid, causing the Yang Qi to become excessive and reckless.
> *(Wei Jing Su Wen)*
> *(Ni (trans) 1995: p. 11)*

This may be due to a deficiency of Yin fluids such as blood or body fluids arising from blood loss in haemorrhage, or depletion of Yin fluids following febrile disease, through excessive sweating or diarrhoea. Accordingly, two main patterns are associated with a pathological Rapid pulse:

Repletion of Yang (rapid and forceful)

An increase in Yang supplements the body's Yang Qi in moving Qi and blood. Consequently, the pulse rate increases (changes in other parameters such as contour and possibly arterial width and length may also be present). Repletion of Yang is often attributable to external variables, such as the presence of an external pathogenic factor producing fever. Dietary factors such as alcohol, herbs and spices may also supplement the body's Yang. In this situation the pulse will be Rapid and forceful (see section 6.8.1 for further information).

Yin vacuity producing heat (rapid and forceless)

Yin vacuity may occur as the result of loss of Yin fluids through excessive sweating, vomiting, diarrhoea or blood loss. As the relative amount of Yin (in the form of fluids) has decreased then there is a relatively excessive amount of Yang producing heat. As such, the term, 'Yin vacuity producing heat' refers to the creation of heat in the body because Yin is vacuous. Poor sleep and overwork are lifestyle factors which have an cumulative affect over time of depleting Yin.

From a biomedical perspective Yin vacuity can be associated with a relative increase in the sympathetic nervous system due to an inability of the parasympathetic nervous system to maintain appropriate control over these aspects. For example, stress can cause palpitations (see section 6.5.4) and digestive disturbances (Wood attacking the Earth); conditions such as irritable bowel syndrome (IBS) are affected by stress, producing bouts of either constipation or diarrhoea. Additionally, Guyton & Hall (2000) note that the 'contractile strength of the heart often is enhanced temporarily by a moderate increase in temperature, but prolonged elevation of the temperature exhausts the metabolic systems of the heart and eventually causes weakness' (p. 106).

There are two possible effects on the pulse wave when Yin becomes vacuous. These are:

– If Yin is vacuous then it is no longer able to control (or constrain) the movement and function of Yang. Therefore the flow rate of Qi and Blood in the arteries increases, manifesting as an increase in heart rate.
– As Yin's function of anchoring Yang may be affected, the pulse could also present relatively stronger (but overall is not actually forceful) at the superficial level as Yang 'floats', moving upwards and outwards, in addition to an increase in heart rate.

6.4.2.5 Biomedical perspective

Tachycardia or tachyarrythmia is defined as an abnormally fast heart rate (>100 bpm) that may be transient or ongoing. When heart rate increases there is ineffi-

---

Box 6.3

Racing pulse 疾(急)脉

There is a subcategory of the Rapid pulse called the Racing pulse. The Racing pulse is defined by a pulse rate greater than 120 bpm, or seven or more beats per respiration cycle. According to Deng (1999: p. 113), the pulse was first described in the *Zhen Jia Shu Yao* around 1000 CE, and expanded on in the Ming dynasty text *Zhen Jia Zheng Yan*. The Racing pulse is similar to the biomedical definition of tachycardia, with a similar description of aetiology and conditions in which it manifests such as thyrotoxicosis and high fevers reflecting an increased metabolic rate. It may be associated with some forms of compromised cardiac function.

Box 6.4

Heart rate and temperature

Guyton & Hall (2006: p. 197) assert that heart rate increases by 18 bpm for each °Celsius increase in body temperature to 40.5°Celsius. Beyond this the heart weakens and so pulse rate may slow. HR increases with fever because the increased temperature stimulates the SA node's metabolic rate, excitability rate of rhythm.

---

cient filling of the left ventricle during diastole and stroke volume is diminished. Whether due to poor refill during diastole or shortened ejection duration with systole, the result of tachycardia is often a compromised circulation of blood affecting tissue perfusion, especially over the longer term (Box 6.3).

Guyton & Hall (2006: p. 147) note three general causes of tachycardia:

- Increased body temperature
- Sympathetic nervous system stimulation of the heart
- Toxic conditions of the heart.

Tachycardia may also result from acute emotional stress such as anxiety, increased body temperature associated with fever or exercise (Box 6.4), blood loss and anaemia reducing effective blood volume or medication stimulating the pacemaker, or as a reflexive response from heart disease in an attempt to maintain normal circulation. Box 6.5 lists some conditions associated with tachycardia.

The body's response to stress is a common cause of tachycardia. Stress initiates neuroendocrine processes, leading to the release of epinephrine (adrenaline) and norepinephrine (noradrenaline), as well as other

Box 6.5

Conditions associated with tachycardia

- Sinus tachycardia
- Atrial and ventricular fibrillation (heart Qi or Blood stagnation; heart shock)
- Hyperthyroidism (which may equate to Yin vacuity)
- Febrile diseases (Yang excess)
- Haemorrhage
- Pregnancy. In the third trimester normal resting heart rate increases by 10 bpm and cardiac output increases by 40% due to increased stroke volume (Braunwald et al 2001: p. 25)
- Chronic rheumatic heart disease may result in damage to the heart structure such as heart valves, as well as conduction defects leading to atrial fibrillation

From both CM and biomedical perspectives, the conditions listed above are accompanied by changes in other pulse parameters, not just pulse rate alone.

hormones from the pituitary and adrenal glands ('fright, flight or fight' response). Norepinephrine (noradrenaline) constricts smooth muscle in all blood vessels and therefore plays a major role in peripheral vasoconstriction. Epinephrine (adrenaline) is responsible for increasing heart rate and also for the force of myocardial contraction.

Atrial fibrillation is a form of tachycardia, involving increased impulses affecting the contraction of the atria. (A number of the CM pulse qualities are due to atrial fibrillation.) As atrial fibrillation can also result in irregular rhythm, it is discussed in section 6.5 on Rhythm.

Hyperthyroidism increases heart rate considerably because the thyroid hormone appears to directly cause heart excitation. Thyroid hormone may also increase cardiac output and blood flow (Guyton & Hall 2006: p. 937).

Haemorrhage may also cause an increase in heart rate, as part of a cardiovascular compensatory mechanism to increase circulating volume by pulling fluids from the interstitium. This dilutes the viscosity of blood, resulting in faster blood flow. In addition, hypoxia results in vasodilatation of blood vessels, also increasing blood flow. As a result venous blood return is increased and the heart needs to pump faster and harder to get oxygenated blood to the body and prevent cardiopulmonary congestion (McCance & Huether 2006: p. 929).

6.4.3 Moderate pulse (Huǎn mài) 缓脉

6.4.3.1 Alternative names

Leisurely, Slowed Down, Relaxed, Retarded or Languid pulse.

6.4.3.2 Requisite parameters

The Moderate pulse is a simple pulse that has changes in two pulse parameters:

- Rate: There may be either an increase or decrease in rate dependent on the individual's 'normal' resting heart rate.
- Contour: The pulse shape is rounded (see Slippery pulse, section 7.9.1).

The Moderate pulse is initially identified by the pulse rate (Table 6.4) and further differentiated from the standard Slow pulse by the shape of the pulse contour.

6.4.3.3 Clinical definition

The Moderate pulse has a pulse rate of 60 bpm, with a distinctly rounded contour felt under the palpating fingers.

6.4.3.4 Classical descriptions from the Nei Jing and Mai Jing

> A pulse that is neither too strong nor too weak, that comes and goes in a rhythmic fashion, flowing like a stream . . . (*Nei Jing*)
> (Ni 1995: p. 32).

> The moderate pulse is also a pulse slow in coming and going but a little faster than the slow pulse . . .' (*Mai Jing*)
> (Wang, Yang (trans) 1997: p. 3)

6.4.3.5 CM indications

The Moderate pulse can be either healthy pulse or pathological, depending on the signs and symptoms accompanying it.

Health

It is a normal pulse rate in a healthy person if no other change in pulse characteristics accompany it, or when there are no other presenting pathological signs and symptoms. In this situation it is a sign of a strong constitution. When this occurs, it could be classified both as a Slow pulse, due to the rate, but also a Slippery pulse, and would be a sign of sufficient Qi and blood.

Pathology

The Moderate pulse is often associated with the presence of Damp or vacuity of the Stomach and Spleen, especially Spleen Yang Qi deficiency. Therefore, it would occur in conjunction with signs and symptoms associated with such patterns. This could include digestive symptoms such as loose stools, fatigue and tiredness, cold limbs, fluid retention and an aversion to cold.

Pathogenic damp is broadly seen as a Yin condition and tends to injure Yang. In addition, damp is heavy,

Table 6.4 ● Summary of definitions for the pulse qualities defined by pulse rate

Pulse rate (bpm)	Pulse quality/category	Biomedical	Possible indications	Traditional (Beats per respiration)
<60	Slow pulse	Bradycardia	Health Cold EPA Heath Damp	3
60	Moderate pulse Slow pulse		Yang vacuity	4
61–80	Normal pulse rate	Normal pulse rate	Health	4–5
81–89	Borderline normal to rapid		Health Unhealthy heart Blood vacuity Recovery phase Progression of illness	5–6
90–119	Rapid pulse	Tachycardia	EPA Heat Vacuity Heat	7–8
>120	Racing pulse		Heat/Fire Infections Dehydration Extreme fevers	≥8

slowing down and impeding the flow and circulation of Qi and blood. 'Phlegm and Dampness lead to Qi obstruction; Qi obstruction leads to Qi stagnation' (Flaws 1994: p. 79).

6.5 Rhythm

Pulse rhythm is an expression of the heart's functional capacity to contract and relax in a consistent fashion. Rhythm as such is not how frequently the heart contracts – this is pulse *rate* – rather, it is whether the heart is sufficiently contracting at all.

A normal pulse has a regular rhythm, with a consistently even interval between each pulsation. When the intervals between pulsations vary in length or there appears to be 'missing' beats or an interruption, this is said to be an irregular rhythm. Any pulse occurring with an irregular rhythm is termed an arrhythmia or dysrhythmia, or simply a pulse lacking a regular rhythm.

Arrhythmic pulses may have an interruption to their normal rhythm occurring at irregular or regular intervals. Interruptions range from pulses with occasional 'missed' beats or rapid beats, to serious rhythmic disturbances that impair the pumping action of the heart.

Three specific CM pulse qualities are associated with the rhythm parameter:

- Skipping pulse (section 6.6.1)
- Bound pulse (section 6.6.2)
- Intermittent pulse (section 6.6.3).

The Skipping pulse and Bound pulses have *irregular* interruptions to their normal rhythms and are further differentiated by pulse rate. The Intermittent pulse has *regularly spaced* interruptions to the normal rhythm and is defined only by the rhythm parameter.

6.5.1 Pulse rhythm and its assessment

The method for assessing pulse rhythm requires the pulse to be felt for an interval of at least 60 seconds. This is because irregularly interrupted pulses, with only occasional interruptions to normal heart rhythm, may not be detected in any shorter time frame. With the fingers placed on the artery, the practitioner notes the presence of pulsations and whether these are occurring at regularly spaced intervals.

When an irregularity in rhythm is detected, such as a 'missed' beat, the practitioner next needs to determine the nature and frequency of the interruption to normal pulse rhythm:

- Is the interruption to heart rhythm occuring regularly (that is, is it occurring at a consistent interval between each beat?)
- If so, how often does this occur? (number of rhythmic beats between each interruption to heart rhythm)
- Or, is the interruption to heart rhythm occurring only at irregularly spaced intervals: is there a

Box 6.6

Clinical questions to ask your patient

- Are you aware of what your normal heart rate is?
- Are you aware that it is slower or faster than usual?
- If you have noticed changes to your HR does this occur suddenly or gradually?
- How long has this been happening?
- Is this happening all the time?
- Does this occur with any other symptoms?
- Is it better when you rest?

Box 6.7

Sinus arrhythmia

- Sinus arrhythmia is a normal occurrence often seen in young adults where the heart rate slightly speeds up during inspiration due to activation of neural input to the brain when the lungs are expanded (for example, deep breathing), and then slows down during expiration.
- Sinus arrhythmia often results from alteration of the strength of the nerve signal to the heart sinus node affecting the heart rate (Guyton & Hall 2000: pp. 134–135). Specifically, the mechanism affecting heart rate occurs during deep breathing when neural receptors in the lungs are activated.
- McCance & Huether (2006) state that the increase in heart rate during inspiration is caused by the stretching (activation) of vagal fibres in the lungs that cause heart rate to speed up by inhibiting the cardioinhibitory centre of the medulla. Inhibition of this centre allows unopposed sympathetic acceleration of heart rate (p. 1049).
- Sinus arrhythmia needs to be carefully differentiated from arrhythmia or dysrhythmia. A pulse is described as arrhythmic when there are pauses in the heart's normal conduction system resulting in a perceived missed beat. With sinus arrhythmia there are no missed beats but rather a change in the length of time between beats. This is not deemed a pathological occurrence.
- The phenomenon of sinus arrhythmia was likely clinically observed by the authors of the *Nei Jing*, as evidenced by the following lines of text.

If the vessels exhibit five movements,
this is an intercalation [of a fifth movement] because of a deep breathing.
That is called a 'normal person'.
(Su Wen)
(Unschuld 2003: p. 257)

This partial description of the normal pulse appears be an early reference to sinus arrhythmia and was clearly viewed as a variation of the normal healthy pulse rate.

missed beat only occasionally (no regular interval or specific number of beats between each missed beat)?

When assessing pulse rhythm, it is also important to inquire if the patient is aware of any irregularity in their heart rate, as this may not be apparent at the time of consultation (Box 6.6). Changes in heart rhythm may include palpitations and this will be discussed in 6.5.4.

Sometimes an interruption to the pulse rhythm can be due to a blockage in the conduction of the pulse wave from the heart to the periphery (Box 6.7). It is therefore also important to compare the left and right radial pulses. Differences in rhythm between the two sides may indicate some type of problem with the arterial system, such as arterial blockage or aortic coarctation, rather than specific heart-related pathology (Constant 1999).

6.5.2 Regulation of pulse rhythm: CM perspective

In CM the Heart governs the movement of blood. Heart Qi maintains the functional ability of the heart to contract. Rhythm is affected when Heart Qi is affected. In this context, changes in pulse rhythm occur when the heart Qi is exhausted or obstructed.

Changes in heart rhythm, especially rhythm changes associated with cardiovascular damage, can be the final common pathway for a number of diseases (AtCor Medical 2006: pp. 1–3.1). These include:

- Hypertension
- Left ventricular hypertrophy and failure
- Diabetes mellitus
- Renal disease
- Hyperlipidaemia.

Differentiation of the cause and aetiology are further elucidated on other presenting signs and symptoms and medical history. In a pulse diagnosis context, the parameter of pulse rate is used to identify aetiological factors of heat and cold affecting heart rhythm. This includes internal aetiologies arising from vacuities of Yin and Yang , and external pathogenic factors of heat and cold.

In CM terms, the Heart also governs the Mind or Shen. Physical heart damage will, theoretically, affect the clear expression of the Shen and be associated with Blood stagnation. The relationship is seen in the incidence of depression and heart disease. Severe shock or pain, anxiety and stress also affect the Shen, which in turn can affect heart rhythm.

6.5.3 Regulation of pulse rhythm: biomedical perspective

The ability of the heart to contract rhythmically is due to both an intrinsic conduction system and extrinsic innervation of the autonomic nervous system, as noted in section 6.3.5. The sinoatrial (SA) node is the pacemaker of the heart, whose rhythm determines the heart rate. It initiates action potentials that spread throughout the heart muscle, causing it to contract in a coordinated manner (see section 6.3.5).

The pulse rhythm will be affected if cardiac function is impaired. Abnormal heart rhythm may be due to problems with the electrical conduction system through the heart, affecting both the rate of the pulse and the intervals between each pulsation. For example, 'heart block' refers to problems with the AV node, affecting the transmission of impulses to the ventricles from the atria. Although the ventricles have their own pacemaker, it is too slow to maintain sufficient circulation and arrhythmias may develop (Table 6.5). This is a chronic cause of arrhythmias. Transient functional irregularities, arising from stimulants and emotions can similarly affect heart rhythm (see section 6.5.5).

6.5.4 Palpitations

Palpitations are defined as an abnormal awareness of the heart beating, which may be momentarily stronger, faster or irregular in rhythm (Box 6.8). Palpitations can be an indicator of interruption to normal heart rhythm, an arrhythmia, but not all palpitations are necessarily arrhythmic or cardiac related. For example, palpitations can be a prominent symptom in fever, hypoglycaemia or thyrotoxicosis (Lee 2001: p. 64).

Palpitations are a subjective feeling that may occur as:

- The heart beating abnormally fast or irregularly
- The heart momentarily beating more forcefully than normal
- Ectopic beats (extra beats or extra systoles).

In CM, palpitations are normally associated with the Heart. They can occur in any pattern involving Heart disharmonies, whether physiological, psychological or emotionally based. This includes patterns ranging from vacuity patterns of Yin, Yang, Qi or Blood, to repletion patterns involving Heat or Phlegm. In addition to palpitations, pathology is further differentiated by:

Table 6.5 ● Heart block and associated conditions affecting the normal conduction of electrical impulses through the heart with related changes in the arterial pulse wave

Type of heart block	Effect on heart activity	Cause	Manual palpation
First degree	Atrial depolarisation becomes prolonged, there is a delay in the in normal conduction from atria to the ventricle but no 'dropped beats'	Local hypoxia, damage to heart conduction pathways, digitalis toxicity, Rheumatic fever, electrolyte imbalances such as hypo- or hyperkalaemia	No change to normal rhythm or rate
Second degree	Atrial depolarisation becomes prolonged or occasional loss of atrial depolarisation, and corresponding loss of ventricular depolarisation, i.e. 'dropped beats'	Problems with AV node, complications of endocarditis, hypokalemia, digoxin toxicity, coronary artery disease, myocardial infarction (MI), diabetes, antidys rhythmics, cyclic antidepressants	Interrupted rhythm. Occasional missed beat followed by larger beat – ectopic beats. Some transient variation in pulse force. Severity increases as HR increases
Third degree	Complete block of the normal signal in the heart: atrial depolarisation not coordinated with ventricular systole. Pacemaker cells in the ventricles take over but at a much slower rate	Hypokalaemia, myocardial infarction, problems with conduction pathway (bundle of His)	Decreased cardiac output, decreased (slow) heart rate 41–59 bpm, consistent decrease in pulse force. Electrocardiogram records the atrial contraction at 100 bpm and the ventricle at only 40 bpm

Modified from Table 30–12 McCance & Huether 2006 Pathophysiology: the biologic basis for disease in adults and children, 5th edn. Elsevier/Mosby, St Louis, p. 1137.

Box 6.8

Clinical questions to ask your patient

- Are you aware of any palpitations?
- Is arrhythmia occurring on a regular basis (that is, is the patient aware that this is occurring or is this the first time that they've been made aware of this)?
- Is it old or new; if old, is it worsening in regards to duration and/ or frequency?
- How often is it occurring: daily, weekly, occasionally, no pattern to occurrence?
- What type of sensation does the subject experience?
- Previous history or family history of heart disease?
- Are the palpitations associated with stress, anxiety, exercise, fever, caffeine or nicotine intake, medication, alcohol or chocolate? Or do they occur at rest?
- What medication are you taking, including vitamin and herbal supplements?
- Do palpitations occur during the day or at night?

Additionally, always note the onset, duration, associated symptoms and circumstances in which arrhythmias/palpitations occur. Also ask the patient to tap out the rhythm of the arrhythmia or palpitations that they are feeling.

Box 6.9

CM patterns associated with the occurrence of palpitations

CM Zang Fu patterns associated with palpitations usually involve the Heart:

- Heart Yin vacuity
- Heart blood vacuity
- Heart Yang vacuity
- Heart fire
- Phlegm heat misting the heart
- Heart blood stasis

Box 6.10

Flutters and fibrillations

Fibrillations and flutters occur when segments of the heart contract far more than normal. Because the contraction is associated with only a certain area of the heart, or because the contraction is not complete, this is a situation in which the pulse rate will not correlate with what's occurring in the heart. Instead there will be changes in other pulse parameters such as pulse force which is decreased, reflecting incomplete filling of blood in the ventricles and subsequent volume of blood ejected into circulation.

- Atrial flutter: Rapid atrial contractions (240–360 bpm) occur in conjunction with 2nd degree atrioventricular (AV) block resulting in some missing beats due to the electrical impulses not always reaching the ventricles.
- Atrial fibrillation: Asynchronous contraction of atrial muscle fibres, leading to cessation of atrial contraction. Regardless, blood can still flow from the atria into the ventricles, so cardiac output continues but is decreased by 20–30 percent. This can occur for a number of reasons such as myocardial infarction, hyperthyroidism or rheumatic heart disease (Tortora & Grabowski 1996).
- Ventricular fibrillation: Associated with heart rate of >300 bpm, as different areas of the ventricles are stimulated. The ventricles do not contract properly, which quickly leads to unconsciousness and likely death if the fibrillation is not stopped within 2–3 minutes (Information from Guyton & Hall 2006: pp. 152–6).

- Other accompanying signs and symptoms
- Additional changes in other pulse parameters.

Patients who report experiencing palpitations and have a psychiatric disorder are known to report longer-lasting periods of palpitations and ancillary symptoms than patients without a psychiatric disorder (Lee 2001: p. 64). In CM this is seen to be associated with conditions affecting clear expression of the Shen. The Shen or Mind resides in the Heart; disturbance of the Shen can disturb Heart function (Box 6.9).

6.5.4.1 Ectopic beats

Ectopic beats are a premature contraction of the heart due to an impulse generated outside the SA node or abnormally generated by the SA node, interrupting the normal cardiac rhythm. They can occur regularly or irregularly.

Ectopic beats can be relatively benign and occur in healthy individuals with no apparent cause. They also occur when the heart is excessively irritated through either metabolic or chemical stimulus (see section 6.5.5 for further details).

6.5.4.2 Ectopic beats – pulse presentation

Because the heart contracts prematurely there is incomplete filling of the left ventricle, resulting in less blood volume being ejected than would normally occur if the left ventricle had completely filled (Box 6.10). Consequently a pulse wave arising from an ectopic beat is felt weaker or absent than other pulsations, sometimes mistaken for a 'missed beat' (Guyton & Hall 2006).

Following an ectopic beat, there is a compensatory pause or a longer interval before the heart contracts

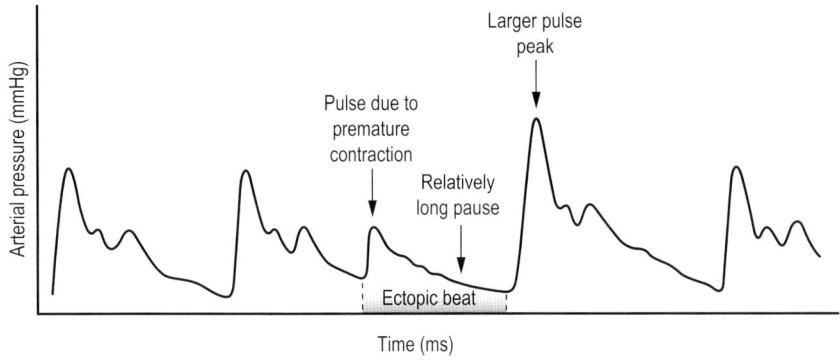

Figure 6.3
Schematic of the variation in pulse amplitude and regular rhythm as occurs with an ectopic beat.

again. This can result in a stronger pulse beat because there is an increased filling of the left ventricle; a greater volume of blood is expelled into circulation when ventricular contraction next occurs (Fig. 6.3).

On a more serious note, ectopic beats may indicate some type of metabolic damage leading to excessive irritability of the heart muscle. This can occur as a result of viral or bacterial infection affecting the heart such as rheumatic fever, or may result from damage due to myocardial infarction (Epstein et al 1992: p. 7.30).

6.5.5 Pulse rhythm: Clinical perspective

Arrhythmias, palpitations and ectopic beats can be signs of a serious heart condition involving the conduction system in the heart; Heart Qi and Yang maybe seriously impaired (Box 6.11).

The presence of arrhythmia is seen as part of a pathological process; however, the regularity of interruptions to normal heart rhythm can indicate the severity of the process. The increasing regularity of missed beats indicates a worsening of the condition, and a decreasing occurrence of missing beats indicates a continuing resolution of the condition. The timing of the commencement of missed beats also has prognostic value. If they start with the onset of a new illness then the prognosis is better than if arrhythmia occurs during a chronic or critical disease.

The same factors that affect heart rate may also cause arrhythmias, palpitations and ectopic beats, including:

- Excessive intake of stimulants such as nicotine, coffee and other beverages containing caffeine
- Alcohol
- Acute periods of stress, tension, anxiety and panic attacks

---

Box 6.11

Arrhythmia: summary

- Palpitation: A subjective abnormal awareness of heart beating, reported by the patient
- Arrhythmia: A general term to describe any irregularity in the heart rhythm, also called dysrhythmia
- Arrhythmias range in severity from occasional missed beats (which may be normal in the absence of any other symptoms), to changes in speed (rapid beats), extra beats (ectopic), to extremely irregular with no rhythm (e.g. atrial fibrillation – 240–360 bpm)
- From a CM perspective, arrhythmias are associated with primary exhaustion of heart Qi, Yin or Yang in nature. This has secondary effects on circulation
- From a biomedical perspective, arrhythmias are due to abnormal rate of impulse generation or the abnormal conduction of impulses
- Possible causes of arrhythmias include stress, anxiety, exercise, fever, caffeine or nicotine intake, medication and herbs, alcohol, chocolate, hyperthyroidism, potassium deficiency and certain heart diseases.

- Hypoxia (resulting in less oxygen supply to the body)
- Lack of sleep
- Increased basal body temperature (Prolonged increase in the basal body temperature eventually weakens the heart)
- Medications such as epinephrine, ephedrine, aminophylline, and atropine which are responsible for palpitations (Lee 2001: p. 65)
- Toxic reactions to some drugs and herbs which have cardiostimulatory affects and can cause palpitations and arrhythmias

87

6.6 CM pulses defined by rhythm

6.6.1 Skipping pulse (Cù mài) 促脉

6.6.1.1 Alternative names

Hasty, Abrupt, Hurried, Running, Agitated, Accelerated or Rapidly Irregularly Interrupted pulse.

6.6.1.2 Requisite parameters

The Skipping pulse is a simple pulse quality with changes in two pulse parameters:

- Rhythm: The Skipping pulse has irregular pauses in heart rhythm
- Rate: The pulse rate is greater than normal (>90 bpm).

6.6.1.3 Clinical definition

The Skipping pulse has *irregular* pauses or interruptions in normal heart rhythm, accompanied by a pulse rate of more than 90 bpm (Box 6.12). The pauses or interruptions may occur with any interval of pulse beats. However, the more often (that is, closer together) they occur, the more severe the condition.

6.6.1.4 Classical description from the *Mai Jing*

> The skipping pulse is a pulse coming and going rapidly with occasional interruptions but having the ability to recover
> (Wang, Yang (trans) 1997: p. 3).

6.6.1.5 CM Indications

The Skipping pulse always indicates disharmony involving heat-related conditions affecting the main-tainence of the regular rhythm by Heart Qi, or Heart dysfunction.

There are three main CM patterns associated with the formation of the Skipping pulse:

Internal heat

Internal heat from EPAs producing fever agitate Qi and blood, supplementing Yang Qi and increasing pulse rate. The heat agitation of the Qi and blood also obstructs the smooth flow of these to the heart. The heart function becomes arrhythmic. Prolonged incidence of internal heat may give rise to consumption of Yin fluids and weaken the Heart Qi (see below).

Consumption of Yin fluids

With internal heat, over time this may be complicated by the consumption of Yin fluids – the fluids are consumed and thus cannot flow continuously. This situation is associated with febrile conditions such as rheumatic fever, consumed Yin resulting in heart damage. An increase in heart rate caused by heat, if prolonged, eventually exhausts the heart and arrhythmias can result.

Exhausted heart Qi and blood

The pulse is usually seen in critical diseases such as organic heart disease that is due to exhausted Heart Qi and Blood. This can arise as a complication of internal heat and Yin fluid consumption. The pattern refers primarily to the heart's inability to maintain a rhythmic contraction required for appropriate circulation, or is representative of the body's attempt to maintain circulatory integrity of blood and fluids when it is no longer capable of doing so. Prognosis is poor, and indicates end-stage aetiology involving heart failure.

6.6.1.6 Biomedical perspective

The Skipping pulse may be associated with:

- Hyperthyroidism (thyrotoxicosis)
- Heart valve problems (damage from rheumatic fever)
- Hypertension.

6.6.2 Bound pulse (Jié mài) 结脉

6.6.2.1 Alternative names

Knotted, Nodular, Adherent or Hesitant pulse.

6.6.2.2 Requisite parameters

The Bound pulse is a simple pulse quality with changes in two pulse parameters:

- Rhythm: There are irregular pauses in heart rhythm resulting in varying intervals between subsequent beats.
- Rate: The pulse rate is less than normal (<60 bpm).

Box 6.12

Irregular pauses without changes in pulse rate

Irregular pauses in the rhythm occur in healthy people without changes in the rate. This is often seen in individuals with high levels of tensions/stress. In these situations the irregular pauses are transient and often resolve when the stressor has been removed. From a CM perspective, irregular pauses accompanying stress or anxiety are often associated with a stagnation of the Liver's physiological function of maintaining the free flow of Qi and Blood.

6.6.2.3 Clinical definition

The Bound pulse has *irregular* pauses in heart rhythm accompanied by a pulse rate of less than 60 bpm.

6.6.2.4 Classical description from the *Mai Jing*

> The bound pulse is a pulse slow in coming and going with occasional interruption but the ability to recover
> *(Wang, Yang (trans) 1997: p. 5).*

6.6.2.5 CM indications

The Bound pulse always indicates pathogenesis involving the Heart. Three patterns are associated with the Bound pulse:

- Pathogenic Cold obstructing the smooth flow of Qi and blood to the heart
- Obstruction of Qi and Blood
- Yang vacuity and Vital (Yuan) Qi vacuity.

Pathogenic cold

The Bound pulse as a result of pathogenic Cold is probably a relatively acute onset associated with exposure of the previously healthy individual to environmental Cold. This is described as a Cold pathogen invasion. In a biomedical context this is termed hypothermia. The description of the pulse type in the classical literature was probably a direct reflection of the environmental conditions in the Chinese winter, and thus a relatively common presentation in traditional clinical practice in China. Hypothermia is still a relatively common occurrence at high latitudes, with children and the elderly particularly susceptible.

Physiological changes occurring with hypothermia depend on the severity of exposure to cold and also on the individual's core body temperature. In terms of the Bound pulse, arrhythmic changes occur when the core body temperature decreases to 32.2 28 °C (or 90–82.4 °F) (Danzl 2001: p. 108). This is considered moderate hypothermia.

Moderate hypothermia is associated with both atrial and ventricular arrhythmias. Additionally, the decrease in body temperature causes decreased contractility of the cardiac muscles, so there are accompanying changes in the strength of cardiac output as well as decreases in heart rate. In a CM context this is the Cold's constraining effect on the Heart Qi and Yang, associated with secondary obstructions in the normal Qi and blood flow in the vessels.

Obstruction of Qi and Blood

A number of authors (Lu 1996, Deng 1999, Guangzhou College notes 1991) note that the Bound pulse may be associated with phlegm, food retention or masses (concretions). These pathogenic factors impede both Qi and blood circulation. In these cases the pulse would also be forceful, however there may also be additional parameter changes. For example, in phlegm conditions the pulse may also have a rounded contour (the Slippery pulse).

Yang vacuity and vital (Yuan) Qi vacuity

The Bound pulse may also arise due to the vacuity of Yang Qi, which can be the result of constitutional factors or damage caused by lifestyle, emotional disturbance or dietary habits. As noted by Lyttleton (2004: p. 17) an invasion of pathogenic Cold (albeit a milder form than the hypothermia described above) may happen readily in the Western lifestyle, via the ingestion of overly cold foods and drinks or excessive consumption of raw food, living or working in a cold damp environment or as a result of overwork and insufficient sleep. Although this may not cause significant problems in the short term, prolonged damage to Yang will have inevitable effects on the normal functioning of the organs. In particular, the heart's ability to contract sufficiently is affected by Heart Yang Qi vacuity, so heart contraction is weak. This results in a pulsation that is forceless.

The significance of the Bound pulse occurring with Cold is not in diagnosing Cold as a causal agent but rather that the body's Qi and Yang were weak to have allowed Cold penetration in the first instance, and in particular, for it to have affected the heart function at all. Irrespective of the cause, there are a considerable number of processes involved in the underlying pathogenesis in the formation of this pulse. Lifestyle, genetic and dietary factors all predicate towards the formation of the pulse once the appropriate causal agent activates the triggers. As such, although the pulse can present in an acute situation, it is nearly always preceded by other aetiologies.

6.6.2.6 Biomedical perspective

The Bound pulse may indicate problems with normal heart function such as pacemaker dysfunction, for example second- and/or third-degree heart block or more seriously, it may indicate heart failure (see Table 6.5).

6.6.3 Intermittent pulse (Dài mài) 代脉

6.6.3.1 Alternative names

Regularly interrupted, Replacement or Changing pulse.

6.6.3.2 Requisite parameters

The Intermittent pulse is a simple pulse quality defined solely by pulse rhythm: there are regular pauses in the heart rhythm.

6.6.3.3 Clinical definition

The Intermittent pulse has an interruption to heart rhythm occurring at regular intervals. This may occur every few beats (indicating a more severe illness) or less frequently. There is no accompanying change in heart rate from normal (60–90 bpm)

6.6.3.4 Classical description from the *Mai Jing*

> The interrupted pulse is a pulse with regular interruption and inability to recover itself, resuming to beat (only after a long pause). The bound pulse is prognosticative of survival but the interrupted one of death.
>
> *(Wang, Yang (trans) 1997: p. 5).*

6.6.3.5 CM indications

The Intermittent pulse is almost always a sign of pathogenesis, usually involving the heart and other vital organs. A footnote in *The Lakeside Master's Study of the Pulse* (Li, Flaws (trans) 1998: pp. 122–123) states that this pulse is associated with serious heart disease. How frequently the interruptions occur is used to indicate the relative severity of the condition. The more often pauses occur with the Intermittent pulse, the more severe the condition.

An Intermittent pulse can occur in individuals without accompaniment of other apparent signs and symptoms. In such cases, the regular interruptions to rhythm are probably more widely spaced (Table 6.6).

Three patterns are associated with the Intermittent pulse:

Table 6.6 ● Comparison of the three CM pulse qualities defined by the rhythm parameter

Specific CM pulse quality	Rhythm	Heart rate
Bound	Irregular: occasional irregular interruption to rhythm	Slow: ≤60 bpm
Skipping	Irregular: occasional irregular interruption to rhythm	Rapid: ≥90 bpm
Intermittent	Regular interruption: a interruption to rhythm between a consistent number of beats	Normal: 60–90 bpm

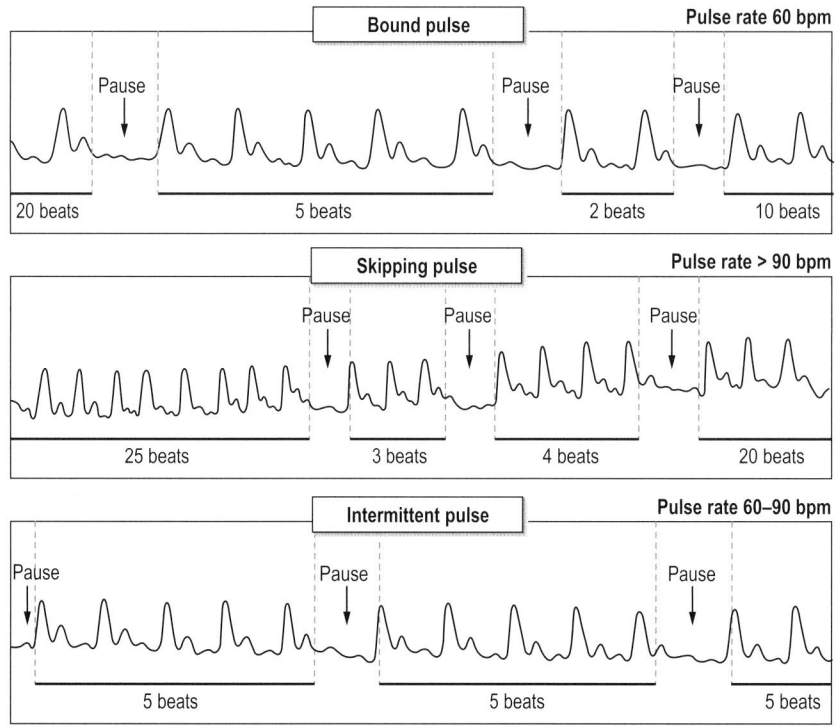

Note that the above diagrams are for illustrative purposes only. The number of beats between each pause will vary between patients depending upon the pathogenesis and severity. The lessening of beats between more frequent pauses indicates a more severe condition.

Exhaustion of Heart Qi

This is a primary pattern specifically relating to the Heart and its physiological function. It may be associated with congenital defects in the heart's conduction system or organic disease of the heart muscle such as dystrophies, or may develop as a result of damage associated with fevers and infarction.

Severe vacuity of essential substances

The Intermittent pulse occurs in response to vacuity of Yuan Qi and Jing Qi. This is a pattern with systemic origins rather than originating solely from the heart, even though the heart is eventually affected. For example, Yuan Qi and Jing Qi are essential components in the production of Qi and blood, therefore affecting the supply of both Qi and blood to the organs.

In a sick person the Intermittent pulse is considered serious but can be treated. The logic being that since the person is already sick then an arrhythmic pulse is a 'natural' progression of prolonged illness consuming Yuan Qi and Jing Qi and so affecting visceral Qi.

Pain

The traditional pulse literature lists this pulse occurring in conditions of severe pain, usually the result of obstruction of blood and Qi, thus affecting circulation. In light of the involvement of the heart in the formation of this pulse, severe pain may incorporate angina as a related cause.

6.6.3.6 Biomedical perspective

The Intermittent pulse usually occurs as a result of heart disease, severe pain or severe traumatic injury. If it occurs in the elderly or develops during chronic disease, it is viewed as a critical situation. From a CM perspective this would be viewed as a severe depletion of Heart Qi.

6.7 Depth

The parameter of depth is a simple pulse parameter used to indicate the level of depth at which the pulse is felt as being the strongest. Three levels of depth are used in the Cun Kou system of pulse palpation, each found by using incremental pressure applied to the radial artery by the palpating fingertips. (See Chapter 5 for further informa-

tion on technique used for finding and assessing the levels of depth.) The three levels of depth are termed the superficial, middle and deep levels of depth.

A great proportion of the traditional 27 pulse qualities are felt strongest at one of the three levels of depth and so are defined as either superficial, middle or deep level of depth pulses (Fig. 6.4, Box 6.13). For example, several CM pulse types are located at the superficial

---

Box 6.13

Normal pulse strength with level of depth

- Superficial level of depth: Often felt as the least strongest in healthy individuals
- Middle level of depth: Often has the most pulse strength
- Deep level of depth: Equal to or slightly less strong than middle level of depth

---

Box 6.14

Revision of assessment technique for determining pulse depth

- Superficial pulse depth: Found by resting the fingertips lightly on the skin surface without pressure. Superficial level is *not* the depth at which the pulse is first felt.
- Deep pulse depth: Found by occluding the radial artery (pressing firmly on the artery against the radial bone) and then releasing the pressure gently and slowly until the pulse can be felt again. This pressure should be maintained. This release of pressure creates an initial rush in blood flow; therefore a few seconds should be allowed to enable the pulse to equalise before assessing it.
- Middle pulse depth: Found by applying a moderate pressure to the radial artery (not sufficient to occlude it); somewhere between superficial and deep. The middle depth is examined after palpating the superficial and deep levels to determine the pressure required to reach each level of depth.

91

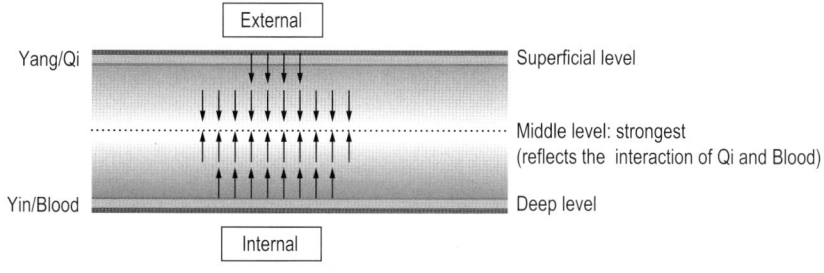

Figure 6.4
Diagrammatic representation of a healthy pulse and the relative pulse strength at the three levels of depth. The middle level of depth should be strongest, representing the interaction of Qi and Blood.

level of depth (which can be felt by resting the fingers on the skin) or are palpated most forcefully at the superficial level of depth. These may be classified as superficial pulses, so this is defining the pulse by its level of depth (Box 6.14).

The *Floating pulse* is one such pulse that is commonly defined as a superficial pulse (but it should be noted that not all superficial pulses are classified as Floating). Similarly, there are several CM pulses that can be felt only with heavy pressure, or are felt strongest at the deep level of depth and are consequently termed deep pulses.

There are three simple CM pulse qualities that are solely defined by the parameter of depth alone:

- Floating pulse (section 6.9.1)
- Sinking pulse (section 6.9.2)
- Hidden pulse (section 6.9.3).

There are other CM pulse qualities that can also be felt strongest at the superficial or deep levels of depth; however, they are accompanied by changes in other pulse parameters and may be more appropriately defined by that pulse parameter. For this reason, pulses found at a particular level of depth are listed in other pulse parameter sections relating to their most defining rubric, and are not listed here under the depth parameter.

6.7.1 Pulse depth and its assessment

As discussed in section 5.6 (locating the pulse depth), the parameter of pulse depth may be interpreted in two ways:

- The level of depth where the radial arterial pulsation is found to be the strongest, regardless of the overall intensity of the pulsation (that is, assessing relative strength)
- The level of depth at which the radial artery is physically located.

Assessing the level of depth requires palpation at each of the three levels of depth and judging at which level of depth the pulse wave is felt most strongly or most distinctly. Sometimes the pulse can only be felt at one level of depth and so defining the pulse by the level of depth is easy. At other times the pulse is felt at more than one level of depth and the practitioner needs to make a decision about the level of depth where it is strongest. Alternatively, the pulse may be felt equally strongly at all three levels of depth, and this is diagnostically relevant too: this is the Replete pulse, which is discussed in section 7.7.1.

Diagnostically, the level of depth may be affected by pathological processes occurring within the body, resulting in either a pulse that can be felt strongest at the superficial or deep level of depth, or perhaps equally

strong at all three levels of depth. Other factors affecting where the pulse can be felt include the strength of cardiac contraction (see pulse force, section 7.6). Pathological processes may also result in anatomical structural variations and so vary the perceived level of depth. This arises when there are physiological changes in the subcutaneous layer of tissue overlying the radial artery, or anatomical variations in the musculature and tendinous insertions around the forearm and wrist area. This causes the actual arterial structure to 'sink' or 'float', altering the level of pulse depth as well.

6.7.2 The normal pulse depth

In order to determine whether the pulse is felt pathologically relatively stronger or weaker at a specific level of depth, it is first necessary to know what the 'expected' relative strength of each level of depth should be.

Generally, the radial arterial pulse should be palpable at all the three levels of depth. However, the strength of the pulse at each of the three levels of depth may differ. In terms of relative strength, the pulse will usually be less palpable at the superficial level of depth and most forceful in the middle level of depth. At the deep level of depth, the pulse should be either equally forceful or slightly less forceful than the middle level of depth. This is what would be expected for a healthy pulse. From a CM perspective, as the pulse is formed by the interaction of both Yang (external, movement, function) and Yin (internal, Blood, form), the balance of these two dynamic forces results in a pulse that should be palpable at all levels of depth but felt with most strength in the middle level of depth.

Changes in strength at individual levels of depth are used to identify pathology and provide information about the location of disease and functional status of Yin and Yang. When describing the level of depth with regard to a specific pulse we are talking about the level of depth at which the pulse is felt relatively strongest (meaning that it may still be felt at other levels of depth but it is not as strong.)

6.7.2.1 Physiological response of the circulatory system to climate – when changes in the normal level of depth are appropriate

According to the CM classical pulse literature, seasonal effects impact on the presentation of the pulse in many aspects (see section 5.12.2). With regard to pulse depth, the classical literature notes the level of depth where the pulse is felt strongest varies depending on the season. For example, in summer the pulse is described as more superficial, and in winter the pulse is deeper. The change in the level of depth where the pulse is felt strongest is

A 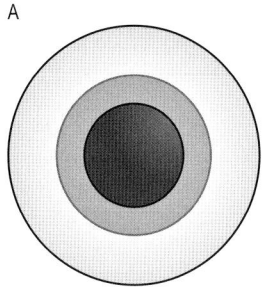   B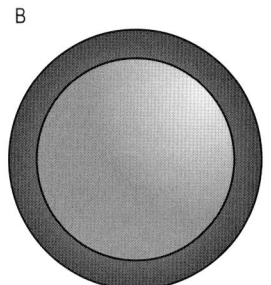

Figure 6.5

(a) Cold is associated with cutaneous vasoconstriction and normal or increased blood flow to many organs. The white area represents the skin, which serves as a shell of insulation because it receives almost no flow. The darkest regions (the body core) have the highest blood flows and the stippled regions (e.g. muscle) receive relatively low flows. (b) Hot conditions cause high surface (cutaneous) blood flow (dark region), causing loss of thermal insulation and reduced flow to the body core (stippled region) so that less heat is stored centrally and thermal insulation is lost (no white regions). (After Fig. 5.1 in Rowell LB 1986, Human circulation regulation during physical stress, with permission of Oxofrd University Press.)

explained with respect to the body's Qi, retreating in winter and expanding in summer. This is alternatively viewed as the body's attempt to maintain a stable core body temperature, varying the degree of exposure the blood vessels have to the environment and so mediating the retention or loss of body heat (Fig. 6.5).

In a clinical context, a deeper located pulse in winter or a more superficial pulse in summer is then viewed as an appropriate response of the body to climatic influences and not necessarily always related to pathology.

6.7.3 Levels of depth and their meaning: CM perspective

The level of depth of the pulse may provide information about:

- Location of disease
- Quality and quantity of Qi, particularly Yang, and its ability to move outwards
- Integrity of Yin and its ability to balance and anchor Yang.

6.7.3.1 Pulse depth and location of disease

In the *Mai Jing* (Wang, Yang (trans) 1997: p. 26) Wang noted that 'a floating pulse is ascribed to the exterior, and a sinking one to the interior'. If the pulse is felt relatively strongest at the superficial level of depth, this generally indicates an external condition or a condition that has affected the superficial layers of the body such as the skin, muscles and channel systems. A pulse strongest at the superficial level of depth may also refer to disharmony affecting the Yang organs that are theoretically assigned to the superficial level of depth.

> **Box 6.15**
>
> ### Levels of depth and diagnosis
>
> A specific example of the use of level of depth as a diagnostic tool is the theory of the Eight Principles. The Eight Principles are a foundational framework that is used in diagnosis to determine the location and nature of a disharmony or illness. This thereby assists in formulating a treatment plan (Maciocia 1989: p. 179). There are a myriad of different pattern identification methods, but they are all based on the Eight Principles: Internal, External, Replete, Vacuity, Hot, Cold, Yin and Yang. From this perspective, the level of depth at which the pulse can be felt the strongest informs us simply about the location of disease.

93

A pulse that is felt relatively strongest at the deep level of depth is usually related to an internal disorder, affecting the interior of the body or the Yin organs. For example, a pulse that can be felt forcefully at the deep level of depth may indicate obstruction or stagnation of Qi and blood. In this situation the pulse cannot be felt at the superficial level of depth because Yang is being obstructed in the interior of the body, unable to move outwards towards the exterior of the body and so the pulse remains in the deep levels of depth (Box 6.15).

6.7.3.2 Yang Qi

The superficial level of depth of the radial pulse represents the exterior or the Yang aspect of the body. In this respect, the superficial level of the pulse also represents the quality of Qi, in particular Yang. Where the pulse can be palpated may also inform us about the capacity of Yang Qi to motivate the pulse and lift it to a palpable depth. If Yang is vacuous (deficient) this can result in a deeply located pulse, with Yang insufficient to raise the pulse to the surface. Parameters such as pulse force and rate may provide additional information about the quality of Yang. For example, when Yang Qi becomes vacuous, it would be expected that the pulse would present without strength, possibly with a slow rate and an increase in *relative* strength at the deep level of depth.

If the pulse is strongest at the superficial level of depth, this may indicate that Yang is more active than normal. This may occur when an external pathogenic agent (EPA) such as Wind, Heat, Cold or Damp enters the body and lodges in the skin and muscle layers. In response to this invasion, *Wei Qi* (the body's defensive Qi) rushes to the body's surface to fight this EPA. This is reflected in the radial pulse as a relative increase in strength at the superficial (external) level of depth. (Wei Qi is considered to be the relatively Yang manifestation of *Zhen Qi* (True Qi) or meridian Qi, circulating outside the channels on the exterior of the body, protecting and warming the body. *Ying Qi (Nutritive Qi)* is the Yin manifestation of Zhen Qi, circulating in the blood vessels, channels and internal organs.)

Excess Yang, in the form of Heat, which may arise internally or externally, may lead to the pulse being palpated forcefully at the superficial level of depth as occurs with the formation of the Surging pulse (along with notable changes in the pulse contour, force and width. The Surging pulse is discussed in more detail in section 7.9.3.)

6.7.3.3 Yin

In terms of pulse depth, the quality of Yin energy is symbolised by the deep level of depth. Yin has the effect of cooling and nourishing the body. It encompasses the numerous fluids that circulate around the body such as Blood, Body Fluids (Jin-Ye) and Essence (Jing). It also plays a role in helping to control and balance Yang; this is the 'functional Yin'. If Yin and its various aspects become vacuous, then Yang becomes relatively hyperactive. This results in the pulse being felt relatively stronger at the superficial level of depth because the Yin is no longer able to restrain Yang, so Yang moves outward to the exterior of the body.

Yin vacuity also affects other pulse parameters such as pulse force, width and rate, resulting in a pulse that is decreased in strength and arterial width but with an increase in pulse rate (dependent upon the strength of the deficient heat produced).

Conversely, excessive Yin in the form of pathogenic Cold or Damp (Yin pathogenic factors) may attack the body from the exterior and enter via the skin, muscles and channels or move directly into the interior of the body via certain internal organs such as the stomach, intestines or uterus. In the former case, the pulse would

be felt strongest at the superficial level of depth, and in the latter example, the pulse would be strongest at the deep level of depth.

Internal Cold (also Yin in nature) may develop from qi causes such as deficiency of Yang affecting the Yin organs, notably the Spleen, Lung, Kidneys and Heart. This may develop as a consequence of a weak constitution, chronic illness, hypo-functioning metabolism or inappropriate diet. The pulse would be felt relatively stronger at the deep level of depth, indicating both an internal condition and the involvement of the Yin organs.

6.7.4 Levels of depth and their meaning: biomedical perspective

The ease with which the radial artery can be palpated may be affected by the person's constitutional body type. For example, a slim person's radial artery may be more easily accessible because of the thinner layer of subcutaneous tissue, while someone with a higher proportion of body fat may have an artery that is more difficult to palpate because of the thicker subcutaneous tissue layer. Alternatively, difficulty palpating the pulse may also be due to a pathological process occurring in the body. For example, oedema or accumulation of fluids in the connective tissue layer (in the interstitial spaces between cells and outside the blood vessels) may affect the ease with which the radial artery can be palpated.

Arterial blood pressure and the strength of cardiac contraction equally influence the level of depth at which the pulse is felt strongest. An increase in volume in the pulse is described as 'full and bounding' while a decrease in volume is described as 'weak and thready' (Funnell et al 2005: p. 267). Full bounding pulses are associated with strong cardiac contraction and are felt more readily at the superficial levels of depth where weak thready pulses may be hard to discern.

6.8 CM pulse qualities defined by level of depth

6.8.1 Floating pulse (Fú mài) 浮脉

6.8.1.1 Requisite parameters

The Floating pulse is a simple pulse quality defined solely by pulse depth. It is felt most forcefully at the superficial level of depth, with fingers resting lightly on the skin, exerting no pressure except the weight of the fingers.

6.8.1.2 Clinical definition

The Floating pulse is felt relatively strongest at the superficial level of depth, compared to the other levels

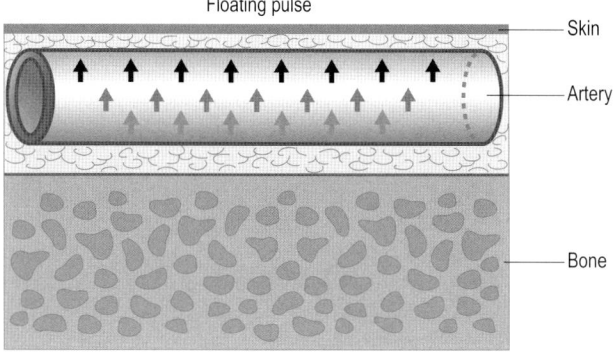

Floating pulse

— Skin

— Artery

— Bone

Figure 6.6
Floating pulse and relative strength differences within the arterial pulsation relative to pressure applied by the fingers. The pulse wave is felt strongest at the superficial region. The strength of the pressure wave is symbolised by arrows. Note the arrows lessen at the deeper levels of depth reflecting the relative decrease in strength.

of depth. With increasing finger pressure there is a decrease of force, the pulsation cannot be felt at the depth deep level of depth. In order to identify the Floating pulse, each level of depth must be examined and the relative strength of each level determined.

6.8.1.3 Identifying whether the Floating pulse is present

Step 1: When the fingers are placed over the radial artery pulsation with only the pressure of the resting fingers exerting pressure, the pulse may be easily palpated (Fig. 6.6).

Step 2: With increasing finger pressure exerted over the radial pulsation, there is a resulting decrease in the pulse force. With increasing finger pressure the pulsation disappears and the pulse at the deep level of depth cannot be felt.

The term 'floating' is also used as a general descriptor of any pulse type that can be palpated strongest at the superficial level (the level at which the fingers rest gently on the artery without pressure), regardless of changes in other parameters. This should not be confused with the Floating pulse, a distinct CM pulse quality. Describing a pulse as being felt strongest superficially or at the superficial level of depth should help to prevent such terminological confusion.

6.8.1.4 Classical description from the *Shang Han Lun* and *Mai Jing*

A pulse that is felt when light pressure is applied is called 'Floating' (*Shang Han Lun*) (Mitchell et al 1999: p. 34).

Box 6.16

Summary of the Floating pulse
- Floating and forceful = Replete condition externally: EPA
- Floating and forceless = Vacuous condition internally: Vacuity of Yin fluids
- Floating, forceless and narrow arterial diameter: Severe vacuity of Yin → Soggy pulse
- Floating, forceless and wide arterial diameter: Qi and Blood vacuity → Vacuous pulse

---

The floating pulse is a pulse potent when felt with no pressure applied but impotent when felt with pressure applied
(Wang, Yang (trans) 1997: p. 3).

6.8.1.5 CM indications

The Floating pulse is always considered to be indicative of pathogenesis (Box 6.16). There are two primary patterns where the Floating pulse may occur:

- Replete condition, indicating an external pathogenic agent (EPA)
- Vacuous condition, involving vacuity of Yin fluids causing Yang to 'float'.

They are differentiated by changes in the pulse parameter of force, accompanying signs and symptoms and whether the disharmony is an acute or chronic condition.

A replete condition indicating the presence of an external pathogenic agent (EPA)

The Floating pulse is relatively strongest at the superficial level, with an accompanying increase in the parameter of pulse force. The EPA may take the form of a Yin or Yang type pathogenic factor such as Wind, Heat, Cold or Damp. This pattern could be further differentiated by the accompanying changes in pulse rate or arterial wall tension. For example, an EPA of Heat may also cause an increase in pulse rate, or an EPA of Cold may slow the pulse rate and increase arterial wall tension. In this scenario, the formation of the Floating pulse may be accompanied by a Rapid pulse or Slow pulse (if the rate changes were great enough). Additional signs and symptoms such as body aches, fever, aversion to cold and sudden onset of illness further differentiate the pathogen type.

Mechanism

The EPA enters the body via the skin, nose, and mouth and Wei Qi (defensive Qi), which usually circulates through the skin and muscles to defend the body, rushes to the exterior of the body to fight off the pathogen. Where the Qi goes blood goes. Therefore, the pulse can be felt strongest at the superficial level of depth, reflecting the location of the pathogen. If the Floating pulse also presents with increased pulse force, this signifies the ability of the healthy immune system (also known as the Zheng Qi or Upright Qi in CM terms) to respond strongly to the pathogenic factor.

Clinical relevance

From a clinical perspective, the formation of the Floating pulse in response to an EPA would be associated with the rapid onset of an acute condition such as a cold or flu-type viral infection. Other signs and symptoms such as fever, sore throat, sweating, headache and quesion to cold may accompany this pulse depending upon the nature of the EPA.

Exception

The Floating pulse when forceful may not occur in someone who has an underlying vacuity condition (such as a compromised immune system or chronic illness) as their Wei Qi or Zheng Qi is too deficient to respond strongly to the pathogenic factor. Therefore the Floating pulse may still occur, being relatively stronger at the superficial level, but it may not be accompanied by an increase in pulse force.

Vacuous condition involving vacuity of Yin fluids

In this pattern the formation of the Floating pulse would be accompanied by changes in other parameters such as pulse force. In this case, the Floating pulse is forceless, reflecting the underlying vacuity. This pulse quality may appear as a result of internal disease, manifesting as a vacuity of Yin substances. This may take the form of deficiency of Yin, blood or body fluids. It is the accompanying signs and symptoms that further define the disharmony.

- Mechanism: This pulse is formed when the insufficient Yin is unable to control and anchor the relatively excessive Yang, whose natural inclination is to move outward. Therefore, Yang rises to the surface, resulting in a pulse that is felt strongest at the superficial level of depth. However, because Yin is deficient the pulse is lacking in force and decreases significantly in strength as finger pressure is exerted on the artery.
- Clinical relevance: This may be the result of the consumption of Yin due to lifestyle issues such as overwork, irregular eating patterns and insufficient sleep. The loss of body fluids due to excessive sweating or vomiting may also result in the formation of this pulse type.

6.8.1.6 Further differentiation of the Floating pulse

As noted, the Floating pulse can be further differentiated on the basis of changes in parameters other than level of depth. The parameter of pulse force provides information about whether the Floating pulse is caused by repletion or vacuity. Similarly, changes in pulse width can inform us about the condition of Yin and blood or the hyperactivity or relative hyperactivity of Yang (Lu 1996: p. 33). It is the combination of changes in other pulse parameters, in addition to a pulse that feels strongest at the superficial level of depth, which results in the formation of other CM pulse qualities. For example:

- A forceless, superficial and narrow pulse indicates Yin vacuity: this becomes known as the *Soggy pulse* rather than the Floating pulse. (The difference is that the Soggy pulse is only felt at the superficial region while the Floating pulse has decreasing levels of strength with increasing finger pressure; that is, it can still be felt in the middle level but not as strongly as the superficial level.)
- A forceless, superficial and wide pulse indicates both Qi and blood vacuity: this then becomes termed the *Vacuous pulse*.

6.8.2 Sinking pulse (Chén mài) 沉脉

6.8.2.1 Alternative names

Sunken, Deep or Submerged pulse.

6.8.2.2 Requisite parameters

The Sinking pulse is a simple pulse quality with a change in the pulse parameter of depth. It is felt relatively strongest at the deep level of depth.

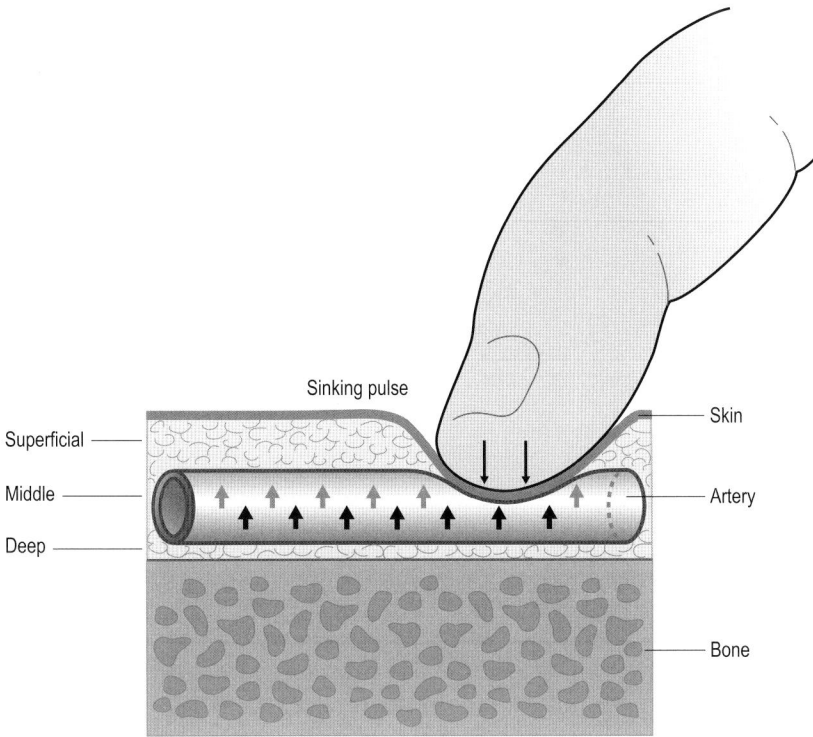

Sinking pulse

Superficial
Middle
Deep

Skin
Artery
Bone

Figure 6.7
Sinking pulse and relative strength differences within the arterial pulsation relative to pressure applied by the fingers. The pulse wave is felt strongest at the deep region. The strength of the pressure wave is symbolised by arrows moving up while the pressure of the finger pressure is symbolised by arrows moving in.

97

6.8.2.3 Clinical definition

The Sinking pulse can be felt relatively strongest at the deep level of depth. With increasing finger pressure over the radial pulsation, there is an increase in pulse force as the deep level of depth is approached (Fig. 6.7). The formation of the Sinking pulse means that the arterial pulsation cannot be felt at the superficial level of depth, but may be felt slightly at the middle level of depth. It is strongest and clearest at the deep level of depth. (The Sinking pulse is considered to be opposite to the Floating pulse. This is based on the depth parameter and their relative opposite locations according to the levels of depth.)

6.8.2.4 Identifying whether the Sinking pulse is present

Step 1: The pulse is best identified by first placing the fingers gently on the skin overlying the radial artery, with only the weight of the palpating fingers exerting

downward pressure. At this superficial level of depth, the radial pulsation cannot be felt.

Step 2: The deep level of the pulse is next examined by increasing finger pressure so that the radial artery is occluded for a few seconds and then the finger pressure is slightly eased so that the pulsation can once again be felt. The radial pulsation will appear at its strongest at this level of depth.

Step 3: Once the deep level of the pulse has been located, the middle level of the pulse should then be assessed. The radial pulsation may be able to be palpated at the middle level of depth but will be felt with less intensity than the pulsation felt at the deep level of depth.

Once the three levels of depth are located, the fingers can be gradually moved from the superficial level of depth to the deep level of depth. In doing this the radial pulsation will sequentially increase in relative strength as the fingers move deeper into each level of depth.

Summary of Sinking pulses

- Sinking and forceful: Internal pathogenic factor or obstruction of Qi and blood
- Sinking and forceless: Vacuity of Qi and blood, especially Yang

6.8.2.5 Classical description from the Nei Jing and Mai Jing

A deep pulse is where one must press all the way to the bone to find it (*Su Wen*)
(Ni 1995: p. 70).

The deep pulse is a pulse impotent when felt with no pressure applied but potent when felt with pressure applied [said in another version to be absent unless heavy pressure is applied] (*Mai Jing*)
(Wang, Yang (trans): p. 3).

6.8.2.6 CM indications

Pulse depth provides information pertaining to where disease is located, differentiated further by additional changes in other pulse parameters. The *Nei Jing* says 'when there is an imbalance in the body's interior, one should examine the pulse at the deepest level'. In this sense, the Sinking pulse indicates disharmony in the interior. We have already noted that pulse depth provides information about Yang Qi, characterised by the superficial level of depth. Therefore, if a pulse cannot be palpated at the superficial level it may suggest that either Yang Qi is deficient or that disharmony is occurring internally. The Sinking pulse is always indicative of pathogenesis (Box 6.17).

The Sinking pulse can indicate two primary patterns that are further differentiated by changes in the parameter of pulse force:

- Internal replete condition
- Internal vacuous condition.

Internal replete condition

The Sinking pulse due to repletion (excess) in the interior will be forceful at the deep level of depth. It indicates the presence of a pathogenic factor such as Cold, Heat, Damp or Phlegm depending on the accompanying signs and symptoms. In these cases, changes in other pulse parameters may be apparent. For example, the pulse rate may be slow in the presence of Cold or rapid in the case of Heat.

The Sinking and forceful pulse may also imply the obstruction of Qi and blood. This may result from the aforementioned pathogenic factors or from retention of food (Lu 1996). The pulse presents forcefully and would be accompanied by some type of pain. (Pain is symptomatic of obstruction, irrespective of the cause of the obstruction.) Pain often results in an increase in arterial tension (another of the pulse parameters), resulting in a distinctly palpable arterial wall (see section 7.3 for further details).

- Mechanism: The deeply located pulse signifies the location of the disease, while the forcefulness of the pulse infers that the body's defensive Qi has responded to the presence of the pathogenic factor and moved inwards to fight it.

Internal vacuous condition

The Sinking pulse due to vacuity (deficiency) will present with decreased pulsatile force. The main pattern associated with the Sinking and forceless pulse is Vacuity of Qi and blood, and in particular Yang Qi.

- Mechanism: Yang Qi is unable to lift the pulse so that it can be palpated at the superficial level of depth.
- Clinical relevance: Cold signs and symptoms such as aversion to cold, lethargy and cold extremities usually accompany the Yang vacuity pattern. Clinically this may be seen in hypothyroidism or in severe exhaustion.

6.8.3 Hidden pulse (Fú mài) 伏脉

6.8.3.1 Alternative names

Deep-lying or Recondite pulse.

6.8.3.2 Requisite parameters

The Hidden pulse is a simple pulse quality defined only by changes in pulse depth. It can only be palpated below the deep level of depth (Fig. 6.8).

6.8.3.3 Clinical definition

The Hidden pulse cannot be palpated at the superficial or middle levels of depth. It is located very deeply, situated just above the bone, requiring extremely heavy pressure with the palpating fingers. It is not necessarily a forceless pulse.

The formation of the Hidden pulse probably results from the actual anatomical location of the physical arterial structure deep in the flesh next to the bone or under other anatomical structures such tendons. In this sense, the Hidden pulse is not about the actual pulse wave, it is about anatomy.

6.8.3.4 Identifying whether the Hidden pulse is present

Step 1: First place the fingers gently on the skin overlying the radial artery, with only the weight of the palpating fingers exerting downward pressure. At this superficial level of depth the radial pulsation cannot be felt.

Step 2: As increasing finger pressure is exerted downwards through the epidermis and dermis and the

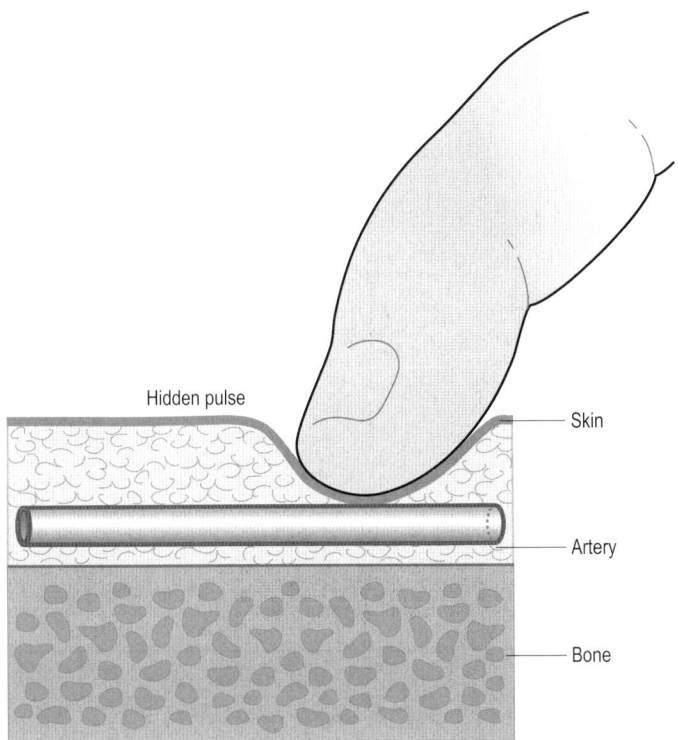

Figure 6.8
The Hidden pulse. The anatomical structure of the artery is located adjacent to the bone, deep in the tissue. This means the pulse cannot be felt at the superficial or middle levels of depth simply because there is no arterial structure for the pulse to occur in at these levels.

subcutaneous layer of the hypodermis, the radial artery pulsation may still not be obtained. This is the expected 'deep' level of the pulse. Finger pressure is further increased, so that the radial bone can be felt just below the palpating finger tips. At this point the pulsation should be able to be felt.

Step 3: Once the pulse is located, determine its overall strength and rate.

6.8.3.5 Classical description from the *Mai Jing* and *The Lakeside Master's Study of the Pulse*

The hidden pulse is a pulse imperceptible till the fingers touch the bone with extremely heavy pressure . . . (*Mai Jing*)
(*Wang, Yang (trans) 1997: p. 4*).

The pulse moves under the sinews (*Bin Hue Mai Xue*)
(*Li, Flaws (trans) 1998: p. 114*).

6.8.3.6 CM indications

The Hidden pulse is always indicative of pathogenesis, representing a more severe form of internal illness than

> ### Box 6.18
> **Summary of Hidden pulses**
> - Hidden and forceful: Severe obstruction of Yang Qi due to internal pathogenic factors or retained food
> - Hidden and forceless: Severe vacuity of Yang Qi leading to internal cold

the Sinking pulse (Box 6.18). The two patterns associated with the Hidden pulse are:

- An internal replete condition
- An internal vacuity condition.

The two patterns can be differentiated by the parameter of pulse force.

Internal replete condition
The Hidden pulse when forceful indicates a severe obstruction of Yang Qi internally by either pathogenic Cold, retained food, Phlegm or toxic Fire. This pulse has historically been seen in 'sudden turmoil' or epidemic illnesses such as cholera like diseases causing severe vomiting and diarrhoea (indication from the *Bin Hue Mai Xue*, Li, Flaws (trans) 1998: pp. 114–115).

Internal vacuity condition

The Hidden pulse when forceless denotes a severe vacuity of Yang causing chronic internal cold, for example vacuity of Kidney Yang.

- Mechanism: The decreased Yang and resulting nature of the Cold that is produced by the severe vacuity of Yang results in the pulse being located at a very deep level, unable to lift the pulse to the exterior. The internal Cold may also impact on the pulse causing stasis and decreasing the flow of Qi and blood. This may also result in a decrease in pulse rate, the Slow pulse and potentially, an increase in arterial wall tension due to the contracting nature of cold.

6.9 Length (longitude)

Pulse length is categorised as a simple pulse parameter that reflects the quantity of Qi and blood circulating in the organs, blood vessels and channels and its smooth unimpeded flow. The parameter of pulse length refers to the presence or absence of a *palpable* arterial pulsation at the three traditional positions of Cun, Guan and Chi and beyond the Cun and Chi positions. There are two CM pulse qualities that utilise length solely as the defining pulse parameter:

- Long pulse (section 6.11.1)
- Short pulse (section 6.11.2).

The Long and Short pulses are defined only by their length. The palpable pulse length can also increase or shorten with other traditional CM pulse qualities, but this is in combination with changes in other pulse parameters. For example, the Stirred pulse can also be described as a 'short' pulse, commonly felt in the Guan position only. However, there are additional changes in the pulse contour, and the Stirred pulse is consequently categorised under the pulse contour parameter.

6.9.1 Pulse length and its assessment

Pulse length is evaluated by checking for the presence of pulsations at each of the three traditional pulse positions and at the pulse positions beyond Cun and beyond Chi, at all levels of depth:

- Beyond Cun is defined as the area of skin on the wrist crease one finger breadth distal, medial and lateral to the Cun position (Box 6.19).
- Beyond Chi is defined as the skin region one finger breadth proximal to the Chi position, above the radial artery (Box 6.20).

The three pulse positions are located according to the usual procedure. Each position is then palpated

Box 6.19

Presence of pulsations beyond Cun

The presence of the pulse beyond Cun extending into the palmar thenar eminence on the right hand side is said to indicate a constitutional Lung deficiency. This 'special' Lung position is found distally and medially to the Cun position where the Lung is represented (Maciocia, 2004: pp 503–504)

Box 6.20

Tibetan pulse diagnosis

Traditional Tibetan medicine has a form of pulse diagnosis that requires palpation far beyond the Chi position along the radial artery. Pulse examination as a diagnostic tool has been used by a number of different cultures (see section 2.5). While in CM use of the radial pulse has taken precedence, this wasn't always the case. The Nine Continents pulse system (using various pulses located on the head and upper and lower limbs) was the main method discussed in the *Nei Jing* (see section 9.5 for detailed information), until CM theoretical developments in the *Nan Jing* led to focus upon the radial artery pulsation.

individually at all three levels of depth and the absence or presence of pulsations noted. The same procedure is then carried out at the positions beyond Cun and beyond Chi (Box 6.22).

When examining the three traditional positions, it should be noted that there are differences in how 'easy' each position may be to palpate. This is associated with the physical characteristics of the radius, with the Cun and Guan pulse positions on the artery being better supported by underlying bony structures than the Chi position and beyond Chi position, so pulsations are more apparent. Note that pulsations can readily be felt beyond Chi position and can also denote health (Table 6.7).

6.9.2 Pulse length: CM perspective

The concept of a continuous circulation throughout the body, introduced in the *Nei Jing* was expanded upon in the *Nan Jing* (Unschuld 1986) where the First Difficult Issue discusses the movement through the vessels during each inhalation and each exhalation. The contents of the vessels are said to progress six inches with each complete respiration, resulting in fifty complete cycles throughout the body in the 'course of one day

Box 6.21

Questions to consider when assessing pulse length

When looking at the length of the pulse we need to consider the following:
- Under how many fingers is the pulse felt? (exerting even pressure with all three fingers)
- Can the pulse be felt as a continuous length of pulsation under all three fingers?
- Can the pulse be felt beyond the three traditional positions?
- What other factors are associated with the Long and Short pulses? (Hint: deficiency or excess?)
- Are there other signs and symptoms? In an otherwise healthy person the Long pulse can be a sign of abundant Qi and blood.

Box 6.22

Summary of definitions of the pulses defined by the length parameter

- Long: Felt at Cun, Guam and Chi and felt beyond the three positions, beyond the Cun and/or Chi positions (i.e. can be felt closer to thenar eminence and/ or towards the elbow). Classified as Yang.
- Short: Felt in only one or two of the three positions. Usually felt in the guan position plus one of the other two positions. Classified as Yin.

and one night'. Therefore the presence of pulsation at all three pulse positions and beyond is a sign of abundant Qi and blood circulating through the channels and vessels.

The length of the pulse reflects the relative amount of Qi and blood and the circulation of this within the arterial system, organs and channels. Wang noted in the *Mai Jing* (Wang, Yang (trans) 1997: p. 25) 'Since the pulse is the mansion of the blood, the Qi is in a good state if the pulse is long, but diseased if the pulse is short'.

Accordingly, changes in pulse length occur as a reflection of health or change as the result of disease. When pathogenic agents or internal disharmony impact on Qi and blood, then Qi and blood can become overactive, obstructed or vacuous (deficient).

The length of the pulse can indicate:

- The overall 'health' of an individual
- The relative quality and quantity of Qi and Blood
- The presence of pathogenic heat
- Obstruction of Qi and blood.

6.9.3 Pulse length: biomedical perspective

The presence of arterial pulsations depends on the underlying support of the arterial structure at the point of palpation (by the radial bone in this case) in order to establish an internal/external pressure equilibrium that enables the pulsation to be felt. Additionally, there needs to be sufficient volume for the vessels to be filled. Where the artery is not supported or volume is lessened so the artery and pulsations become less distinct with finger pressure.

6.10 CM pulse defined by length

6.10.1 Long pulse (Cháng mài) 长脉

6.10.1.1 Requisite parameters

The Long pulse is a simple pulse quality with changes in the pulse parameter of length. It can be palpated at Cun, Guan and Chi and beyond Chi and/or beyond Cun.

6.10.1.2 Clinical definition

With the Long pulse we are only interested in whether we can feel the pulsation of the radial pulse at each of the three traditional positions and beyond these positions, that is, distal to the wrist crease, in the area of the thenar eminence and beyond the Chi position (defined as one finger breadth proximal to Chi, towards the direction of the elbow). The Long pulse can be palpated at Cun, Guan and Chi, beyond the Chi and maybe beyond the Cun position.

Note: Li (Flaws (trans) 1998: pp. 85–86) describes the Long pulse as not only 'a pulse which extends beyond its position' but '(It) is not only bowstring but full and distended.' This description encompasses much more than length, incorporating increased arterial tension, width and an increase in pulse force.

6.10.1.3 Identifying whether the Long pulse is present

Step 1: The radial pulse is examined for the presence or absence of pulsations at the superficial and deep levels of depth and at each of three positions, using the radial styloid process as the anatomical landmark for the Guan position (see Box 6.21 for further information).

Step 2: The positions beyond Cun and beyond Chi are examined for the presence or absence of pulsations at all levels of depth.

101

6.10.1.4 Classical description from *The Lakeside Master's Study of the Pulse*

'The long pulse is neither large nor small,
Far, far, calm and at ease.
A pulse which extends beyond its position is called long . . . is not only bowstring but full and distended
(Li, Flaws (trans) 1998: pp. 85–86).

6.10.1.5 CM indications

The Long pulse is a simple CM pulse quality defined primarily on the presence of pulsation beyond Cun and/or Chi pulse positions. It is not always considered to be a pathological pulse quality, occurring in individuals with abundant Qi and blood and as well as those who are unwell.

Four patterns are associated with the Long pulse; one is a sign of health, but three represent pathology:

- Abundant Qi and blood (healthy)
- Heat
- Phlegm
- Liver disharmony.

Healthy

In the absence of abnormal signs and symptoms, the Long pulse indicates a normal flow of abundant Qi and blood filling the radial artery. In someone who is not sick, it is a sign of good health. When indicating good health, there is usually no corresponding change in other parameters – that is, the presence of the pulse is simply there. When there is an increase in arterial tension or contour changes then the increase in pulse length probably reflects pathology (see below).

Heat

The Long pulse occurs when Heat agitates the blood causing the blood to expand longitudinally. When Heat pathogens occur there are likely to be changes in other pulse parameters and these need to be assessed in relation to the increase in pulse length. Clinically, an increase in pulse length occurs in fever, but if the Heat is strong then the pulse rate may also increase.

Phlegm

A number of authors mention the Long pulse in connection with the presence of Phlegm or Phlegm fire, relating this clinically to epilepsy and manic symptoms: Deng (1999), Maciocia (2004). However, this would also usually include changes in accompanying pulse parameters.

Liver disharmony

The Long pulse is associated with Liver disease by a number of authors: Deng (1999), Lu (1996) and Maciocia (2004). However, this is not strictly a pattern that is solely associated with the classical Long pulse,

as another pulse parameter, arterial wall tension, is also involved. If the Long pulse is accompanied by an increase in arterial tension so that the arterial wall feels increasingly 'harder' than usual, and the artery retains this rigidity on increased pressure, then this indicates that there is Liver disharmony. Associated Liver signs and symptoms would be expected to accompany this pulse.

6.10.2 Short pulse (Duǎn mài) 短脉

6.10.2.1 Requisite parameters

The Short pulse is a simple pulse quality defined only by the parameter of length. It has a decrease in length, indicated by the absence of a pulsation in at least one of the three traditional pulse positions.

6.10.2.2 Clinical definition

The Short pulse is defined as a pulse that cannot be felt across the three pulse positions of Cun, Guan and Chi, or beyond Cun or beyond Chi. It is usually felt at the Guan position and/or at the Cun or Chi position.

6.10.2.3 Classical description from *The Lakeside Master's Study of the Pulse*

A short pulse does not reach its position *(Mai Xue).*
It responds to the fingers (as if) wound up.
It is not able to fill its position *(Mai Jing).*
(Li, Flaws (trans) 1998: pp. 87–88).

The literature records conflicting views about the application of the term 'short' to the radial arterial pulse and the physical manifestation of a Short pulse. For example, authors such as Maciocia, when defining the Short pulse, imply that the pulsation can be short within each position. That is, even when the pulse is clearly felt at the three pulse positions, the pulse can be simultaneously described as 'short' for a particular position, because it does not expand across the whole position as it should.

In contrast, Li Shi-zhen, who often described the clinical significance of specific qualities within the Cun, Guan or Chi pulse positions, does not attribute the term short to the pulse in the same sense that Maciocia has. Rather, Li Shi-zhen's use of the term 'short' appears to imply that the Short pulse is used only to describe the situation when there is a total absence of a discernable pulse at one of the three pulse positions Cun, Guan or Chi.

6.10.2.4 CM indications

The Short pulse indicates two main patterns:

- Vacuity of Qi
- Obstruction and stagnation of Qi

Table 6.7 ● Evaluation of pulse length. The ✓ indicates the presence of the pulse at a particular position

Presence of pulse	Normal length	Long pulse	Long pulse	Firm pulse	Wiry pulse	Short pulse	Short pulse	Stirred pulse
		Possible pulse patterns				Possible pulse patterns		
Beyond Cun		✓						
Cun	✓	✓	✓	✓	✓	✓		
Guan	✓	✓	✓	✓	✓	✓	✓	✓
Chi	✓	✓	✓	✓	✓		✓	
Beyond Chi	possible	✓	✓	✓	✓			
Simultaneously felt under all three fingers?			✓	✓	✓			
Increased arterial tension?				✓	✓			

The two patterns are further differentiated by the parameter of pulse force.

Vacuity of Qi (Short and forceless)

The Short pulse that is also forceless indicates Qi vacuity. As Qi leads blood, and accordingly if Qi is vacuous, then blood will not have the motive force to be propelled along the arteries as usual.

One possible interpretation of the Short pulse relates to the relationship between the Cun, Guan and Chi positions and their respective relationship to the upper, middle and lower Heaters of the body. In a situation where pulsations are absent from both the Cun positions, for example, and present in the Guan and Chi positions, then an upper Heater vacuity (deficiency) would be indicated.

Obstruction or stagnation of Qi (Short and forceful)

The Short pulse due to stasis presents with an increase in pulsatile force. Generally this indicates Qi obstruction due to the presence of phlegm or retained food. To relate the three pulse positions to the upper, middle and lower Heaters, it can be seen if there is obstruction in one of the heaters, this can affect communication between the three regions of the body and consequently the formation of the Short pulse. For example, a lack of a pulse in the Cun positions with a strong pulse in the Guan positions and forceless pulses in the Chi positions could indicate an obstruction in the middle Heater; Qi is not being distributed to the upper and lower Heaters.

When the Short pulse only manifests on either the left or right side, and the pulse on the other side is felt normal, then obstructive circulatory disorders disrupting the flow wave within the artery on the affected side need to be considered. From a CM perspective, this may also reflect an organ type disharmony or vacuity according to where the pulsation can not be felt (see section 9.4 on Five Phase pulse diagnosis).

When the Short pulse occurs bilaterally with strength then systemic causes arising from obstruction in the digestive tract need to be assessed.

6.11 Width (latitude)

Pulse width is classified as a simple pulse parameter, which is concerned with the actual tactile presentation of the radial artery across the lateral plane. It is the diameter of the radial artery or the lateral displacement of the pulse wave acting on the radial artery that is examined to determine whether the artery is thinner or wider than would be expected relative to that individual.

Assessment of pulse width provides information mainly pertaining to the volume of circulating Yin fluids. Pulse width may also indicate the level of activity of Qi; the ability of the Qi to move blood outward, and also 'Qi' in the broader sense as relating to the presence of Cold or Damp pathogenic factors. In these cases, there are usually accompanying changes in other pulse parameters in conjunction with specific pathological signs and symptoms. In a CM context, pathogenic factors are seen as affecting the pulse width.

Only one CM pulse quality is solely defined by its width; the Fine pulse. The Fine pulse is associated with a decrease in pulse width and is defined as a 'thin' pulse quality. Three other CM pulse qualities can be defined as 'thin':

- Faint pulse (section 7.7.4)
- Weak pulse (section 7.7.5)
- Soggy pulse (section 7.7.6).

The Fine pulse can be seen as the template or prototype pulse of these narrow pulses. It is the presence of

Box 6.23

Further differentiation of pulses presenting with narrow arterial diameter

Any pulse with a narrow diameter can be defined as the Fine pulse. However, if changes in other pulse parameters are also present then this may become another CM pulse quality. For example:

- Narrow + forceless + superficial: Soggy pulse
- Narrow + forceless + deep: Weak pulse
- Narrow + extremely forceless + lack of arterial tension: Faint pulse
- Narrow + increased arterial tension: Stringlike pulse

changes in other pulse parameters that further differentiate the Soggy pulse, Weak pulse and Faint pulse from the Fine pulse. For example, the Weak pulse, while also a thin pulse, is found at the deep level of depth and is defined primarily by its decrease in pulse force (Box 6.23).

At the other extreme of the pulse width parameter are several pulse qualities that are associated with an increase in pulse width: Replete pulse, Firm pulse, Tight pulse, Scallion Stalk pulse, Drumskin pulse, Scattered pulse, Vacuous pulse and Surging pulse.

These pulse qualities also have important changes in other pulse parameters such as pulse force or contour and flow wave, and are therefore discussed in the sections on the more relevant pulse parameter to which they relate.

6.11.1 Pulse width and its assessment

The width of the artery is identified manually by determining the proportion of the total arterial circumfer-

ence that can be palpated under the fingertips. In this way, the pulse or artery is categorised 'thin' or 'not thin' by the area that the arterial wall displaces laterally on the palpating finger.

The arterial width is examined by using all three fingers to apply pressure simultaneously over the three pulse positions. The pulse is examined at the deep and superficial levels.

There are two basic subdivisions: thin and not thin (Fig. 6.9).

Thin

A pulse that is 'thin' is defined as having a very narrow arterial diameter, with a definite edge-like feel to it. It does not displace a wide surface area of the fingertip laterally. A greater proportion of the total arterial wall circumference is palpable, indenting the fingertip. Classical descriptions often compare the narrow pulse with a piece of sewing cotton or thread, giving the impression that the arterial wall is definitely palpable within the confines of the fingertips, the artery does not need to be 'rolled' to feel the entire arterial width. Alternatively, the artery is seen occupying a relatively small space between the styloid process and the flexor carpi radialis tendon.

The underlying aetiology of a thin pulse means that irrespective of the degree of pressure applied to it, the thin pulse should retain its 'thin' classification. For example, a thin pulse felt superficially does not become a 'wide' pulse when further finger pressure is applied. If this does occur, then this would not be categorised as a 'thin' pulse. It is simply the uppermost level of a wider pulse that is not being sufficiently palpated.

Not thin

A pulse that is 'not thin' is any pulse with a diameter wider than the 'thin' pulse and this may encompass a pulse width that is neither narrower nor wider than expected, being the norm for that individual. It may

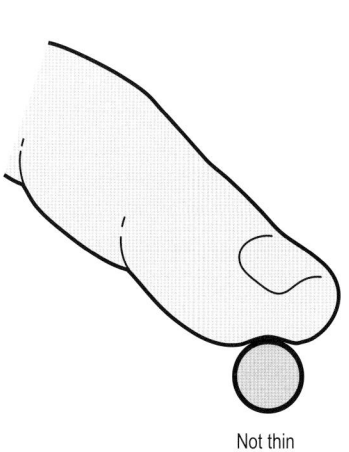

Not thin

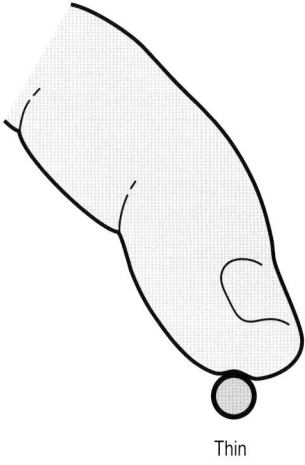

Thin

Figure 6.9
Cross-sectional schematic of the radial artery and diameter variations with finger palpation.

also describe a pulse that is broader or wider than it should be, with the pulse expanding both laterally and longitudinally. The category of 'not thin' includes those pulses that displace a broad area under the fingertip and possess a distinct arterial wall. It also includes pulses where the arterial wall is not distinctly felt, with the artery felt as an area of pulsation with no clear separation of artery from the surrounding connective tissue, yet the pulse displacement across the finger is wide. The artery occupies a relatively larger space between the styloid process of the radius and the flexor carpi radialis. 'Not thin' pulses can equally be forceful or forceless.

Additional palpatory technique

An additional method of palpating the width of the radial artery involves moving the fingers medially and laterally across the artery to check the width (Fig. 6.10). To do this:

- First place the fingers on the skin surface overlying the radial artery.
- Next, feel for the level of depth where the pulsation is felt strongest.
- Maintaining the amount of pressure to locate the pulsation, move the fingers consecutively from medial to lateral (or from left to right) 'rolling' the arterial structure under the fingers.

This method is also used to determine if there is any increased tension in the arterial wall.

When a thin pulse is palpated and the rolling method applied there is very little more that can be felt of the arterial structure. When the pulse is 'not thin', the rolling technique further reveals areas of the arterial wall that could not be readily palpated initially. When the arterial wall tension is not distinct, assessment of pulse width is best done by assessing the displacement of the pulse wave across the finger tip.

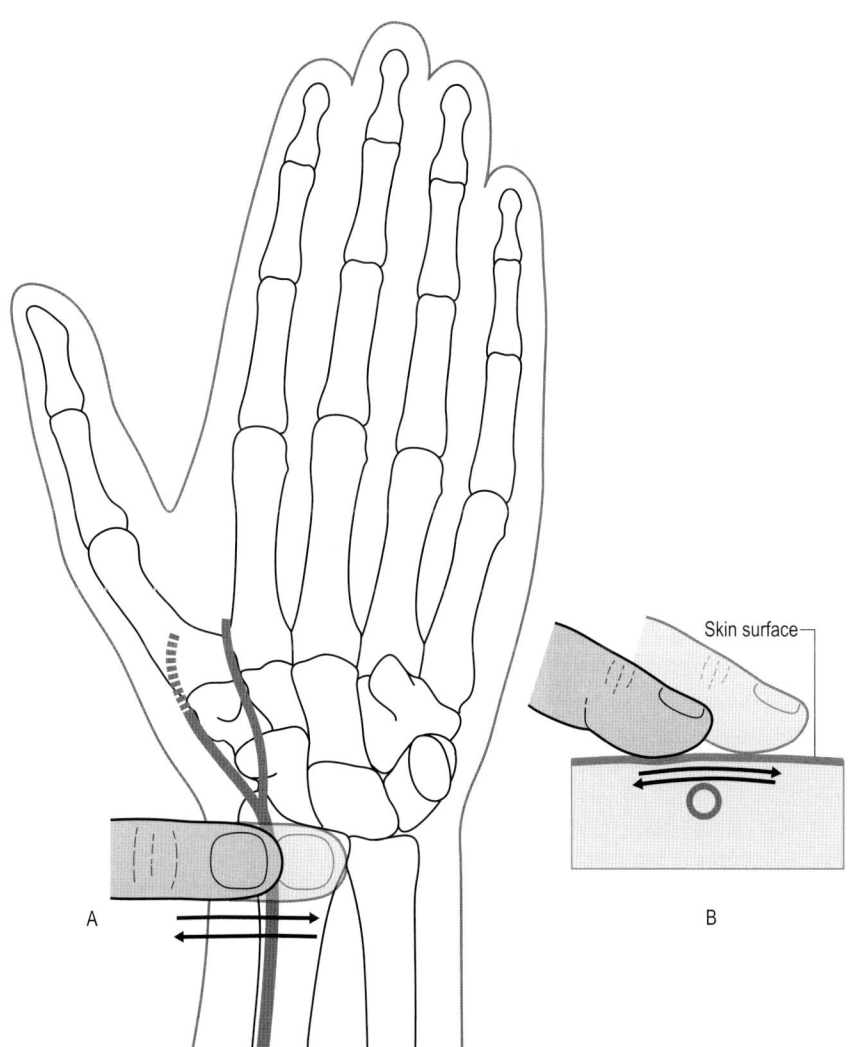

Skin surface

A

B

Figure 6.10
The rolling technique for assessing arterial width. (The technique is also used for assessing arterial wall tension).

6.11.2 Normal pulse width

There is no standard quantifiable measure for the normal pulse width, nor consequently a definitive measurement of a thin or not thin pulse, in spite of an objective measurement being obtainable using Doppler ultrasound. The average diameter of the muscular arteries, of which the radial artery is one, is approximately 4 mm (Stables & Rankin 2006: p. 227) but this will vary from individual to individual according to the height and body type.

Broadly speaking, pulse width is considered normal so long as the artery is wide enough to allow sufficient blood flow for tissue perfusion to maintain healthy normal function. In this sense, the pulse width is described in terms of 'appropriateness'. In terms of the radial artery, 'appropriateness' of normal pulse width can be assessed in two ways:

- Response of the peripheral circulation to return to capillary beds when tissue is compressed
- Degree of warmth in the extremities, skin and muscle.

The idea of the pulse width as 'appropriate' occurs in a number of classical CM literature sources. For example, the *Mai Jing* discusses the necessity of taking into consideration a person's physique:

> Large or small, long or short, and whether their nature's Qi is moderate or impetuous . . . if the pulse . . . is in agreement with the form and nature of the person, it is auspicious. Otherwise it is ominous . . . if the person is small, a female, or thin, the pulse is (accordingly) small and limp.
> *(Wang, Yang (trans) 1997: p. 10).*

6.11.3 Variables affecting pulse width

When assessing the appropriateness of pulse width there are several factors to consider, including:

- An individual's physique
- Temperature
- Body fluids.

6.11.3.1 Physique

A tall person should have a wider pulse than a short person, and someone who is slim would have a smaller arterial width than someone of a larger build. This correlates simply to the relative size of the individual: small, slender individuals have proportionally smaller arteries than individuals of a large build.

6.11.3.2 Temperature

With increased heat in the body, the blood vessels in the skin dilate in an attempt to decrease the core body temperature, leading to an increase in arterial width.

Box 6.24

Body fluids

In an average 70 kilogram person body fluids account for about 42 litres (L). This is mainly composed of ICF (inside cells) 28 L, while BCF constitutes the remaining 14 L and is composed of interstitial fluid, plasma and transcellular fluid (fluids found in the synovial, peritoneal, pericardial and intraocular spaces as well as cerebrospinal fluid constituting about 1–2 L in total) (Guyton and Hall 2006: p. 292–3).

This is controlled by inhibition of the sympathetic centres in the posterior hypothalamus that canse vasoconstriction (Guyton & Mall 2006: p. 895).

Variations in the environmental temperature can also cause regulatory changes in the arterial width. For example, climatic cold may cause the blood vessels in the skin to constrict to conserve body heat, thereby decreasing blood vessel width.

6.11.3.3 Body fluids

Body fluids play an important part in the circulatory system, comprising about 60% of the total body weight (Box 6.24). The term 'body fluids' refers to both the body water and solutes (substances such as electrolytes) dissolved in it (Tortora & Grabowski 2000: p. 956). An important part of homeostasis involves regulation of body fluids, which helps to maintain the proper functioning of cellular activity. These body fluids consist of intracellular fluid (ICF) fluid and extracellular fluid (ECF). The ECF in blood vessels is called *plasma* and the ECF that surrounds the cells of tissues is known as *interstitial fluid*.

Capillary exchange between plasma and interstitial fluid takes place so that nutrients, oxygen, ions and other nutrients can reach cells and waste material such as carbon dioxide and other metabolic by-products can be removed. More fluid moves slowly out of capillaries by filtration than is removed by reabsorption, so this excess interstitial fluid moves into the lymphatic system to become lymph which eventually moves back into the blood. Lymphatic vessels also carry lipids and lipid-soluble vitamins (A, D, E, K) absorbed through the gastrointestinal tract to the blood. About 20 litres of fluid filters out of capillaries each day. Of this, 17 litres is reabsorbed and the remaining 3 litres enters the lymphatic capillaries and becomes lymph.

6.11.4 Regulation of pulse width: CM perspective

The parameter of width refers to arterial diameter. Normal pulse width requires appropriate volume of Yin fluids (Blood, body fluids and Essence) to fill the vessels.

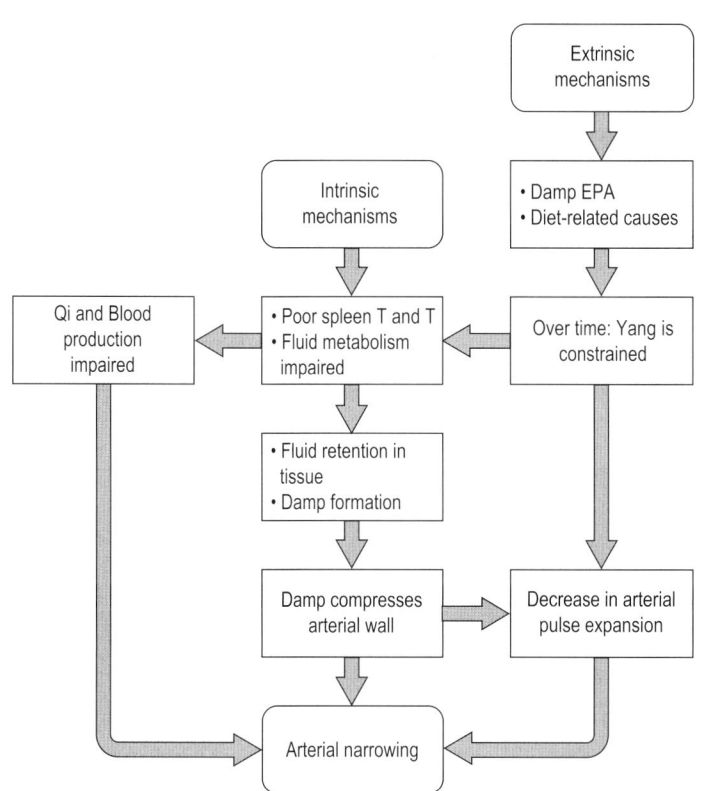

Figure 6.11
Extrinsic and intrinsic mechanisms associated with the formation of pulses with a narrow (thin) arterial width.

The secondary component determining pulse width is sufficient Qi. Sufficient Qi is required to cause the Yin fluids to move in the vessels. This causes the arterial wall to expand, leading to changes in the arterial width. The pulse width is primarily affected when the Yin fluids are affected. This can occur in a number of ways: as a primary problem affecting the fluid volume, or secondary effects on the volume such as quality of Qi and pathogenic factors which affect this (Fig. 6.11). In this context, changes in pulse width occur when the Yin fluids are affected by:

- Internal factors affecting blood volume; fluid can decrease or increase and accordingly the pulse width may also increase or decrease
- External factors such as EPAs affecting blood volume; the Yin or Yang nature of the pathogen determines the effect this will have on pulse width and lateral expansion of the flow wave.

6.11.4.1 Volume of Yin fluids

In CM there are three distinct 'elements' that are incorporated under the concept of 'Yin fluids'. These are blood, Yin Ye (thick and thin fluids not associated with blood) and Essence.

Blood and arterial width

Blood is the primary Yin fluid associated with the arterial pulse. From a palpatory perspective, Chapter 53 in the *Nei Jing* (Ni 1995: p. 190) states:

When the pulse is large and full, there is an abundance of blood. When the pulse is small, thready and weak, there is not enough blood. These conditions are normal; their opposites indicate abnormality.

Blood pathologies affecting pulse width are primarily associated with vacuities (deficiencies). Blood vacuity is associated with either increased or decreased changes in arterial width. The body's response to blood vacuity often depends on the cause or pathogenesis of the vacuity and the presence of complicating factors such as Damp or Qi vacuity. Primary blood vacuities are associated with an increase in arterial width. When there are Qi and/or Damp complications then arterial width decreases. Table 6.8 lists the association between blood and the CM organs.

Body fluids and arterial width

Body fluids are the second component of Yin fluids. Clavey (1995) refers to 'body fluids' or *Jin Ye* as:

All the normal physiological fluids in the body, including internal fluids which may be secreted by the Zang organs, such as tears, saliva, sweat, normal nasal mucus and stomach or Intestinal fluids, and also the fluids which act to moisten the various tissues within the body, such as the skin, the flesh, the tendons, the bones and the marrow (p. 1).

Table 6.8 ● Yin organs and their relationship to blood

Yin organ	Relationship with blood	Production	Function
Spleen	Blood production	The Spleen converts food and drink into Gu Qi that is sent up to the Lungs	Spleen holds the blood in the vessels – easy bruising occurs when this function is impaired
Lung	Blood production	The Lung moves Gu Qi received from the Spleen to the Heart	
Heart	Blood production	The Heart converts Gu Qi from the Lungs into Blood	The Heart governs the Blood and blood vessels
Kidney	Blood production	The Kidneys provide Kidney Essence and Yuan Qi for the conversion of Gu Qi into Blood in the Heart	
Liver	Storage and replenishment of Blood	At night the Blood returns to the Liver to be replenished	The Liver helps Blood to move smoothly through the body by ensuring the smooth flow of Qi

Body fluids are classified as Yin, being substantial (in the form of liquids) in comparison to Qi. They play an important part in nourishing and moistening the various tissues of the body and maintaining the fluidity and volume of blood. They are further differentiated into Jin and Ye, with differing functions and textures. Ye fluids have a thicker and more viscous form, lubricating the organs, bones, joints, marrow and brain, for example the synovial fluids lubricating the joints or cerebrospinal fluid bathing the spinal cord and brain comparable to the transcellular component of ECF described in Box 6.24. Jin fluids are thin, clearer and able to flow swiftly, and are responsible for nourishing and moistening the skin and muscles of the exterior body. Sweat is a clear example of a Jin fluid. These fluids can be used for thermoregulation and are able to be transformed into sweat or urine, in order to regulate the level of fluids in the body. Jin fluids flow with Qi and blood within the blood vessels and can be transformed into blood when necessary. Therefore, both blood and Jin contribute to filling out the blood vessels and expanding the arterial diameter.

The relationship between blood and fluids is apparent in dehydration where fluid moves from the blood to replenish tissue fluids. This is reversed in the case of haemorrhage, where fluids move from the tissues to the blood vessels, in order to maintain a functional blood volume for continuing blood supply to the vital organs.

Vomiting, diarrhoea and excessive sweating or urination are ways in which fluid is also lost from the body. As Jin fluids contribute to blood volume, any loss of body fluids may also result in decreased blood volume and thus decreased arterial width.

Fluid pathologies affecting pulse width are often vacuity related, especially in chronic conditions, but may also result from acute viral or bacterial infections (EPAs). Of the two fluid types, 'thick' or Ye and 'thin' or Jin, it is the Jin fluids which are primarily involved.

Essence and arterial width

Kidney Essence (also known as Kidney Jing) is considered to be one of the fundamental substances that contribute to an individual's overall health. It is involved in our constitutional health, development and reproductive ability and is also responsible for marrow (the brain) and the material foundation of the Shen or Mind (Maciocia 1989). Kidney Essence is closely related to Yuan Qi, considered as Essence in the form of Qi, and has an integral role in the transformation of fluids by the various Zang Fu organs via the Three Heaters. Kidney Essence and Yuan Qi both play an important part of the transformation of blood in the Heart.

Vacuity of Essence affects pulse width, causing a Fine pulse. This can be seen in a vacuity of Kidney Essence/Jing leading to problems with the production of blood or the transformation of fluids. The natural decline of Kidney Jing occurs with age, therefore, as noted in *The Lakeside Master's Study of the Pulse*, the Fine pulse is not unusual in elderly people, but it always indicates a vacuous (deficient) condition.

6.11.4.2 Activity of Qi and arterial width

Qi provides the vitality for the functional operation of the various organs, including the Heart. The Heart is seen as governing or controlling both the blood and the blood vessels. The ability of the Heart to contract and pump blood through the arterial system is dependent on both the condition of Heart Blood and strength of Qi. When the Qi is affected so the heart is affected. This occurs with:

- Qi vacuity
- Pathogenic factors affecting Qi.

Qi vacuity

Vacuity of Qi may affect the strength of the cardiac contraction, resulting in a reduced volume of blood being expelled into the arterial system. This causes a decreased expansion of the radial artery and so can affect the perception of pulse width.

Qi vacuity can also play a role in the accumulation of body fluids and so affects arterial width. Yuan Qi is an important catalyst in the transformation and transportation of Qi and fluids. Therefore vacuity of Yuan Qi can affect any of those steps in the transformative process of fluids.

Pathogenic factors

The presence of a pathogenic factor may impact on the arterial width, causing it to be either narrower or wider than usual.

- Decrease in width: The presence of an internal Yin pathogenic factor such as Damp can decrease arterial width by compressing the artery so that is unable to expand laterally. This may occur due to an abnormal increase in fluid in the connective tissues surrounding the artery, that is, oedema. When Damp causes pulse width to narrow, there is often an underlying vacuity of the body's Qi and blood allowing this to occur. When Qi and blood are strong and Damp is present, pulse width will not decrease.
- Increase in width: The presence of a Yang pathogenic factor such as Heat or Fire can affect the arterial width by agitating Qi and blood, causing it to expand and thereby increasing the arterial diameter. Heat also affects the contractility of the heart with an increase in cardiac contraction causing greater expansion of the vessel by the resultant pulse wave.

6.11.5 Regulation of pulse width: biomedical perspective

The width or size of the pulse, generally speaking, is related to the circulatory blood volume, the cardiac contractility . . . Insufficient filling of blood, weak contraction of the heart and the arteries may cause lowering of blood pressure, which will in turn lead to a small or thready pulse.
(Lu 1996: p. 179).

The circulating blood volume has an effect on the size of the arterial width. A decreased strength of cardiac contraction leads to less blood entering the arterial system, resulting in a decreased expansion of the arterial walls.

Other factors may also influence the arterial width by causing vasoconstriction and vasodilatation of the arteries. This may occur as part of the normal regulation of the body's metabolic processes known as homeostasis. Homeostasis maintains the body's internal environment within set physiological limits (Tortora & Grabowski 2000: p. 6). There are several factors that attempt to maintain or regulate homeostasis, including hormonal influences and other processes regulated by the nervous system.

6.11.5.1 Hormonal influence

The endocrine system produces hormones that can influence the action of the heart, blood vessels and blood volume. This is used to maintain a stable blood pressure and ensure the continuous flow of blood throughout the circulatory system to the vital organs, particularly the brain.

Epinephrine (adrenaline) and norepinephrine causes vasoconstriction of the vessels supplying the abdominal cavity and the skin, while causing vasodilatation of vessels to the brain, lung, heart and skeletal muscles. This comes into play during 'fright, flight or fight' reactions (Tortora and Grabowski 2006: p. 600).

Antidiuretic hormone (ADH) can affect blood volume especially when there has been excessive blood or body fluid loss due to haemorrhage, dehydration, vomiting, diarrhoea or excessive sweating. Its main action is to decrease urine output, thereby retaining extra fluid that can be returned to the blood to maintain blood pressure. Other effects of ADH include decreasing sweat production and constriction of arterioles, which helps to further retain fluids and increase blood pressure.

The cortex of the adrenal gland secretes aldosterone, a hormone that also helps to maintain body fluid balance by controlling the concentration of sodium and potassium ions. By retaining sodium ions (Na^+), this also leads to retention of water and can affect blood volume and arterial width.

Relationship between Qi and Blood

There is a dynamic balance between Qi and blood. Blood depends on the activity of Yang Qi to move it through the blood vessels and Qi depends upon Blood for its nourishing and stabilising influence. When blood becomes vacuous, then the Yang aspect of Qi can become relatively hyperactive. Yang's nature is to move upward and outward and once the anchoring effect of Yin has been eroded then Yang is more difficult to contain. This is reflected in the pulse by the movement of Yang to the superficial level of depth and may also lead to an increase in pulse width.

6.12 CM pulse qualities defined by arterial width

6.12.1 Fine pulse (Xì mài) 细脉

6.12.1.1 Alternative names

Thin, Thready, Minute or Small pulse.

6.12.1.2 Requisite parameters

The Fine pulse is a simple pulse quality with a change solely in the parameter of arterial width, which is decreased.

6.12.1.3 Clinical definition

The Fine pulse is primarily concerned with the physiological presentation of the arterial width, irrespective of the presentation of the arterial flow wave. The Fine pulse has a narrow arterial width. It has a distinctly palpable arterial wall that retains its form with increasing finger pressure. This is not necessarily a forceless pulse and may be a difficult pulse to occlude, even with heavy pressure. It would be expected that the Fine pulse would be relatively strongest at the middle level of depth. If it is felt strongest at either the deep or superficial level of depth, this would respectively suggest the development of either the Weak pulse or Soggy pulse.

6.12.1.4 Identifying whether the Fine pulse is present

Step 1: The pulse is examined at each level of depth. The arterial width is noted at all levels of depth. It would be expected that the pulse should be narrow at all levels of depth where it can be palpated and probably strongest at the middle level of depth.

Step 2: As the deep level of depth is examined, note whether the pulse is easily occluded or whether it takes considerable pressure to stop the pulsations. This information is used to further differentiate the pathogenesis of the pulse.

6.12.1.5 Classical description from the *Mai Jing*

> The fine pulse is a little larger pulse than the faint pulse, a pulse constantly present yet thin.
> *(Wang, Yang (trans) 1997: p. 4).*

Note that the term 'fine' is often used in the literature to denote a specific CM pulse quality, the Fine pulse, or, may also be confusingly used as a descriptive term meaning 'narrow' that is applied to other CM pulse qualities. For example, when a pulse is fine, superficial and lacking in force it is classified as the Soggy pulse.

Box 6.25

Blood vacuity signs and symptoms

Signs and symptoms of Blood vacuity will depend on which Zang organs are affected. In addition to changes in pulse parameters, Blood vacuity signs and symptoms may include:

- Pale face and lips
- Dizziness
- Pale inside lower rim of eye
- Slow return of blood to nail bed following digital pressure
- Dizziness on rising quickly
- Pale tongue colour

In addition to the general signs and symptoms of Blood vacuity there are other signs and symptoms which occur when Blood vacuity involves certain organs. These are:

- Heart: Palpitations, poor memory, anxiousness, trouble falling asleep
- Liver: Numbness or tingling in limbs, cramping in limbs, blurry vision, floaters in the eyes ('spots'), ridges on nails
- Spleen: Digestive disturbances, lighter than normal menstruation or even absent period, weakness of muscles

---

6.12.1.6 CM indications

The Fine pulse is always seen as a pathological pulse quality. Three main patterns are associated with the Fine Pulse:

- Blood and Qi vacuity
- Depletion of body fluids
- Internal pathogenic Damp

All three patterns are vacuity-type disorders, as the pathogenic Damp is the result of an underlying failure of fluids to be transformed properly.

Blood vacuity and Qi vacuity (Box 6.25)

Insufficient blood volume circulating through the arterial system leads to an inadequate expansion of the radial artery, resulting in a narrower than normal arterial diameter. This may be the result of decreased blood volume occurring due to loss of blood or through poor production of blood. In addition, vacuity of blood adversely affects Qi, resulting in Qi vacuity. Qi vacuity affects the strength of cardiac contraction and this in turn affects the capacity of the pulse wave to expand the radial artery.

Blood vacuity arises from dysfunction in the production and storage of blood or vacuity due to the loss of blood (Box 6.26).

Box 6.26

Causes of Blood loss and vacuity contributing to the formation of the Fine pulse

- Menorrhagia (excessive menstrual bleeding)
- Metrorrhagia (uterine bleeding outside menstruation)
- Nosebleeds
- Haemorrhage (for example, due to trauma or childbirth)
- Haemoptysis
- Gastrointestinal bleeding (for example, stomach ulcer, ulcerative colitis, coeliac disease)
- Poor production of blood can arise as a result of organ-based dysfunction (not producing blood) or through dietary causes (organ functioning well but there are insufficient sources of dietary iron or vitamin B_{12}).

Box 6.27

Vacuity of body fluids as a compensatory response to blood loss

- If excessive blood loss occurs, then compensatory mechanisms draw on body fluids outside the blood vessels to replace the fluid within the arterial system. This can then result in deficiency of body fluids, with signs and symptoms such as thirst, dry mucous membranes (such as nose, mouth and eyes, dry throat), cracked lips, decreased urine output, lack of sweating, and dry skin. Depending on the organs affected, menstrual bleeding may become lighter and constipation may occur.
- If there is excessive loss of body fluids, then fluids may leave the arterial system to help replace the lost body fluids. This results in the blood vessels 'empty and deficient, a condition known as 'jin withered and blood parched'. As Clavey notes, this can result in severe Shen disturbances, as blood is considered to be the residence of the Shen (Clavey 1995: p. 14).

- Dysfunction in the production or storage of blood: The production of blood involves the interaction of the Spleen, Lung, Heart and Kidney (as noted in Table 6.8) and the Liver plays an important part in the storage of blood. Therefore, although blood vacuity can involve dysfunction any of these organs, it usually involves dysfunction of the Spleen, Heart or the Liver (Maciocia 2004, Wiseman & Ye 1998).

- Loss of blood through abnormal bleeding: If blood vacuity continues to occur untreated then eventually the loss in Yin fluids via blood will lead to a relative imbalance between Yin and Yang, with Yang becoming relatively excessive. Yin is no longer able to exert a stabilising and constraining effect on Yang, resulting in Yang following its natural behaviour of moving outwards and upwards. This results in a pulse that can be felt wider and at a more superficial level of depth than usual and may see a progression of the fine pulse into a Scallion stalk or Vacuous pulse.

Depletion of body fluids

As previously described, there is a close relationship between blood and body fluids, with body fluids moving into the blood vessels when necessary to replenish blood and maintain its volume and vice versa. The causes of body fluid loss are varied and include excessive sweating, vomiting, diarrhoea or urination (Box 6.27).

If there is an excessive loss of body fluids this can also affect the quality and quantity of blood, as there are insufficient body fluids to replenish blood. If severe, body fluids will move from the blood volume to replenish the fluids in the tissue. This may also result in a decreased arterial diameter.

A consequence of movement of fluid in and out of the arterial system would be a change in the viscosity of the blood. An increase in the viscosity of blood can lead to changes in blood viscosity and the smoothness of blood flow (see section 2.3).

Depletion of Kidney Essence may also result in a narrow arterial wall, due to its contribution to the formation of both blood and body fluids via Yuan Qi and Kidney Yang. Depletion of Kidney Essence may arise from natural decline with age, constitutional weakness, or excessive sexual activity.

Internal pathogenic Damp

Pathogenic Damp may arise from dysfunction of the Spleen, which is unable to transform and move fluids correctly. If fluids are not transformed properly, then excessive fluid may leak into the area under the skin (connective tissue layer) exerting increased pressure on the vessels in this layer. This compresses the radial artery so that it cannot expand to its normal width. This also results in a pulse that is not necessarily forceless, as the volume of Blood is being compressed into a smaller arterial diameter.

6.12.1.7 Other literature descriptions

There appears to be differences in the pulse literature regarding the severity of the pathology underlying the Fine pulse:

- Maciocia (2004: p. 480) describes this pulse as indicating a severe deficiency of blood and Qi. It is seen as reflecting a more severe deficiency of blood

Box 6.28

Summary of causes of change in arterial width

A decrease in pulse width or size can indicate:

- Vacuity of Yin fluids such as blood, body fluids or Essence resulting in insufficient blood or Yin fluids to sufficiently fill the vessel
- Insufficient Qi to propel the blood to the periphery of the body and expand the vessel
- Pathogenic damp compressing the vessel.

An increase in the width of the pulse can indicate:

- The presence of a Yang pathogen which can agitate or cause excessive movement of Qi and Blood. Heat has an expansive quality
- Blood vacuity causing a relative hyperactivity of Yang – floating and wide due to Yin being unable to contain or anchor Yang

Box 6.29

Effect of acupuncture on radial artery width

In a study by Boutouyrie et al. (2001) looking at the effect of acupuncture on radial artery haemodynamics, in subjects with previous experience of acupuncture, real acupuncture was shown to statistically significantly increase the radial artery diameter (pulse width). There was no change during the sham acupuncture. It was suggested in this study that, 'acupuncture might be able to decrease smooth muscle tone at the site of a muscular artery'. This occurs due to inhibition of sympathetic vasoconstriction. It hypothesized that this may occur via numerous mechanisms: endogenous opioids (because naloxone counteracted this effect), a centrally mediated reflex response and a presynaptic inhibition of sympathetic nerves. The inhibition of sympathetic vasoconstriction will also have an effect upon arterial tension, resulting in an arterial wall that does not feel as 'hard' on palpation. (Refer to arterial wall tension parameter in Chapter 7.)

Interestingly, in this study in naive subjects (subjects that had never had acupuncture before) the radial arterial diameter did not change during real or sham acupuncture. Clinically, the results of the study may have implications for practitioners that use perceived changes in the radial pulse to successfully gauge treatment effects, in regards to using this technique with naive (first time) acupuncture clients.

than the Rough pulse (defined by Maciocia as the Choppy pulse).

- Lu (1996: p. 101) describes the Fine pulse as indicating a mild deficiency while the 'Feeble' pulse (known in this text as the Faint pulse) indicates 'severe deficiency' such as collapse of Yang due to profuse sweating or massive haemorrhage.
- Li Shi-zhen notes that this pulse would be appropriate if seen in a weak or elderly person.

A common thread linking these opinions is that a vacuity condition of Qi and Yin fluids is the underlying mechanism for the formation of this pulse (Box 6.28). It is the presentation of varying accompanying signs and symptoms that can assist in further differentiating the pathogenesis.

6.13 Summary

This concludes the chapter on the simple pulse parameters of rate, rhythm, depth, length and width and their associated CM pulse qualities. These are considered to be simple pulse qualities because they are defined by changes in either a single pulse parameter or, at most, two pulse parameters (Table 6.9).

If there is one message to take from this chapter it is that changes in the pulse parameters are always happening and this is considered normal or healthy when those changes are in response to maintaining homeostasis or Yin/Yang balance through day-to-day activities. It is when the changes in the pulse parameters are sustained that dysfunction is often indicated, and it is only when the change in the parameter is excessive that it warrants categorisation as a CM pulse quality. For example, an increase in pulse rate does not necessarily mean that the pulse is Rapid. It is only a Rapid pulse when the pulse rate exceeds 90 bpm. So with this in mind, it is acceptable not to feel a CM pulse quality as is defined in the literature, and not all changes in the pulse parameters will always form a CM pulse quality.

Thus, rather than always focusing on the CM pulse qualities it is just as important to understand the diagnostic meaning of pulse parameter changes, how and why these occur and the related diagnostic meaning. In this way the information provided by parameter changes is very important for diagnostic purposes.

In the following chapter we move on to the more complex pulse parameters such as arterial wall tension, pulse force, pulse occlusion and pulse contour. It is the various combinations of these complex parameters in conjunction with the simple parameters that produce the more complex CM pulse qualities such as the Firm pulse or the Soggy pulse, to name but two.

Table 6.9 ● Summary of the simple CM pulse qualities and their related parameters and indications

CM pulse quality	Pulse parameters involved	Change in parameter	Indications
Rapid pulse	Rate	Increase in rate: >90 bpm	Pathogenic Heat or Fire, heart dysfunction, Yin vacuity
Slow pulse	Rate	Decrease in rate: <60 bpm	Pathogenic Cold or sign of health, Yang vacuity
Moderate pulse	Rate	Rate of 60 bpm	Pathogenic Damp or sign of health
Skipping pulse	Rate Rhythm	Increase in rate: >90 bpm Irregular pause in rhythm	Pathogenic Heat or Fire Heart arrhythmia due to heart dysfunction, e.g. pacemaker, Hyperthyroidism
Bound pulse	Rate Rhythm	Decrease in rate: <60 bpm Irregular pause in rhythm	Pathogenic cold Heart arrhythmia due to heart dysfunction, e.g. pacemaker, Hypothyroidism
Intermittent pulse	Rhythm	Regular interruption to rhythm, the closer the pauses, the more severe the condition.	Serious heart disease Severe pain Chronic disease
Floating pulse	Level of depth at which pulse is felt relatively strongest	Felt relatively strongest at the superficial level of depth Cannot be felt at the deep level of depth	External Replete condition: Attack of EPA such as Wind Heat or Wind Cold Internal Vacuous condition: Yin Vacuity
Sinking pulse	Level of depth at which pulse is felt relatively strongest	Felt relatively strongest at the deep level of depth	Internal replete condition: pathogenic factor of cold or damp, retention of food, phlegm Internal vacuous condition: Yang Qi vacuity, vacuity of Yin organs
Hidden pulse	Level of depth at which pulse is felt relatively strongest	Very difficult to palpate, requiring extremely strong digital pressure. Felt relatively strongest beyond the deep level of depth Cannot be felt at the superficial or middle levels of depth	Internal Replete condition: pathogenic factor of cold or damp, retention of food, phlegm, toxic Fire Internal vacuous condition: severe Yang vacuity leading to strong internal cold
Long pulse	Length	An increase in length: can be felt at Cun, Guan and Chi and beyond Chi and/or beyond Cun	Internal Heat or Fire Sign of good health: abundant Qi and Blood Liver disharmony
Short pulse	Length	A decrease in length: can be felt only in one or two pulse positions	Vacuity: Vacuity of Qi Repletion: Stagnation of Qi
Fine pulse	Arterial width	Decrease in arterial diameter: narrow	Deficiency of blood, body fluids or Kidney Essence

References

AtCor Medical 2006 A clinical guide: pulse wave analysis. AtCor Medical, West Ryde, NSW

Boutouyrie P, Corvisier K, Azizi M et al 2001 Effects of acupuncture on radial artery haemodynamics: controlled trials in sensitized and naive subjects American Journal of Physiology-Heart and Circulatory Physiology 280: 628–633.

Braunwald E, Fauci A, Kasper D et al (eds) Harrison's principles of internal medicine, Volume 1, 15th edn. McGraw-Hill, New York

Clavey S 1995 Fluid physiology and pathology in traditional Chinese medicine. Churchill Livingstone, South Melbourne

Constant J 1999 Bedside cardiology. Lippincott Williams and Wilkins, Philadelphia

Deng T 1999 Practical diagnosis in traditional Chinese medicine. Churchill Livingstone, Edinburgh

Danzl D 2001 Hypothermia and frostbite. In: Braunwald E, Fauci A, Kasper D et al (eds) Harrison's principles of internal medicine, Volume 1, 15th edn. McGraw-Hill, New York, Ch 20

Epstein O, Perkin G D, de Bono D P, Cookson J 1992 Clinical examination. Mosby-Wolfe, London

Estes M 2006 Health assessment and physical examination, 3rd edn. Thomson Delmar Learning, Southbank, Vic

Flaws B 1994 Statements of fact in traditional Chinese medicine. Blue Poppy Press, Boulder, CO

Funnell R, Koutoukidis G, Larence K 2005 Tabner's nursing care: theory and practice, 4th edn. Elsevier, Sydney

Guangzhou Chinese Medicine College April, 1991 Inspection of the tongue and pulse taking. Guangzhou, China.

Guyton A, Hall J 2006 Textbook of medical physiology, 11th edn. Elsevier Saunders, Philadelphia

Katz A 2000 Heart failure pathophysiology, molecular biology and clinical management. Lippincott Williams and Wilkins, Philadelphia

Lee T 2001 Chest discomfort and palpitations. In: Braunwald E, Fauci A, Kasper D et al (eds) Harrison's principles of internal medicine, Volume 1, 15th edn. McGraw-Hill, New York, Ch 13

Li S Z, Flaws B (trans) 1998 The lakeside master's study of the pulse. Blue Poppy Press, Boulder, CO

Lu Y 1996 Pulse diagnosis. Science and Technology Press, Jinan

Lyttleton J 2004 Treatment of infertility with Chinese medicine. Churchill Livingstone, Edinburgh

Maciocia G 1989 The foundations of Chinese medicine. Churchill Livingstone, Edinburgh

Maciocia G 2004 Diagnosis in Chinese medicine: a comprehensive guide. Churchill Livingstone, Edinburgh

Marieb E N 2001 Human anatomy and physiology, 5th edn. Benjamin Cummings, San Francisco

McCance K L, Huether S E 2006 Pathophysiology: the biologic basis for disease in adults and children, 5th edn. Elsevier/Mosby, St Louis

Mitchell C, Feng Y, Wiseman N 1999 Shang han lun on cold damage: translation and commentaries. Paradigm, Brookline, MA

Ni M (trans) 1995 The Yellow Emperor's classic of medicine: a new translation of the neijing suwen with commentary. Shambala, Boston

Perk G, Stressman J, Ginsberg G et al 2003 Sex differences in the effect of heart rate on mortality in the elderly. Journal of the American Geriatrics Society 51(9);1260–1264

Stables D, Rankin J (editors) 2005 Physiology in childbearing with anatomy and related biosciences. Elsevier, Edinburgh

Tortora G J, Grabowski S R 2000 Principles of anatomy and physiology, 9th edn. John Wiley and Sons, Inc., New York

Townsend G, De Donna Y 1990 Pulses and impulses. Thorsons, Wellingborough

Unschuld P 2003 Huang di nei jing su wen. University of California Press, Berkeley

Unschuld P 1986 Nan ching: the classic of difficult issues. University of California Press, Berkeley

Wang S H, Yang S (translator) 1997 The pulse classic: a translation of the mai jing. Blue Poppy Press, Boulder, CO

Wiseman N, Ye F 1998 A practical dictionary of Chinese medicine, 2nd edn. Paradigm Publications, Brookline, MA

Complex CM pulse qualities and associated pulse parameters

7

Chapter contents

7.1 Introduction 115
7.2 The complex pulse parameters 115
7.3 Arterial wall tension 116
7.4 Pulse occlusion 120
7.5 CM pulse qualities defined by arterial wall tension and ease of pulse occlusion 123
7.6 Pulse force 137
7.7 CM pulse qualities defined by pulse force 142
7.8 Pulse contour and flow wave 154
7.9 CM pulses defined by pulse contour 158
7.10 Revision of the 27 CM pulse qualities 170
7.11 Using the pulse parameter system 170

7.1 Introduction

This chapter introduces the more complex CM pulse qualities and the pulse parameters associated with them. The complexity of these CM pulse qualities is related to:

- The increased number of changes in pulse parameters associated with each CM pulse quality
- The complexity of each of the associated pulse parameters.

The complex CM pulse qualities are characterised by changes to *two or more* of the pulse parameters. For each to be defined as a specific CM pulse quality, it is necessary for changes in all the requisite parameters to be present.

7.2 The complex pulse parameters

In this chapter we examine four complex pulse parameters:

- Arterial wall tension
- Ease of occlusion
- Force
- Flow wave and pulse contour.

Although there may be changes in a number of pulse parameters for a complex CM pulse quality, usually one key parameter is considered to be the defining aspect of that particular CM pulse quality. This key parameter is often used to loosely categorise the CM pulse qualities. It should be noted that different CM texts may utilise different ways of grouping the CM pulses, according to differing pulse parameters.

Changes in these pulse parameters are associated with 15 of the 27 traditional CM pulse qualities. The CM pulse qualities associated with each of the complex pulse parameters are:

- Defined primarily by arterial tension and ease of occlusion: Stringlike (Wiry) pulse, Scallion Stalk pulse, Drumskin pulse, Tight pulse, Scattered pulse

- Defined primarily by pulse force and ease of occlusion: Replete pulse, Firm pulse, Weak pulse, Vacuous pulse, Soggy pulse, Faint pulse
- Defined primarily by flow wave and pulse contour: Slippery pulse, Rough pulse, Surging pulse, Stirred pulse.

As noted above, the pulse parameter of pulse occlusion plays an important role in the differentiation of the traditional CM pulse qualities associated with both arterial tension and pulse force.

The complex pulse parameters are so named because, unlike the simple parameters such as rate or rhythm, there is no single objective measurement to definitively evaluate these parameters. They encompass a number of different physiological characteristics involving the actual structure of the artery and the manner in which it responds to the pressure wave that is produced from cardiac contraction. The quality and quantity of blood volume and blood flow, cardiac function and the variability of smooth muscle tone within the arterial wall are equally important factors that impact on the radial artery pulsation. It is the degree to which these factors are involved that determines the specific CM pulse quality produced.

7.3 Arterial wall tension

The parameter of arterial wall tension is a complex pulse parameter, primarily concerned with the physical structure of the artery wall. The degree of arterial wall tension informs us about the functional state of Qi (particularly Yang) in the body. It is necessary to have some tension in the arterial wall. It is when the degree of arterial tension varies from the norm that this is seen as a diagnostic indicator of pathology. For example, variations in tension can result from the stasis or obstruction of Qi and/or blood, an underlying vacuity of Yin fluids and/or blood, or the vacuity of Qi (especially Yang).

The specific CM pulse qualities associated with this parameter are differentiated by the degree of arterial wall tension, ranging from greatly increased tension to a marked reduction. In this sense, it is not the pulse wave that is being assessed but rather the arterial structure. The tension, or lack of tension, in the artery is assessed distinctly differently from the actual shape of the pulse wave.

Five CM pulse qualities are defined primarily by the parameter of arterial wall tension:

- Stringlike (Wiry) pulse (section 7.5.1)
- Tight pulse (section 7.5.2)
- Scallion Stalk pulse (section 7.5.3)
- Drumskin pulse (section 7.5.4)
- Scattered pulse (section 7.5.5).

7.3.1 Differentiation of the CM pulse qualities primarily defined by changes in arterial wall tension

The five CM pulse qualities primarily defined by the degree of tension in the arterial wall range greatly in their presentation. At one extreme is the Stringlike (Wiry) pulse that resists deformation with finger pressure because of the significant increase in arterial wall tension. At the other extreme, the Scattered pulse is characterised by its distinct reduction in arterial tension, which makes it difficult to manually detect the presence of the arterial wall at all. The Drumskin pulse and Scallion Stalk pulse are also defined by the increased tension in the arterial wall. However, when increasing finger pressure is applied to the artery, the arterial wall has only momentary resistance before succumbing to the pressure, a result of their underlying vacuity. In this sense, they are 'empty'. Further, a distinguishing feature of the Scallion Stalk pulse is the ability of the arterial wall to remain distinct and pliable even when the pulsation in the artery has been occluded.

In addition to changes in arterial wall tension, accompanying changes in other pulse parameters, such as pulse width, force and depth, further differentiate these five CM pulse qualities. However, it is the increase or decrease in tension in the arterial wall of these five pulses that predominantly differentiates them from the other traditional CM pulse qualities.

To further qualify this: the term 'arterial wall tension' has been used to encompass a range of different mechanisms that result in the arterial wall being able to be felt distinctly on palpation. The differing mechanisms influence how the increased arterial wall tension manifests in each pulse quality, depending on the involvement of other pulse parameters. For example, the Stringlike (Wiry) pulse and Tight pulse tend to arise due to increased smooth muscle tension within the artery wall, while the Tight pulse may additionally include sclerotic changes to the arterial wall, causing stiffness and a decreased ability to expand easily. So the underlying condition of the arterial wall may well influence how changes in pulse parameters manifest. For the Scallion Stalk pulse, a combination of increased arterial tension and decreased blood viscosity lead to its distinctive manifestation of pliable arterial wall and easy occlusion. This is replicated in the Drumskin pulse but complicated further by the presence of pathogenic Cold.

Constitutional body types may also influence the manner in which changes in pulse parameters present. For example, in an slim individual with a small build, who has smaller arteries than someone with a taller, larger build, increased arterial wall tension may result in a more typically Stringlike (Wiry) type pulse than it would in someone with a wider artery. However, it is the maintenance of this tension with increasing finger pressure, regardless of the width, that signifies the Stringlike (Wiry) pulse.

7.3.2 Definition of arterial wall tension

The degree of arterial wall tension is denoted by the level of clarity or distinctness felt in the artery wall with the palpating fingers.

Three factors are involved in the parameter of arterial wall tension:

- The distensibility and compliance of the arterial wall to pressure changes, whether this occurs internally from the pulse wave or externally from the pressure exerted by the practitioner's fingertips
- The tone of the smooth muscle component in the arterial wall structure
- Secondary tensile changes occurring in the arterial wall structure unrelated to vascular smooth muscle.

Arterial tension contributes to the perceived 'hardness' of the arterial wall on palpation. When arterial tension is present, the artery can be easily distinguished from the tethering support of the surrounding connective tissue. Equally, a lack of arterial tension makes it difficult to distinguish the artery from the surrounding tissue.

Increased arterial wall tension can occur in both replete or vacuity conditions as a result of different physiological mechanisms. For example, increased arterial wall tension may occur in response to Yin vacuity or loss of Yin fluids, resulting in the relative hyperactivity of Yang and accordingly, increased arterial tension. The Scallion Stalk pulse is a good example of a vacuity-type pulse quality, where tension is not associated with vascular smooth muscle contraction but with tension in other parts of the rigid arterial wall structure (see section 7.3.5.2 Alternative mechanism for increased arterial wall tension). Alternatively, a Cold pathogen may lead to increased arterial wall tension by its contracting nature, obstructing Qi and blood flow. This pathogenic factor is considered to be an excess pattern, reflected in an increase in pulse force and arterial width and an increase in arterial wall tension associated with increased smooth muscle tone. The Tight pulse and the Firm pulse are good examples of excess-type CM pulse qualities with increased arterial tension due to contraction of vascular smooth muscle. Qi stasis may also result in hyperactivity of Yang Qi thus leading to increased tension

7.3.3 Arterial wall tension and its assessment

Assessing the arterial wall tension requires the use of two separate techniques:

- Assessment of the physical characteristics of the radial artery wall to determine the degree of arterial tension
- Assessment of pulse occlusion.

7.3.3.1 Assessment of arterial tension

Assessment of arterial wall tension employs the same technique as used in assessment of arterial width. This is initiated by placing the fingers on the skin surface above the radial artery at the three traditional pulse positions and moving them laterally from side to side, using a rolling type motion. This technique has been previously described in section 6.12.1 (see Fig. 6.10 depicting lateral sideways movement of fingers). When the artery is located deeper in the flesh then further finger pressure is required to locate this before moving from side to side. Be careful not to use excessive pressure when assessing for arterial wall tension, because the parameter is associated with both vacuity and replete-type pulses. If too much pressure is applied, then for the vacuity patterns the arterial wall becomes deformed and assessment of the arterial tension is compromised. Pressure needs to move over the artery without compressing it.

7.3.3.2 Assessment of pulse occlusion

Assessment of pulse occlusion requires compression of the arterial wall; in particular, this involves determining what happens to both the arterial wall and the pulsation when increasing pressure is exerted on it by the fingers. That is, does the wall retain its distinctive shape or is it easily deformed, does it easily regain its original form when pressure is released and how easy is it to occlude the arterial pulsation? (Box 7.1)

To assess ease of pulse occlusion, the fingers are placed at the three traditional pulse positions and finger pressure is gradually increased over the radial artery until pulsations can no longer be felt. This is held for five seconds. There are two subcategories for ease of occlusion:

- Easy to occlude: A pulse that is classified as easy to occlude requires little pressure exerted on it to halt

---

Box 7.1

Hints for assessing arterial tension
When assessing arterial tension, don't focus on any pulsatile movement. Rather, your attention needs to focus on the actual arterial structure. The lateral movement of the assessing fingers will help you in this, disguising arterial movement while assisting in feeling the artery.

the pulsations, with either the arterial walls easily compressed or the arterial pulsation being easily stopped. The level of depth at which the pulsation can be felt strongest does not affect pulse occlusion. That is, both superficially and deeply located pulses may be easily occluded.

- Difficult to occlude: Significant pressure is required to occlude the pulse, equal to the pressure that is needed to palpate to the deep level. In some cases, the pulse may be still felt under the fingers. Sometimes the pulse can still be felt at the side of the proximal side of the ring finger. This is seen as an indicator of pulse strength

7.3.3.3 Interpretation of findings

When arterial wall tension is increased above normal, the artery feels very distinct and can still be clearly felt under the fingers when pressure is applied into the deeper levels of depth. In the extreme case it is even difficult to indent the arterial wall at the deep level of depth. At the other extreme, a lack of tension often means that only a pulsation can be felt; there is no evidence of the arterial wall. In this situation when the fingers are moved from side to side on the wrist where the artery is situated, only the soft skin of the wrist can be felt; there is no indication of the artery. Of course, between these two extremes there is a range of degrees of arterial tension.

7.3.3.4 Normal levels of arterial tension

Ideally, some tension in the arterial wall is required for a pulse to be classified as healthy. Such a phenomenon is due to sympathetic vasomotor tone, which will be discussed in more detail shortly. When considered healthy, arterial tension should be felt so that there is a distinct 'impression' of the arterial wall so that the width can be ascertained, but it is not 'hard'.

7.3.4 Regulation of arterial tension: CM perspective

From a CM perspective, arterial tension is particularly related to Yang Qi. Therefore factors that affect Yang Qi affect arterial tension. Variations in arterial wall tension may arise as a result of hyperactivity of Yang Qi due to obstruction or stasis, vacuity of Yang Qi or damage to Yin fluids, or as the result of emotional stress.

7.3.4.1 Role of Yang Qi

Pulse tension depends on the functional state of Yang Qi. Lu (1996: p.109) quotes from the *Nei Jing* 'When Yang Qi functions normally, it can maintain the flexibility of the tendons and vessels.' This is explained

further, that arterial tension increases when Yang Qi is hyperactive and decreases when Yang Qi is deficient. A good example of this is the Stringlike (Wiry) pulse that results from a hyperactivity of Liver Yang Qi. Conversely, when Yang Qi is deficient the arterial wall may be difficult to feel clearly, as in the Scattered pulse.

7.3.4.2 Effect of Yin and Blood deficiency on arterial tension

Both Yin and Blood, as a Yin fluid, not only act as carriers for Qi but also have a balancing, cooling and nourishing effect on Yang, allowing it, among other responsibilities, to maintain the normal tension in the arterial walls. If that harmonising effect is impaired through loss of Yin (in numerous ways such as acute or chronic loss of blood or body fluids through sweating, vomiting or diarrhoea) then this may have a number of effects on the pulse. In the case of arterial tension, Yang Qi becomes relatively hyperactive, leading to an increase in arterial wall tension.

7.3.4.3 Emotions and arterial wall tension

In CM, emotional stress is considered to be a major cause of disease due to the flow-over effect on the physical body. The expression of a range of emotional responses is considered to be a healthy part of the normal psyche, but if any of these becomes prolonged or excessive in nature, or is not expressed freely, this may have an adverse effect on the individual's health. Most commonly this may affect the normal flow of Qi, which, if sustained, may lead to problems of Qi stagnation.

In particular, the Liver is susceptible to emotional disturbance, particularly anger or frustration or the inhibition of emotional responses. As the Liver has a vital role in maintaining the free flow of Qi and consequently blood, factors impacting on the Liver may also affect arterial tension.

7.3.5 Regulation of arterial wall tension: biomedical perspective

The nervous system is responsible for controlling general blood flow to different regions of the body, heart activity and arterial blood pressure regulation as discussed by Guyton & Hall (2006: pp. 204–215) in Chapter 18. It does so via the autonomic nervous system in which the sympathetic nervous system plays an integral role. Most of the blood vessels in the body (except the capillaries, precapillary sphincters and metarterioles) are innervated via sympathetic vasomotor nerve fibres that leave the spinal cord through the thoracic and upper two lumbar spinal nerves. These enter the sympathetic chain and then travel to the

Box 7.2

Effects of the autonomic nervous system on blood flow

- Increased sympathetic activity increases heart rate and strength of cardiac contraction
- Increased parasympathetic activity decreases heart rate, but the effect on heart contractility is only minor.

heart and viscera via specific sympathetic nerves, or travel through the spinal nerves to the blood vessels at the periphery of the body. Higher control from the vasomotor centre located in the medulla and pons of the brain transmits sympathetic impulses to the blood vessels around the body and parasympathetic impulses to the heart via the vagus nerves (Guyton & Hall 2006: p. 206). Blood flow is regulated via vasoconstriction or vasodilatation of the blood vessels (Box 7.2).

7.3.5.1 Sympathetic vasoconstrictor tone

The perceived 'hardness' of the radial arterial wall relates to the tone of the vascular smooth muscle in the tunica media of the blood vessels wall and is influenced by the nervous system's effect on the contraction and expansion of the arteries (Lu 1996: p. 179). (See Fig. 2.5 for layers of the muscular arteries.)

Under normal conditions there is a 'partial state of contraction in the blood vessels, called vasomotor tone' caused by the vasomotor centre in the brain sending continual signals to the vasoconstrictor nerve fibres systemically. This helps to maintain pressure within the arterial system (Guyton & Hall, 2006: p. 206).

7.3.5.2 Alternative mechanism for increased arterial wall tension

The distinctness of the arterial wall is not always due to vasoconstriction. The Scallion Stalk pulse and the Drumskin pulse are examples of pulse qualities that have a distinct arterial wall that is not due to increased vascular smooth muscle tone. The maintenance of a distinct arterial wall such as that perceived in the Scallion Stalk and Drumskin pulses in the presence of vascular smooth muscle relaxation causing vasodilatation (as a consequence of compensatory response to blood loss) may be explained as follows. Kelly & Chowienczyk (2002) state that in muscular arteries such as the radial artery, decreased vascular smooth muscle tone usually leads to increased compliance (the ability to accommodate large volumes with little increase in arterial pressure). As vessel diameter increases, compliance usually does too. However, this does not always happen.

Sometimes very large decreases in vascular smooth muscle (i.e. in a fully relaxed state) may result in the stress being transferred to other rigid components of the arterial wall and this then leads to decreased compliance. This may hypothetically explain the appearance of the Scallion Stalk or Drumskin pulses so that even though the arterial diameter is increased (signifying vasodilatation and therefore relaxation of the smooth muscle) the arterial wall still has increased definition.

7.3.5.3 Effects of febrile conditions and the shiver reflex

Febrile disease (caused by factors such as bacterial infection, environmental conditions, dehydration or tissue damage) has an effect on the temperature control centre in the hypothalamus, resetting the body temperature to a higher than normal value (Guyton & Hall 2006: pp. 898–901). As a result, the current body temperature is now below the new set point so a number of mechanisms are activated to help raise the body temperature to the new level. They include skin vasoconstriction, thyroxine secretion and sympathetic nervous system effects to increase cellular metabolism. During this time the individual usually feels very cold, the skin is cold because of vasoconstriction and this stimulates shivering which is experienced as 'chills'. The shivering reflex increases the tone of the skeletal muscles throughout the body.

Hypothetically, the combination of the sympathetic effects on the blood vessels, causing vasoconstriction, in conjunction with the increased muscular tone, may result in increased radial arterial wall tension. This may explain why the Tight pulse is described as appearing in acute conditions such as an attack of EPA of Cold, accompanied by fever and chills.

7.3.5.4 Arterial tension and hypertension

From a biomedical point of view, the specific cause of primary hypertension is largely unknown, with a combination of genetic and environmental factors thought to be responsible for its progression according to Brashes (Chapter 30 in McCance & Huether 2006: pp. 1086–1092). It appears that a number of factors may lead to increased blood volume and increased peripheral resistance including overactivity of the sympathetic nervous system (increased vasoconstriction and cardiac output), overactivity of control of vascular tone and defects in excretion of sodium by the kidneys, leading to increased water retention and therefore increased blood volume. As the cardiovascular system attempts to deal with the increased blood volume, cardiac output increases, then regulatory vasoconstriction occurs. Blood volume remains high and as a result the increased peripheral resistance leads to increased arterial pressure, hence hypertension.

The vasoconstriction of the systemic arteries and resulting increased peripheral resistance may explain why increased arterial wall tension is considered to appear in hypertension, with some authors citing the Stringlike (wiry) pulse or the Tight pulse as occurring in this condition (Maciocia 2004, Wiseman & Ellis 1996). Researchers at the First PLA Medical University, Guangzhou found that 'Most patients suffering from coronary heart disease have string-like pulse due mainly to disorder of cardiac function, lowered arterial compliance and increased total peripheral resistance' (Chen, Lin, Meng et al 1996). Utilising a combination of manual palpation to identify possible CM pulse qualities and biomedical cardiac function indices, they found generally that the coronary disease group were assessed as having 'taut pulses' (113 out of 120 cases) as well as having decreased myocardial contractility, stroke volume, left ventricular and arterial compliance, impaired left ventricular function and increased total peripheral resistance. It was surmised that the formation of the Stringlike (Wiry) pulse was due to a combination of factors such as arteriosclerosis, decreased vascular compliance and increased peripheral resistance. While the majority of patients were considered to have 'taut pulses' it appeared that these tended to appear in combinations with other CM pulse qualities such as Slippery, Slow, Thready and Rapid. However, there was no further breakdown of the group into subcategories. In addition, no concrete definition was provided for the term 'taut' and this seems to have been used interchangeably with the term 'stringlike'.

The Guangzhou College (1991) notes explain that the mechanism of the taut (Stringlike) pulse may be due to increased vasoconstriction or increased blood volume or a combination of both, caused by arteriosclerosis which leads to increased arterial pressure and peripheral vascular resistance.

7.3.5.5 Arterial tension versus arterial hardening

The distensible nature of the vascular system refers to the ability of the arteries and veins to expand and accommodate pressure changes: both those associated with normal moment-to-moment changes with heart contraction and long-term pressure changes with hypertension and hypotension. This reflects the body's normal ability to respond to the nervous system's signals for vasoconstriction or vasodilatation.

As discussed by Brashers (Ch. 30 in McCance & Huether 2006: pp. 1086–1092), factors such as arteriosclerosis can affect the stiffness of arterial walls impacting upon their ability to dilate or constrict. Arteriosclerosis is caused by thickening and hardening within the arterial wall with eventual narrowing of the arterial lumen. While perhaps due to normal aging, it may also play a role in hypertension and other circula-

tory disorders. Atherosclerosis is an inflammatory pathological change to the arterial system that results in the laying down of fatty plaques in the walls of the medium-sized and large arteries. This has effects on blood flow via a decreased lumen due to the presence of atherosclerotic plaques and other changes to the arterial wall. It plays a major role in coronary artery disease and cerebrovascular disease (stroke) by causing obstruction to blood flow. However, it has been noted by O'Rourke et al (1992: p. 98) that despite the obstructive effects on the coronary and cerebral blood vessels, it appears that atherosclerosis has 'little effect on the transmission of the pulse over long lengths of the aorta or other conduit arteries' and the 'contour of the brachial or radial arteries is rarely altered'.

7.3.5.6 Other factors influencing vascular tone

The ability of the vascular walls to dilate and constrict is influenced not only by the nervous system activity but also by substances that are actively produced by the endothelial cells lining the inside of the blood vessels. These substances play a role in influencing the tone and structure of the arterial wall and also influence its susceptibility to damage such as atherosclerosis. Nitric oxide (which causes vasorelaxation) and endothelin (a strong vasoconstrictor) are mediators produced by the endothelium and participate in the regulation of both basal vascular tone and blood pressure (Cockcroft et al 1997: p. 55). It is hypothesised that increased arterial stiffness may therefore result not only from physical changes to arterial wall structure due to ageing and arteriosclerosis, but also from endothelial dysfunction, affecting the availability of nitric oxide.

7.3.5.7 Ageing and arterial changes

Generalised degenerative changes to the arterial tunica media are responsible for arterial stiffness leading to changes in arterial pressure with age, and this is emphasised with arteriosclerosis (O'Rourke et al 1992: p. 98). Arteriosclerosis reduces arterial compliance and affects the ability of the arteries to expand and contract to the changing pressures during systole and diastole. The stiffening of the arteries occurring with ageing is distinct from that of atherosclerosis, which affects mainly the intimal layer of the artery wall.

7.4 Pulse occlusion

Pulse occlusion refers to the method of applying finger pressure to temporarily stop the pulsation in the radial artery by compressing it against the radius. Specifically, we use the term 'ease of occlusion' to refer to the amount of pressure that is required to halt the radial arterial pulsation. Additionally, this parameter encom-

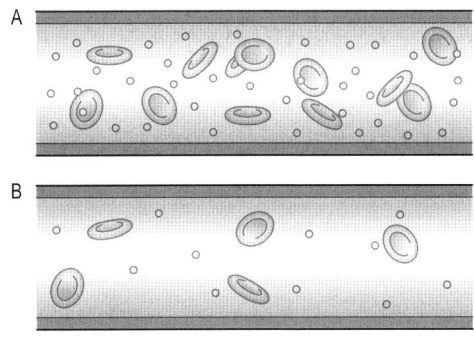

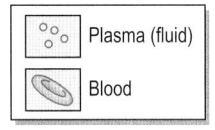

Plasma (fluid)

Blood

Figure 7.1
Schematic representation of variations in density of blood affecting tactile sensation of ease of occlusion.
(A) 'Normal' blood viscosity.
(B) Reduction in blood viscosity.

passes whether pulsation can still be felt at the side of the ring finger once the pulsation has been occluded. This is usually indicative of a pulse that has force and signifies sufficient fluid in the vessel.

The parameter of pulse occlusion is not an actual component of the pulse, such as pulse rate, but rather is used as a diagnostic technique to provide further information about changes in other pulse parameters such as pulse force and arterial wall tension. Accordingly, pulse occlusion is used to further determine the overall strength of the pulse, relative fluid volume and the degree of tension within the arterial wall (Fig. 7.1). As such, it enables us to further differentiate between specific CM qualities that are defined by a number of other parameters.

7.4.1 Pulse occlusion: CM perspective

The parameter of pulse occlusion supplies information about the overall force of the pulse. However, this view is overly simplistic, as the ease with which a pulse is occluded is also influenced by other variables, including:

• The quality and activity of Yang Qi
• The volume of circulating fluids.

7.4.1.1 The quality and activity of Yang Qi

Yang Qi provides the motive force that initiates and sustains cardiac contraction, propelling blood through the arterial system. Yang Qi also plays a role in maintaining the normal tension of the arterial wall. Therefore, Yang Qi vacuity may result in a pulse that lacks force and/or has decreased arterial wall tension, resulting in a pulse that is easily occluded. Conversely, hyperactivity of Yang Qi may result in an increase in arterial wall tension and therefore the perceived 'hardness' of the arterial wall. The overall pulse strength and the volume of blood and Yin fluids may further influence

this. For example, if Blood vacuity develops, then blood no longer cools the Liver, the Liver becomes hyperactive and overall Yang Qi is in relative excess resulting in an increase of arterial tension. In this situation, although tension is increased the pulse is relatively easy to occlude because of the underlying vacuity. There are two or three CM pulse qualities whose formation may be explained in this way.

The stronger the pulse wave the more difficult it is to occlude the pulse against the blood flow. Pulse force relates to both the relative activity of Yang Qi and the presence of sufficient Yin fluids to act as the medium to convey force. If Yin fluids diminish so too does pulse volume; accordingly, the loss of the carrier means that the force of the pulse is not transmitted through the vessels. The artery therefore becomes easier to occlude.

7.4.1.2 Volume of Yin fluids

Yin fluids refers not only to blood circulating in the arterial system but also to body fluids and Essence that reside in other areas of the body (see section 6.11.4.1 for futher information). These are involved in nourishing the organs, skin, muscle and joints and also in the maintenance of blood volume. As Clavey (1995: p. 13) notes, 'In pathological situations, blood and jin ye fluids influence each other considerably'.

Therefore with blood loss, Jin Ye fluids can move into the blood vessels from the surrounding tissues to compensate for the fluid loss and replenish the blood volume, but not necessarily the quality of blood (there is no immediate regenerative effect on the loss of red blood cells). This has the effect of decreasing the viscosity of the blood (due to the loss of red blood cells, and therefore a greater proportion of plasma than usual). This may result in an artery that feels 'empty' (decreased density) and therefore more easily occluded.

Conversely, when there is a loss of body fluids, this can cause fluids from the blood to leave the blood vessels to help replace the lost body fluids. However, this leaves the 'vessels empty and deficient, a condition known in TCM as "jin ku xue zao": jin withered and blood parched. This can lead to severe Shen distur-

121

bance as the blood that would normally nourish the Heart becomes inadequate' (Clavey 1995: p. 14). This also has the effect of increasing the viscosity of the blood (greater proportion of red blood cells than usual due to decreased plasma volume). As a result, this may result in the blood flowing less smoothly, due to increased resistance to the blood flow due to increased ratio of red blood cells to plasma (see Box 7.6).

7.4.2 Pulse occlusion: biomedical perspective

In biomedical terms, the degree of ease with which the pulse can be occluded is considered to be a function of pulse volume. The pulse volume is equated with pulse strength or amplitude, which is reflective of both stroke volume (the amount of blood expelled from each ventricle during systole) and peripheral vascular resistance (Estes 2006: p. 252). The pulse volume (perceived as the strength of pulsation) should be equal with each beat and should be palpable with moderate pressure, being able to be occluded with increased pressure.

Pulse volume is usually assessed via a three- or four-point scale ranging from absence of pulsation through to 'bounding' which is described as being 'difficult to obliterate with pressure' (Estes 2006: p. 254). Terminology that is commonly used to describe pulses with decreased volume includes 'thready' or 'weak', and these pulses are considered to be very easily occluded with light pressure, in accordance with the similarly defined CM pulse qualities (Box 7.3).

Changes in pulse volume from the norm can occur due to changes in either stroke volume or peripheral resistance. The pulse may be easily occluded if the circulating blood volume in the arterial system is decreased. Factors resulting in decreased stroke volume can include heart failure, cardiogenic shock leading to problems with heart contraction or decreased ventricular filling time due to problems with the heart's conduction system.

Peripheral vascular resistance (PVR) is related to the ease with which blood flows through the circulatory system. Increased PVR (due to narrowing of the aorta or inflammation of the pericardium) may lead to a pulse with low amplitude that is easily occluded.

Conversely, the pulse may be more forceful than normal due to fever, infection, exercise, emotional anxiety or hyperthyroidism. Severe anaemia is also considered to be a factor causing a 'bounding pulse' due to the dual effect of decreased blood viscosity leading to decreased peripheral resistance and hypoxia (decreased oxygen to tissues) resulting in increased peripheral dilatation of blood vessels. These both lead to a greatly increased venous return to the heart and therefore greatly increased cardiac output (Guyton & Hall 2006: p. 236).

Box 7.3

Objective measurements of the pulse and ease of occlusion

In a study comparing objective measurements of the radial arterial pulse using applanation tonometry and assessment of the pulse using manual palpation, Walsh (2003) found a significant relationship for two tonometry measurements and the manual evaluation of pulse occlusion. These were PMaxPdt and peripheral systolic pressure (PSP) for the right hand.

The PSP reading was a measure of the maximum pressure exerted by the pulse wave in the radial artery during systole. For ease of pulse occlusion, the results indicated that high peripheral systolic pressure was associated with an increased difficulty in occluding the radial pulse by the pulse assessors using manual palpation (systolic pressure means below 120.2 mmHg for assessor 1 and 117.2 mmHg for assessor 2). Pulses that were selected as easy to occlude were associated with a low peripheral systolic pressure (means below 108.2 mmHg for assessor 1 and 107.7 mmHg for assessor 2).

PMaxPdt relates to the change in pressure with respect to time during systole. Walsh (2003) found that a greater mean value was associated with pulses selected as difficult to occlude (>700 mmHg/s) while a low value was associated with pulse selected as easy to occlude (<600 mmHg/s). This indicates that the quicker maximum pressure is attained during systole (requiring the heart to contract strongly), the more likely the pulse was to be identified as being difficulty to occlude. This indicated a significantly shorter time to reach maximum pressure when the heart contracted for pulses rated as difficult to occlude compared to pulses rated as easy to occlude. Hence pulse force also has a bearing on ease of pulse occlusion.

The relationships as noted by Walsh (2003) must be viewed as a preliminary finding and as such need to be replicated in further studies with the possible investigation of CM descriptions of overall qualities described as easy to occlude, such as the Vacuous and Stringlike (Wiry) pulse, with specific disease states.

7.4.2.1 Factors affecting blood volume

As pulse volume is partially reflective of blood volume then factors affecting blood volume can also impact on how easily the pulse can be occluded. Blood volume can may be impaired as a result of:

Acute blood/plasma/body fluid loss
Blood/plasma loss may occur suddenly such as acute haemorrhaging due to trauma or gastrointestinal bleeding such as a perforated stomach ulcer. Fluid loss

may occur due to excessive vomiting, sweating, diarrhea, dehydration or excessive urination. Hypovolemic shock is a type of circulatory shock that refers to the decreased blood volume resulting from blood or plasma loss. Circulatory shock causes inadequate blood flow around the body. There are usually three stages of circulatory shock (Guyton and Hall 2006: pp. 279–285, Tortora & Grabowski 2000, McCance & Huether 2006):

1. Non-progressive (or compensated) shock: the body's normal compensatory circulatory mechanisms are sufficient to eventually restore normal blood flow.
2. Progressive shock: certain positive feedback mechanisms occur to further weaken the heart and reduce cardiac output so the shock becomes progressively worse.
3. Irreversible shock: the further progression of shock until death.

From a CM perspective the different stages of hypovolemic shock may be the mechanism underlying the traditional CM pulse qualities such as the Faint pulse or the Scallion stalk pulse, relating to sudden acute blood loss (see individual CM pulse qualities for more information).

Chronic blood loss
Chronic blood loss may occur over time due to heavy menstrual bleeding, abnormal uterine bleeding, gastrointestinal bleeding, nosebleeds, hematemesis, hemoptysis, bleeding from haemorrhoids or cancer. Chronic blood loss may mean that blood loss is occurring at a faster rate than haemoglobin can be replaced, resulting in smaller red blood cells containing less haemoglobin (Guyton & Hall 2006: p. 426).

According to McCance & Huether (2006: p. 942) 'haemorrhage that is chronic (occult) produces adaptations that are less prominent and the individual experiences an iron deficiency anaemia when iron reserves become depleted.'

Insufficient blood production
Dietary restraints on eating sources of iron or the poor absorption of appropriate nutrients for the production of blood will also affect blood quality. While plasma volume remains unchanged, the number or size of red blood cells (RBCs) may be adversely affected, leading to a decrease in blood viscosity.

Each of the above situations impacts upon either the number of RBCs, plasma volume or haemoglobin-carrying capacity of the RBCs and therefore affects the circulatory system in varying degrees, hence the appearance of certain CM pulse qualities (see section 7.5.3.7 for more detailed information). These processes may be reflected within the CM pulse qualities such as the Fine, Faint or Scallion Stalk pulse qualities.

7.5 CM pulse qualities defined by arterial wall tension and ease of pulse occlusion

7.5.1 Stringlike (Wiry) pulse (Xián mài) 弦脉

The Stringlike (Wiry) pulse is primarily defined by the physiological presentation of the arterial wall. Specifically, it is the high degree of arterial wall clarity that is of interest. The actual shape of the flow wave through the artery is a consequence of this increased tension in the radial arterial wall (Fig. 7.2).

7.5.1.1 Alternative names

In CM pulse literature the Stringlike (Wiry) pulse is most commonly called the Wiry pulse, but is also variously known as the Bowstring, Stringy or Strung pulse.

7.5.1.2 Requisite parameters

The Stringlike (Wiry) pulse is defined by changes to three pulse parameters:

- Arterial wall tension: The Stringlike (Wiry) pulse has increased arterial tension
- Length: The Stringlike (Wiry) pulse can be felt at all three traditional pulse positions and beyond Chi
- Pulse occlusion: With increasing finger pressure the arterial wall resists deformation, retaining its definitive shape.

7.5.1.3 Clinical definition

The Stringlike (Wiry) pulse has an increase in arterial wall tension and therefore the pulse wave cannot express its normal wave-like fluidity. Rather, it is the distinctness or tension in the arterial wall that inhibits the normal expansion and contraction response to the pressure and flow wave travelling through it. In this sense, it is not the pulse wave that defines the Stringlike (Wiry) pulse, but the actual physical structure of the arterial wall.

The arterial wall is perceived as rigid or dense due to the increased arterial tension, strongly resisting changes to its form when increasing finger pressure is exerted on it. Due to the increased smooth muscle tone in the arterial wall, the pulse is felt as a length of pulsation across the entire arterial segment at the wrist.

7.5.1.4 Identifying whether the Stringlike (Wiry) pulse is present

Step 1: This technique requires assessment of the 'rigidity' of the arterial wall (we are not actually concerned with the pulse wave at this time). Fingers are placed on the skin above the radial artery exerting

123

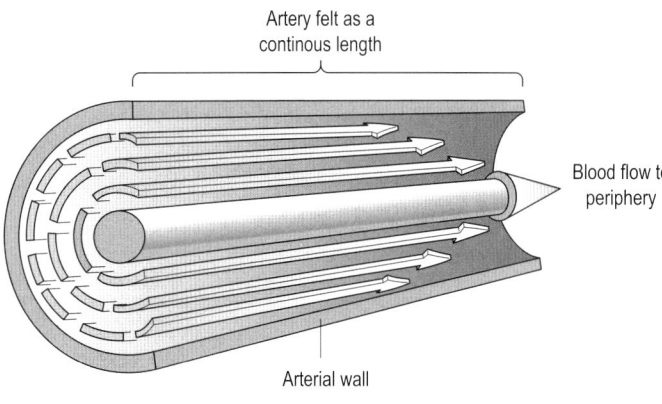

Artery felt as a
continous length

Blood flow to
periphery

Arterial wall

Figure 7.2
Schematic representation of the Stringlike
(Wiry) pulse: Arterial tension constraining
flow wave. The arterial wall is felt distinctly as
a continuous length under all three fingers.
(Adaptal from Figure 29.33 of McCance &
Huether 2006 by permission of Elsevier
Mosby.)

light pressure moving repeatedly over the artery, medially and laterally (rolling side to side). (See Fig. 6.10 showing direction of movement of fingers across the width of the radial artery.)

Step 2: The radial artery is perceived as a distinct tubular structure. The term 'distinct' refers to the increased tension or stress situated in the arterial wall, which means that the arterial wall is clearly felt and it resists easy deformation with finger pressure.

Step 3: It is noted in the pulse literature that the Stringlike (Wiry) pulse retains its form when pressure is exerted on it: 'stiff under the force of the fingers' (Deng 1999: p. 143) and 'press and it does not vary' (Li, Flaws (trans) 1998: p. 100). The often repeated comparison of the Stringlike (Wiry) pulse with the wire string of a musical instrument also brings to mind the image of a pulse that retains its shape even with pressure exerted on it. In terms of the resilience of Stringlike (Wiry) pulse to deformation, two factors should be noted:

- The arterial wall resists deformation to finger pressure possibly even maintaining its shape as the deep level of depth is examined, although it can probably be occluded with sufficient pressure.
- From our experience, when pressure is released from the deep level of depth, the arterial wall quickly regains its original shape.

7.5.1.5 Levels of depth

The Stringlike (Wiry) pulse may be able to be felt at all levels of depth, but is usually strongest at the middle level of depth. However, pulse depth is not an essential component of the Stringlike (Wiry) pulse, rather it is the increased arterial tension. Where changes in both pulse depth and arterial tension occur concurrently, this may develop into a different CM pulse quality such as the Firm pulse which has increased arterial tension but is also found to be forceful and wide at the deep level of depth. Such a pulse type has a different pathogenic

mechanism to that of the Stringlike (Wiry) pulse and therefore a different physical presentation.

7.5.1.6 Classical description from The Lakeside Master's Study of the Pulse

> The bowstring pulse is level and straight like
> the long [description from the *Su Wen*].
> It is like a drawn bowstring [description from
> the *Mai Jing*].
> Press and it does not vary . . .
> Its shape is like the strings of a zither
> [description from the *Mai Jue*].
> Passing through, straight and continuous,
> It is stiff under the fingers'
> *(Li, Flaws (trans) 1998: p. 100).*

7.5.1.7 CM indications

The Stringlike (Wiry) pulse primarily reflects pathology relating to constrained Qi, particularly involving the Liver. This may be transient, reflecting acute stressful situations, or may be indicative of chronic constraint of Qi and consequently associated with pathology. This is termed Qi stagnation and is commonly associated with the Liver. Other CM patterns that can be associated with obstruction of Qi include the presence of pathogenic factors such as Phlegm or Damp. Pain is also usually the result of Qi or Blood stasis (stagnation), so the Stringlike (Wiry) pulse can occur in any condition accompanied by pain.

Liver disharmonies

The Liver is traditionally associated with assisting the free spread of Qi throughout the body, and its movement is considered to have an expansive nature. In addition, the Liver has a major role to play in the storage of blood, providing sufficient blood to circulate through the blood vessels and channels, while returning at night to be stored in the Liver. The patterns of disharmony associated with the Liver therefore involve

Box 7.4

Signs and symptoms associated with Liver/gallbladder disharmonies

These depend on the exact Liver pattern but may be associated with the following:

- Irritability, anger, frustration, depression
- Rib or flank pain
- Sighing
- Flatulence
- Pellet-like stools
- Sore, red eyes
- Bitter taste in the mouth
- Muscular problems such as cramping

obstruction of this normal free flow and spreading of Qi and blood.

Liver disharmonies associated with the Stringlike (Wiry) pulse include Liver Qi stagnation, Liver Yang rising, Liver Fire, internal Liver Wind and Liver Blood stasis (Box 7.4).

- Clinical relevance: Liver patterns can often be seen in patients suffering from emotional stress of some type or actual liver or gallbladder disease. The Stringlike (Wiry) pulse can also result from painful conditions of liver or gallbladder origin such as cholecystitis.
- Mechanism: The Liver is responsible for allowing the smooth circulation of Qi and therefore Blood throughout the body. Liver Qi is easily affected by emotions such as anger, irritability, resentment or the suppression of emotional stress, obstructing Qi flow.

Yang Qi is responsible for maintaining the normal tension of the arterial wall. If Liver Yang becomes hyperactive this can lead to increased tension in the pulse.

Phlegm or Damp

A number of authors agree that the Stringlike (Wiry) pulse can be seen in Phlegm patterns (Deng 1999, Li (Flaws trans) 1998, Lu 1996, Lyttleton 2004, Maciocia 2004). Phlegm is formed by a number of different processes (see Clavey (1995) for a comprehensive discussion on the aetiology and symptomatology of Phlegm) and may occur due to Heat or Fire within the body, causing body fluids to dry up and congeal. Alternatively, Liver Qi stasis can eventually turn to fire, again drying fluids. Flaws (1997: p. 53) describes Yin obstruction (due to Damp, Phlegm, food or blood causing obstruction or stasis) as being capable of impeding the free flow of Qi.

Phlegm/Damp is able to enter and 'choke the circulation both inside and outside of the blood vessels' (Clavey 1995: p. 177) impeding the flow of blood. This can be equated with hypertension in a biomedical context, where there is sclerotic loss of vascular elasticity and therefore increasing hardness of the arterial wall.

Clinically this can be seen in conditions such as epigastric fullness, nausea, vomiting, coughing with production of phlegm. Phlegm/Damp may also result in gynaecological problems such as amenorrhoea and infertility and this may present as a Stringlike (Wiry) pulse, particularly if Liver Qi stagnation is the contributing cause (Lyttleton 2004).

Pain

The Stringlike (Wiry) pulse may be seen in any condition where there is pain. From a CM perspective, pain indicates obstruction of Qi or blood or both. Therefore the lack of free flow is reflected in the increased arterial tension in the pulse. Pain evokes a systemic response, activating the sympathetic nervous system. This will tend to override other pulse variables, with increased arterial tension the predominating change in pulse parameters. Clinically, this pulse may be seen in abdominal or epigastric pain, dysmenorrhoea, headaches and musculoskeletal problems, irrespective of the cause.

Liver attacking the Spleen

Rogers (2000) describes this pattern as Wood energy attacking Earth energy, while Lu (1996) and Deng (1999) briefly mention the pattern of Liver encroaching on Spleen due to an underlying vacuity of the Earth energy. The aetiology is premised on the Five Phase (Wu Xing) arrangement of the organs involving the Ke cycle. The Ke cycle is the controlling cycle and within this cycle the Liver is responsible for keeping in check the functions of the Earth, particularly the Spleen. When the Spleen and Stomach Qi become deficient, or the Wood overexerts its controlling function, this results in digestive problems that present with both Wood and Earth type symptoms. For example, irritable bowel syndrome presenting with alternating diarrhoea and constipation and exacerbated by stress is a classic presentation of the Wood attacking the Earth pattern. Flaws (1997) suggests that a commonly seen pattern is Liver Qi stasis, occurring in conjunction with both Spleen damp and Blood vacuity.

Malaria

A number of authors (Li, Flaws (trans) 1998, Deng 1999, Lu 1996) describe malaria as presenting with a Stringlike (Wiry) pulse. Malaria is a febrile condition and in CM is usually recognised as having an exogenous Cold origin that has entered the body and is located between the interior and exterior. This is equivalent to the Shao Yang stage of Six Divisions (associated with the Gallbladder and Triple Energiser

125

channels). Typical symptoms include fever, chills and severe headaches.

7.5.1.8 Does the Stringlike (Wiry) pulse occur in vacuity patterns?

The Stringlike (Wiry) pulse, in its true form, usually occurs in replete (excess-type) patterns. This is not to say that increased arterial wall tension does not occur in response to Yin or Blood vacuity. Flaws (1997) advises that the Stringlike (Wiry) pulse may evolve as the result of Blood vacuity, which affects the Qi by removing its 'moisture and nourishment'. This, in turn, affects the free flow of Qi, leading to stagnation.

A number of pulses that reflect Blood vacuity do in fact present with increased tension, but these are not necessarily the definitive Stringlike (Wiry) pulse. If Blood vacuity occurs, then one might expect accompanying changes in other pulse parameters refecting the underlying vacuity pattern (such as a decrease in pulse force or change in width) and consequently the formation of another CM pulse quality, for example the Scallion Stalk pulse.

7.5.1.9 Clinical relevance of arterial wall tension

Although the Stringlike (Wiry) pulse in its extreme form may not always be present, there are many instances in which increased arterial wall tension may be identified in the pulse. Rather than trying to fit such a pulse into a certain CM pulse quality definition, and risk disregarding changes in other pulse parameters by doing so, we need to understand what the increase in arterial tension actually means in terms of pathogenesis.

Increased arterial tension may be construed as resulting from obstruction or stasis of Qi and/or blood, remembering that this may have a number of differing causes. This may seem overly simplistic, but it should be remembered that this information should then be incorporated into the bigger picture with the diagnostic information obtained from other aspects of the pulse and the other diagnostic techniques. The example used in the above section on Blood vacuity is a prime example of this. If the pulse information were underutilised to identify the pulse solely as the Stringlike (Wiry) pulse, then information regarding the underlying vacuity (represented by the ease of pulse occlusion in conjunction with the lack of force) would be lost.

7.5.1.10 Increased arterial wall tension as a reflection of stress

An increase in arterial tension in the pulse may be a normal transient response to stressors. This can be seen in the 'fright, flight or fight' response due to the release of epinephrine (adrenaline) and norepinephrine (noradrenaline) mediated through the sympathetic nervous system. CM would see this as a pathological type quality, but it could also be seen as a normal response to an acute situation. Stress in this situation is not considered an adverse reaction, but as an effective mechanism for allowing us to cope with increased demands on the body whether due to physical, emotional or psychological factors. A similar situation is seen in the body's response to pain. In the pulse literature, the pulse qualities often associated with pain have as one of their main defining characteristics, an increase in arterial wall tension, for example the Tight or Stringlike (Wiry) pulses. In this regard, pain is seen as a stressor in the body.

Stress only becomes a problem if this tension remains after the stressor has passed, or if this type of stress becomes chronic. Clinically, if stress occurs – for example preparing for an exam or meeting deadlines at work – then the temporary stress is seen as a useful motivating force, rather than something to be treated. It is when the stress affects the body's ability to be productive or to continue with normal activities, or when stress becomes chronic, that intervention is required. In these cases, levels of cortisol are consistently raised. Cortisol – one of the glucocorticoids produced by the adrenal cortex, useful in helping the body's resistance to stress by increasing the production of ATP (used to produce energy) – makes the blood vessels more sensitive to substances that have a vasoconstrictive effect, which means that it effectively raises blood pressure (Tortora & Grabowski 2000). This is effective if the stress is due to blood loss; however, if it is not and this is happening consistently, then the increased blood pressure may have potentially harmful long-term effects on the heart and circulatory system.

7.5.2 Tight pulse (Jǐn mài) 紧脉

The Tight pulse is a complex pulse quality that is defined primarily by the effect of increased arterial wall tension on the pulse wave.

7.5.2.1 Alternative names

The Tight pulse is also known as the Tense, Intent, Taut or Squeezed pulse.

7.5.2.2 Requisite parameters

The Tight pulse has changes in four pulse parameters:

- Arterial wall tension: The Tight pulse has increased arterial tension.
- Force: There is an increased intensity of pulsation, so that this is a forceful pulse quality.
- Width: The arterial width is increased, so that it is perceived as a wide pulse.

- Length: The Tight pulse is a long pulse, felt in all three pulse positions and beyond Cun and/or beyond Chi.

7.5.2.3 Clinical definition

The Tight pulse, as its name implies, has a decrease in the elastic properties of the arterial wall so that is less able to expand and contract smoothly in response to the pressure and flow waves produced by the contraction of the heart. This is felt as an increase in arterial tension, so that the arterial wall is perceived as 'hard'. The pulse displaces a wide surface area laterally across the finger, being perceived as having a wide arterial diameter. The pulsation hits the finger with increased intensity, and is therefore classified as a forceful pulse.

Although there are no direct references to the length of the Tight pulse, it is often likened to the Stringlike (Wiry) pulse (Li, Flaws (trans) 1998, Lu 1996, Wiseman & Ellis 1996) which is commonly described as long. Additionally, the descriptions often infer length and increased width by equating the Tight pulse with a rope or cord.

While increased width, length and tension are also invoked by the description of 'vibrates to the left and right like a tightly stretched rope' (Li, Huynh (trans) 1981: p.18), this description also gives rise to what is considered to be, by some authors, the distinguishing feature of the Tight pulse; the slight lateral or sideways movement of the artery under the palpating fingers. This is surmised as occurring due to the heightened degree of increased arterial wall tension; the pressure pulse wave causes the artery to 'vibrate' or 'contort' side to side (left to right) due to the arterial wall's inability to absorb and transmit the pulsatile force readily.

7.5.2.4 Confusion over pulse descriptors

There is some confusion in the CM literature over the actual presentation of this pulse quality. While some texts mention a side to side or left to right movement, much of the literature tend to also reiterate the traditional pulse descriptions which describe its similarity to feeling a 'tightly twisted', 'taut' or 'tensely drawn' rope (Deng 1999, Flaws 1997, Kaptchuk 2000, Lu 1996, Wang, Yang (trans) 1997).

Review of the pulse literature reveals that the Tight pulse is generally considered to be a forceful pulse. Li (Flaws trans 1998: p. 93) describes the Tight pulse as 'left and right, pellet-like to the human hand'. The term 'pellet like' is defined earlier in the same text in another pulse definition as being round and hard, but not short. It is also described in the *Mai Jing* (Yang (trans) 1997: p. 3) as feeling 'irregular like a turning rope'. Deng (1999: p. 128) utilises a number of different references, which again address the rope metaphor. However, the idea of an irregularity in form, not rhythm, is also raised, with additional descriptions of the pulse 'with

pressure it is like rolling, not even, but with bumps' and reinforced by the likeness of the Tight pulse to a cord composed of a number of different threads twisted together. There are at least three possible interpretations here: one referring to the physical imperfections of the arterial wall; another to the action of the pulse wave due to the greatly increased tension of the arterial wall causing the artery to appear to slightly 'shake' or 'vibrate' sideways; thirdly, to the actual slipping of the artery from under the fingers due to the heightened arterial tension.

7.5.2.5 Identifying whether the Tight pulse is present

The Tight pulse is formed due to the increased arterial wall tension, which affects how the pressure and flow wave travels through the radial artery.

Step 1: The main feature of the Tight pulse is the significantly increased arterial wall tension, resulting in a tautness that can be felt under the palpating finger. The increased rigidity of the arterial wall results in either: the pressure wave causing the artery to move sideways as it passes through the artery or the artery moves sideways when finger pressure is applied, slipping away from the tips of the fingers.

Step 2: When assessing pulse force, the pulsation hits the fingers with increased intensity, and the artery resists deformation with increasing finger pressure.

Step 3: The pulsation is felt across a broad surface area of the palpating fingers and is therefore defined as wide.

7.5.2.6 Differentiating the Tight pulse from similar CM pulse qualities

There are a number of CM pulse qualities that have increased arterial wall tension. However, these are further distinguished by differences in other pulse parameters and accordingly these changes reflect the underlying pathogenesis (Table 7.1).

The five CM pulse qualities listed in Table 7.1 all present have increased arterial present wall tension. The Scallion Stalk pulse and Drumskin pulse are easily occluded with pressure, whereas the Stringlike (Wiry) pulse clearly retains its form. The Firm pulse has a similar pathogenic mechanism to the Tight pulse, in relation to the presence of pathogenic Cold. In this sense, the Firm pulse and the Tight pulse are interrelated and the Firm pulse could be considered a variation of the Tight pulse but located at the deep level, reflecting the invasion of pathogenic Cold moving directly into the interior. The Tight pulse and Firm pulse have similar changes in pulse parameters and therefore may present in a similar fashion; however, the Firm pulse is always found to be relatively strongest at the deep level of depth. This specifies the location of the disease, which is at the internal level and also reflects the inability of Yang Qi to move outwards due to obstruction, shown by the increased arterial tension. In addition, the Tight pulse as an increase in arterial tension such that the artery gives the impression of slightly moving side to side as a result of the pulse wave moving through the constricted arterial wall.

7.5.2.7 Classical description from the *Mai Jing* and *The Lakeside Master's Study of the Pulse*

The tight pulse is an inflexible pulse like a tensely drawn rope [said in another version to feel like a turning rope]
(Wang, Yang (trans) 1997: p. 3).

Table 7.1 ● Comparison of CM pulse qualities with increased arterial wall tension

	Tight pulse	Firm pulse	Stringlike (Wiry) pulse	Drumskin pulse	Scallion Stalk pulse
Arterial tension	↑ tension	↑ tension	Significantly ↑ tension	Significantly ↑ tension	↑ tension
Response of arterial wall to degree of tension	Arterial wall very distinct, ↑ tension causes slight sideways movement	Arterial wall very distinct	Arterial wall very distinct	Very taut on palpation	Can feel arterial wall distinctly
Pulse occlusion	Retains form with increasing finger pressure due to increased internal resistance within artery. With significant pressure, pulse is occluded.	Retains form with increasing finger pressure due to increased internal resistance within artery. With significant pressure, pulse is occluded.	Retains form with increasing finger pressure due to increased internal resistance within artery. With significant pressure, pulse is occluded.	Retains form with increasing finger pressure but with heavy pressure, the pulse is easily occluded due to the lack of internal resistance (decreased volume)	Retains form even when pulse is occluded but rather than being rigid, it has a pliable arterial wall. The pulsation is easily occluded due to the lack of internal resistance (decreased volume)
Arterial width	↑ width	↑ width	–	↑ width	↑ width
Pulse length	Long	Long	Long	–	–
Pulse force	↑ force	↑↑ force	–	↓ force	↓ force
Pulse depth	–	Deep level of depth	–	Superficial level of depth	Superficial level of depth
Pathogenesis	Pain, food retention, EPA cold or internal cold	Internal cold, internal obstruction due to Qi or Blood stasis and pain	Qi stagnation LV/GB disharmony phlegm/damp malaria pain	Yin vacuity complicated by EPA cold acute profuse Yin fluid loss severe Yin & Essence vacuity	Loss of Blood or Yin fluids (acute or chronic Blood vacuity)

–: not a requisite pulse parameter for this CM pulse quality.

The tight pulse comes and goes with force.
Left and right, pellet-like to the human hand.
(*Su Wen*)

(*Li, Flaws (trans) 1998: pp. 93*)

7.5.2.8 CM indications

It is commonly understood that the Tight pulse is indicative of pain. Pain arises from the obstruction of Qi and/or blood flow. With the Tight pulse, Cold is considered the primary cause of pathogenesis in the pulse literature. This is attributed to the contracting nature of Cold, which is seen as having a constricting effect on the arterial wall. Therefore the Tight pulse can be seen in disharmonies relating to stagnation of Qi and/or blood commonly due to pathogenic Cold, usually presenting with pain as a primary symptom. However, the Tight pulse may be seen in *any* painful condition due to obstruction of the normal flow of Qi and blood. The four patterns associated with the Tight pulse are:

- Pain
- Internal Cold
- EPA of Cold
- Food retention

Pain

Pain is a common symptom associated with obstruction of Qi and/or blood flow. The associated signs and symptoms will depend on the location of the pain and the specific organ affected. The nature of the pain, for example sharp, distending, stabbing or dull, assists in identifying the pattern of disharmony.

Internal Cold (abdominal and pelvic regions)

Three organs are particularly vulnerable to direct invasion by pathogenic Cold: the stomach, the large intestine and the uterus (Maciocia 1989). This can result in strong pain due to the obstruction caused by the contracting nature of Cold on Qi and blood flow.

Clinically, the Tight pulse may be seen in conditions such as sudden stomach pain, abdominal distension and fullness, diarrhoea, loss of appetite or dysmenorrhoea (menstrual pain). Exposure to environmental cold or excessive consumption of cold, raw food such as ice cream, fruit, salad or cold drinks may contribute to the formation of this pulse. In women, exposure to Cold during menstruation, such as swimming or wearing inadequate clothing in cold weather, are also seen as potential causative factors (Lyttleton 2004: p. 17).

EPA of Cold (without abdominal symptoms)

This may be seen in an external invasion of Wind Cold and may occur following exposure to cold weather. Pathogenic Cold has a contracting effect on the blood vessels, causing an increase in arterial tension. As an EPA, it would be expected that the pulse would also be felt relatively strongest at the superficial level of depth, providing the body's Zheng Qi is strong.

Clinically, this may be seen as an acute onset of a cold or flu-type viral infection. Common signs and symptoms include strong body aches, aversion to cold, chills and fever, no thirst or sweating and a sore throat.

Food retention

Food retention may occur when Stomach Qi is deficient or not descending properly or there is excessive food intake. This can cause obstruction of Qi and blood leading to pain, hence the formation of the Tight pulse.

7.5.2.9 Biomedical perspective

The over-distension of a hollow organ, such as the stomach, can result in pain either by overstretching the actual tissue or because the overfilling leads to compression of blood vessels supplying or surrounding the organ. This can lead to pain due to the reduced blood flow to the area (this is known as ischaemic pain) (Guyton & Hall 2006: p. 604).

Intestinal obstruction can occur within or outside the intestines, resulting from fibrous adhesions (postsurgical or from trauma), twisting of the part of the intestine, herniation, inflammatory intestinal disease or diverticulitis. This may lead to distension and pain, depending on the severity and location of the obstruction.

7.5.3 Scallion Stalk pulse (Kōu mài) 芤脉

The main area of focus for the Scallion Stalk pulse is on the physiological presentation of the arterial wall and the manner in which it reacts to increased finger pressure, retaining its clarity and form.

7.5.3.1 Alternative names

Hollow, Onion Stalk, Leekstalk or Split pulse.

7.5.3.2 Requisite parameters

The Scallion Stalk pulse is a complex pulse quality with changes to five pulse parameters:
- Arterial wall tension: There is an increased arterial wall tension
- Depth: The Scallion Stalk pulse is found to be relatively strongest at the superficial level of depth
- Width: The arterial width is increased, resulting in a wide pulse
- Force: The overall pulse force is decreased in intensity

- Pulse occlusion: This pulse is easily occluded with increasing finger pressure.

7.5.3.3 Clinical definition

Two components are involved in defining this pulse: the first relates to the arterial wall tension and the second concerns the pulse wave. There is a distinct and palpable arterial wall at both the superficial and deep levels of depth, reflecting an increase in the arterial wall tension. The pulse wave can be felt relatively strongest at the superficial level of depth, but there is an overall lack of intensity to the pulsation reflecting the underlying vacuity of blood. This means that when finger pressure is applied to the artery the pulsation is easily occluded.

It is the combination of the above two factors which creates the most distinguishing feature of this pulse; the wall of the artery can still be very distinctly felt even when the pulsation within the artery has been occluded. This results in being able to roll the fingers over the arterial wall under the palpating fingers, and 'squash' it, rather like flattening a plastic drinking straw. In this sense, it is not the pulse wave that defines the Scallion Stalk pulse, but the actual physical structure of the arterial wall that can be felt regardless of the pressure exerted on it.

This aspect readily reflects the traditional description of an onion or scallion stalk, indicating a distinct and pliable arterial wall but lacking in substance in the interior. In this case, the substance lacking is Blood. The metaphorical description of the pulse used extensively in the traditional literature in this situation is quite apt in conveying the actual sensation of the pulse as felt.

7.5.3.4 Identifying whether the Scallion Stalk pulse is present

Step 1: The Scallion Stalk pulse should be able to be felt with the fingers resting lightly on the surface of the skin, at the superficial level of depth. The pulsation is decreased in strength and the arterial diameter is relatively wide.

Step 2: This involves feeling for the physical characteristics of the artery wall. The arterial wall is well delineated, being able to be felt easily at the superficial level of depth, with fingers resting on the skin surface. When finger pressure is increased from the superficial level of depth downwards, the arterial wall compresses easily and the pulsation is stopped. However, the arterial wall can be easily rolled underneath the fingers, like squashing a plastic drinking straw, so that the walls are still distinctly felt under finger pressure. This requires moving the palpating fingers from left to right, over the arterial wall.

7.5.3.5 Classical descriptions from the *Mai Jing* and *The Lakeside Master's Study of the Pulse*

The scallion stalk pulse is a floating pulse, large but soft. It is empty in the middle but solid at the sides when pressure is applied. [It is said in another version to be a pulse absent under directly under the (feeling) fingers but present at the sides.]
(Wang, Yang (trans) 1997: p. 3).

Centre is empty, external is replete [or real, i.e. it exists]
Its shape is like an onion stalk.
(Li, Flaws (trans) 1998: pp. 98–99).

7.5.3.6 CM indications

The Scallion Stalk pulse is always considered a pathological pulse quality and is commonly associated with the loss of blood or Yin fluids (Boxes 7.5–7.7). While many authors agree that this is usually due to acute haemorrhage, others describe this pulse appearing due to chronic insidious blood loss, Blood vacuity patterns or in chronic illness affecting the haematological system, such as anaemia or leukaemia (Lu 1996).

Blood vacuity may be due to dietary causes, malabsorption problems or congenital conditions such as pernicious anaemia, thalassaemia or sickle cell anaemia. Anaemia is a complex disease state that can have a number of different causes, affecting both the presentation of the pulse and reflecting the underlying causal factors. Blood vacuity due to iron deficiency anaemia results in a decrease in the number or size of

---

Box 7.5

Blood vacuity signs and symptoms

- Pale white or sallow complexion
- Dizziness
- Floaters in the vision, also called 'flowery vision'
- Pale lips, inner rim of the lower eyelid
- Pale nail beds
- Pale tongue, may have orange sides if severe
- Palpitations
- Dry skin
- Insomnia, particularly trouble falling asleep
- Numbness
- Poor memory

Specific signs and symptoms may differ according to the particular organs involved:

- Liver: Dry eyes, muscle cramping, menstrual problems
- Heart: Shen disturbances such depression or anxiety
- Spleen: Tiredness, loss of appetite

Box 7.6

Body fluid loss versus Blood loss

From a biomedical perspective, the loss of either blood or body fluids (if severe, leading to hypovolemic shock) has a similar effect physiologically on the circulatory system by reducing cardiac output. Body fluid loss may occur due to excessive sweating, excessive urination or failure to replace lost fluids (inadequate fluid intake), while severe vomiting and diarrhoea can also affect both fluid and electrolyte balance. This loss of body fluid is known as *dehydration*.

In body fluid loss, plasma moves from the intravascular (inside the circulatory system) to the extravascular space to compensate for the lost volume. While this has a similar effect on the body's autoregulatory mechanisms as a decrease in blood volume, there is an important difference:

- A decrease in plasma volume means that the viscosity of the blood is greatly increased due to the higher concentration of red blood cells and as such, results in sluggish blood flow (Guyton & Hall 2006: p. 285).
- Blood loss, on the other hand, results in a loss of both plasma volume and red blood cells, therefore the viscosity of blood will tend to decrease. This has the effect of decreasing the resistance to blood flow and increasing the flow rate, as thick fluids cause greater resistance to flow and move more slowly than thin fluids (McCance & Huether 2006: p. 1057).

Box 7.7

Does profuse loss of body fluids lead to the formation of the Scallion Stalk pulse?

Besides blood loss, the profuse loss of body fluids is sometimes implicated in the development of the Scallion Stalk pulse (Maciocia 2004, Townsend & De Donna 1990). From a CM perspective, when body fluids are seriously depleted, fluids (plasma) from the blood can move from the blood vessels into other body tissues to replace lost fluids. From a biomedical pespective the loss of plasma volume results in a decrease in overall blood volume, and an increase in blood viscosity. The increased proportion of red blood cells adds extra resistance to flow as the red blood cells move against each other and the vessel walls. This extra friction causes the blood flow to become sluggish and therefore more turbulent. It is this characteristic of the blood flow that becomes the main defining aspect of the resulting pulsation. As such we could surmise that the Rough pulse, with its fluctuating pulse force reflecting the sluggish blood flow, will tend to manifest as a result of loss of body fluids, while the Scallion Stalk pulse reflects loss of blood.

the red blood cells but no loss of plasma volume. This leads to a decrease in the viscosity of the blood that, with regard to the Scallion Stalk pulse, may partially account for the ease with which the pulse is occluded.

Other causes of Blood vacuity include blood loss through various means: vomiting blood (haematemesis), coughing up blood (haemoptysis), gastrointestinal bleeding, uterine bleeding or abnormally heavy menstrual bleeding. In this case both red blood cells and plasma are lost, resulting in a decrease in overall blood volume as well. In addition, the profuse loss of body fluids may also result in the formation of the Scallion Stalk pulse. There are two main patterns that can result in the formation of the Scallion Stalk pulse both reflecting Blood vacuity but due to different causes. These are:

- Acute: Blood loss due to haemorrhage
- Chronic: Chronic blood loss, vacuity of Blood or Kidney Essence.

Acute, following severe loss of blood (haemorrhage)

From a CM perspective, the acute loss of blood results in an artery that feels 'empty' due to the decreased

volume of circulating blood and is therefore easily occluded. Yang Qi, which is normally anchored and stabilised by Yin blood, moves upwards and outwards causing the pulse to become strongest at the superficial level of depth. Yang Qi becomes relatively hyperactive, having lost the calming aspect of the Yin, leading to an increase in arterial wall tension. This leads to the distinctive arterial wall.

Major blood loss can lead to 'Qi deserting with the Blood' (Wiseman & Ellis 1996: p.151) and may be accompanied by decreased blood pressure, cold sweats or even sudden loss of consciousness.

Chronic: vacuity of Blood or Essence

Vacuity of Blood can occur via the chronic loss of blood due to bleeding from the gastrointestinal tract (for example, ulcerative colitis, stomach ulcers, Crohn's disease or coeliac disease), chronic nosebleeds, abnormal uterine bleeding, haemoptysis or blood in the urine. Although the daily loss may be small in quantity, consistent loss of blood may lead to the body being unable to produce enough blood (haemoglobin to compensate adequately for the continual loss.

Blood vacuity may also occur due to problems with the organs that are involved in blood production such as the Spleen, Heart or Kidneys, so that sufficient blood is not produced. As these organs are also important in the production of Qi, concurrent Qi vacuity signs and symptoms may be present. The Liver helps to replenish blood, so Liver disharmony may also affect the quality of blood.

Chronic illness of any kind can affect the production of both Qi and blood, so that blood and Qi are not replenished. Kidney Yin vacuity can lead to vacuity of Kidney Essence, which in turn affects blood production and nourishment.

7.5.3.7 Biomedical and clinical perspective

The Scallion Stalk pulse can present as a result of:

- Acute blood loss
- Chronic blood loss or reduced iron intake.

Acute blood loss

The Scallion Stalk pulse may be seen in patients following blood loss, usually due to an acute situation. This may result from physical trauma or non-trauma-related blood loss such as acute gastrointestinal bleeding, for example a perforated ulcer. This may cause hypovolemic shock, referring to the decrease in blood volume due to loss of blood (hypovolemic shock also refers to the loss of plasma that may occur due to severe burns, intestinal blockage or the excessive loss of body fluids due to profuse sweating, vomiting, diarrhoea or urination) (see Box 7.6 for further information).

The term 'shock' refers to 'an inadequate cardiac output that results in a failure of the cardiovascular system to deliver enough oxygen and nutrients to meet the metabolic needs of body cells' (Tortora & Grabowski 1996). As previously discussed in section 7.4.2, there are three stages of shock. The Scallion Stalk pulse may possibly arise following either a small amount of blood loss or with increased blood loss (Box 7.7).

If blood loss is less than 10% of total volume then this is known as non-progressive shock and compensatory mechanisms are initiated in the period after the blood loss to return blood volume back to normal (see Box 7.8). This includes the absorption of fluids from the interstitial spaces and intestinal tract. Although this is helpful in increasing the plasma volume back to normal (which takes 1–3 days), it does not compensate for the loss of red blood cells, which may take 3–6 weeks to return to normal. Therefore, following non-progressive blood loss the red blood cell concentration is low while plasma volume returns to normal fairly quickly. This results in posthaemorrhagic anaemia and may help explain why the pulsation is more easily occluded as the blood flow is less dense (lower proportion of red blood cells) and has a decreased viscosity ('thinner' in consistency). This has a number of effects: a decrease in peripheral resistance so blood flow is increased; peripheral vasodilatation to increase blood flow through the tissue because of decreased oxygen supply to tissues due to decreased red blood cell concentration. These both result in more blood returning to the heart and an

---

Box 7.8

Body's response to hypovolemic shock

Nonprogressive shock (compensated shock)

There are certain initial compensatory mechanisms that occur in response to hypovolemic shock to attempt to restore the body's homeostasis, return cardiac output and arterial blood pressure to normal. This includes activation of the sympathetic nervous system and the release of the certain substances that increase heart rate, cardiac contraction and the secretion of certain hormones such as aldosterone and antidiuretic hormone (ADH) that help to retain water and increase vasoconstriction to increase blood volume and blood pressure. This process starts immediately and may continue up to 48 hours if necessary.

Some of the factors than come into play when there is blood loss include the following effects on the circulatory system (Guyton & Hall 2006: p. 279–281):

- Immediate (within 30 seconds): Sympathetic reflexes that cause vasoconstriction of vessels throughout the circulatory system.
- Within 10 to 60 minutes:
  - Release of angiotension and vasopressin, substances that help to constrict peripheral arteries and veins to increase water retention by kidneys.
  - A reverse stress-relaxation of the circulatory system causes the blood vessels to contract down around the decreased volume in order to make it fill the circulartory system more appropriately.
- Longer term (within 1 to 48 hours): Replacing the fluid loss via absorption from the interstitial spaces and intestinal tract and stimulation of thirst and increased desire for salt.

---

increased cardiac output. This may cause the pulse to be more readily palpated at the superficial level of depth, have a wider diameter than usual and be more readily occluded.

If blood loss is more severe, dropping by more than 15% of total volume, then the normal compensatory mechanisms are not sufficient and urgent medical intervention to replace fluids lost is required to return blood volume to normal. This is known as progressive shock, and cardiac output falls dramatically, which is worsened by the instigation of positive feedback cycles. Due to the decreased cardiac output, the heart muscle becomes ischaemic, leading to even lower output and blood pressure. This in turn adversely affects the activity of the vasomotor centre in the brain that controls vasoconstriction. This leads to generalised vasodilatation of blood vessels. The pulse is forceless due to the decreased cardiac output, the arterial width is increased due to vasodilatation and is easily occluded due to the lack of volume in the arterial system and hence, the Scallion Stalk pulse manifests.

The increased arterial wall tension that results in the distinctive pliable arterial wall of the Scallion Stalk pulse (as previously discussed in section 7.3.5) occurs due to tension in other parts of the arterial wall structure, not from contraction of vascular smooth muscle. In fact, the artery wall is in a state of vasodilatation because of the blood loss.

The Guangzhou College notes (1991) state that the Hollow (Scallion Stalk) pulse has been shown to appear experimentally when blood loss is both rapid and heavy (>400 ml) and when the usual compensatory reflexes of vasoconstriction have not resulted in strong contraction of the blood vessels (no specific research study has been cited).

Chronic blood loss or reduced iron intake
Chronic blood loss may result in anaemia, occurring over a period of time due to the body's inability to absorb enough iron from the intestinal tract (mainly the small intestine) to replace the lost haemoglobin. This can result in the production of smaller red blood cells containing insufficient haemoglobin. A loss of 2–4 ml of blood per day is enough to cause iron deficiency anaemia (McCance & Huether 2006: p. 934). Chronic disease such as chronic inflammatory disease, HIV/AIDS, hepatitis and chronic renal failure may also result in anaemia due to alterations to iron metabolism, red blood cell life span, and blood cell production in the bone marrow (McCance & Huether 2006: Ch. 26).

Chronic blood loss may occur due to occult bleeding such as gastrointestinal tract bleeding from ulcers, inflammatory bowel disease, coeliac disease, carcinoma or a range of other gastrointestinal complaints. In addition, menorrhagia (heavy menstrual bleeding) or abnormal uterine bleeding may also contribute to blood loss.

Alternatively, there may be inadequate dietary sources of iron resulting in anaemia due to general decreased food intake, specific dietary restrictions (for example, restrictions on meat) or problems with iron absorption such as coeliac disease or other inflammatory intestinal disease.

As noted by Guyton and Hall (2006), anaemia has a systemic effect on the circulatory system. In anaemia, it is the lowered proportion of red blood cells to plasma volume that results in a decreased blood viscosity. This in turn has a positive effect on the peripheral resistance to blood flow, resulting in an increased amount of blood flowing through the tissues and returning to the heart. The increased blood flow to the heart results in increased cardiac output, which is further enhanced by vasodilatation of peripheral blood vessels due to decreased oxygen supply to tissues (hypoxia). The rate of blood flow also increases. In other words, the cardiovascular system, particularly the heart, has to work much harder to continue to supply the body with sufficient oxygen and nutrients and transport metabolic waste products to be eliminated.

Over time this can have a detrimental effect on the heart, leading to eventual cardiac failure if the underlying cause of anaemia is not addressed. In severe anaemia, the cardiac output may be raised to as much as three or four times normal levels (Guyton & Hall 2006: p. 427).

From a CM perspective, such physiological changes are represented in the pulse by:

- Increased pulse width due to both the peripheral vasodilatation and increased cardiac output
- Distinct presence of the pulse at the superficial level due to the increased cardiac output
- Easy occlusion due to the decreased viscosity and therefore density of blood flow (reflecting the underlying vacuity of blood).

Recent research has shown that *Helicobacter pylori*, bacteria commonly implicated in digestive dysfunction such as duodenal and stomach ulcers, may also lead to iron deficiency anaemia (Russo-Mancuso et al. cited in McCance & Huether 2006: p. 934). *H. pylori* has been shown to impair iron absorption (Ciacci et al. cited in McCance & Huether 2006: p. 934). This has an interesting correlation with CM theory, where impaired functioning of the Spleen and Stomach, integral to digestive functioning, can also lead to the impaired production of both blood and Qi.

7.5.4 Drumskin pulse (Gé mài) 革脉

With the Drumskin pulse, it is the physiological characteristics of the arterial wall that are of primary interest, in particular the significant increase in arterial wall tension, in conjunction with the lack of force.

7.5.4.1 Alternative names

Leather, Tympanic, Leathery or Leather-like pulse.

7.5.4.2 Requisite parameters

The Drumskin pulse is a complex pulse quality with changes in five pulse parameters:

- Arterial wall tension: The Drumskin pulse has increased arterial tension
- Depth: The pulse can be felt relatively strongest at the superficial level of depth
- Width: There is an increase in the arterial width from normal, resulting in a wide pulse
- Pulse occlusion: The Drumskin pulse can be easily occluded with heavy pressure

- Pulse force: There is a decrease in the overall pulse force.

7.5.4.3 Clinical definition

The Drumskin pulse has a wide arterial diameter, so a large surface area is displaced laterally on the fingertip with each pulsation. The Drumskin pulse has a greatly increased arterial tension so that on light palpation the arterial wall feels extremely tense and rigid. Given this, the arterial wall has strong initial resistance to light finger pressure, but with increasing pressure the pulse is easily occluded. This is facilitated by the decrease in blood volume. This also affects the intensity of the pulsation, resulting in a forceless pulse. The Drumskin pulse is felt as a length of pulsating artery, as opposed to distinct wave-like pulsations due to the effect of increased tension in the arterial wall.

When the Drumskin pulse is described in the pulse literature, it is commonly equated with both the Stringlike (Wiry) pulse and Scallion Stalk pulse. For example, Li (Flaws (trans) 1998: p. 103) describes the Drumskin pulse as 'bowstring and scallion-stalk' while Lu (1996) says the pulse is 'felt hard on its walls but hollow in the centre'. Accordingly, we can surmise from this that the important features of the Drumskin pulse relate to:

- Increased arterial wall tension (a common feature of the Stringlike and Scallion Stalk pulse also)
- Decreased volume of either Blood or Yin fluids (common to both the Scallion Stalk pulse and Drumskin pulse), resulting in its forceless pulsation and easy occlusion.

The differentiating feature between the Drumskin pulse and the Scallion Stalk pulse is the degree of increased arterial wall tension: the Drumskin pulse has significantly more tension in its arterial wall, resulting in a more rigid and less pliable artery wall than the Scallion Stalk pulse. Additionally, unlike the Drumskin pulse, the distinct arterial wall is still felt in the Scallion Stalk pulse even when the pulsation within the artery is occluded.

The description and indications for the Drumskin pulse in *The Lakeside Master's Study of the Pulse* are comparatively brief in relation to that of many of the other pulse qualities. This suggests that it only occurs in quite defined situations (as opposed to some of the other pulses that may be seen in a number of different scenarios) and therefore this pulse quality is not commonly seen.

There are also relatively few references to the Drumskin pulse in the *Mai Jing* and these are generally repeated throughout. The *Mai Jing's* description of the Drumskin pulse is identical to more recent definitions of the Firm pulse, being 'replete, large, and long as well as a little bowstring' and somewhat like the deep pulse'. The commentary in the text notes that this is suspected to actually be the Firm pulse rather than the Drumskin pulse (Wang, Yang (trans) 1997: p. 4). If this is the case, the Drumskin pulse, in its current form, was not included as one of the 24 pulse qualities mentioned in the *Mai Jing*.

However, an examination of the *Mai Jing* (Wang, Yang (trans) 1997: p. 343) reveals a further reference to a pulse that is described as 'bowstring and large', further explained as 'modulated bowstring' (as opposed to 'pure bowstring') and 'not so large as scallion stalk'. Pointing out that modulated bowstring indicates cold and scallion stalk means vacuity, the author notes the interaction of these two results in the pulse becoming 'drumskin'. This description closely resembles the definition of the Drumskin pulse as it is known today. Pathogenic Cold has a contracting effect (that is, a vasoconstricting effect on the arterial wall) which may explain why it is described as being not as large (wide) as the Scallion Stalk pulse.

7.5.4.4 Identifying whether the Drumskin pulse is present

Step 1: The Drumskin pulse can be felt relatively strongest at the superficial level of depth, with fingers resting gently on the surface of the skin above the radial artery. However, of primary interest is the significant tautness of the arterial wall. The arterial wall is relatively wide, displacing a wide surface area of the palpating finger. The overall pulsation is forceless.

Step 2: With increasing finger pressure the arterial wall initially resists deformation, maintaining its tenseness. However, as finger pressure is further increased the arterial wall gives in easily, as there is decreased internal resistance within the artery due to the decreased volume of fluids. The pulsation can be completely occluded.

7.5.4.5 Classical description from *The Lakeside Master's Study of the Pulse*

> Drumskin pulse, bowstring and scallion-stalk
> *(Zhong-jing).*

> Like pressing the skin of a drum
> *(Li, Flaws (trans) 1998: p. 103).*

7.5.4.6 CM indications

Although the Drumskin pulse is always considered to be a pathological pulse quality, there is some disagreement in the pulse literature over its aetiology. There is general consensus about blood or fluid loss being the main causal factor, but some authors indicate that this can be complicated by pathogenic Cold, resulting in the greatly increased tension in the arterial wall. There are three main patterns and both are associated with an underlying vacuity of Yin fluids or blood:

- Vacuity of Yin fluids and an acute EPA of Cold
- Acute profuse Yin fluid loss
- Chronic disease leading to severe vacuity of Yin and Essence

Acute: vacuity of Yin fluids complicated by EPA of Cold

This acute pattern of an EPA of Cold occurs on top of an underlying vacuity of body fluids or blood loss. The causes of this blood or body fluid loss are varied and have been discussed previously in the section on the Scallion Stalk pulse. The Drumskin pulse could be interpreted as a further development of the Scallion Stalk pulse, due to the complication of an EPA of Cold.

If the Drumskin pulse is seen in a relatively new illness, this is seen as less critical and therefore has a good prognosis.

- Mechanism of pulse formation: The external pathogenic attack causes the pulse to become relatively stronger at the superficial level of depth as Zheng Qi (antipathogenic Qi) moves to the exterior to fight the pathogen. However, because of the underlying vacuity, the Zheng Qi is not strong and the overall pulse intensity is forceless. The contracting nature of the Cold pathogen causes strong contraction of the arterial wall, thereby greatly increasing arterial wall tension. The underlying loss of Yin fluids enables it to be easily occluded.

From a biomedical perspective, the Drumskin pulse (similarly to the Scallion Stalk pulse) has increased arterial tension but not only due to vasoconstriction (smooth muscle contraction). Due to the loss of blood there is compensatory vasodilatation (relaxation of vascular smooth muscle), so tension/stress in the arterial wall is transferred to other structures within the wall. The additional complication of pathogenic Cold stimulates the body's attempts to maintain warmth, thereby activating vasoconstriction of the arterial walls which has an additive effect on the tension already in the arterial walls, hence the extremely 'hard' presentation of the artery on palpation.

Acute profuse Yin fluid loss (Blood, Essence, body fluids)

The Drumskin pulse may be seen in patients with an acute profuse loss of Yin fluids due to haemorrhage, excessive sweating, diarrhoea or vomiting.

- Mechanism of pulse formation: In this case the pulse can be palpated relatively strongest at the superficial level of depth because the severely decreased Yin can no longer restrain or anchor Yang Qi, which naturally moves upward and outward. This causes Yang Qi to float, becoming more superficial. The extremely vacuous Yin also

results in a hyperactivity of Yang Qi, leading to the increased arterial wall tension. The vacuity of Yin fluids enables it to be easily occluded.

- Clinical relevance: The Drumskin pulse is usually associated with blood loss and in the pulse literature a number of authors (Deng 1999, Li, Flaws (trans) 1998, Lu 1996) note its appearance in abnormal uterine bleeding or miscarriage leading to continuous uterine bleeding in women. The Drumskin pulse can appear postnatally due to abnormal bleeding. Following childbirth, failure of the uterus to contract to compress the uterine blood vessels and stop flow to the placenta can result in primary postpartum haemorrhage. Retention of part of the placenta may also result in abnormal uterine bleeding (Guangzhou Chinese Medicine College 1991) and may be a possible cause of secondary postpartum haemorrhaging, occurring anywhere from 24 hours to 12 weeks postnatally (Stables & Rankin 2005: pp. 575–578).
- In men, the Drumskin pulse may be associated with deficiency of Kidney Essence (associated with lower back pain, nocturnal emissions and other Kidney signs).

Chronic: severe Blood/body fluid loss or Kidney Essence (Jing) consumption due to chronic disease.

The Drumskin pulse may also appear in the course of chronic illness. This is seen as a critical worsening of the disease, indicating the increasing severity of vacuity of blood, body fluids or Kidney Essence, and therefore is considered to have a bad prognosis. The mechanism is similar to the previous pattern.

135

7.5.5 Scattered pulse (Sàn mài) 散脉

Of primary interest in the Scattered pulse is the physiological presentation of the arterial wall (or rather, the lack of presentation in this case).

7.5.5.1 Alternative names

Dissipated or Diffusing pulse.

7.5.5.2 Requisite parameters

The Scattered pulse is a complex pulse quality differentiated by its lack of arterial wall definition. There are changes in five pulse parameters:

- Arterial wall tension: The Scattered pulse has a marked decreased in arterial wall tension.
- Force: There is a decrease in the overall forcefulness of the pulse.

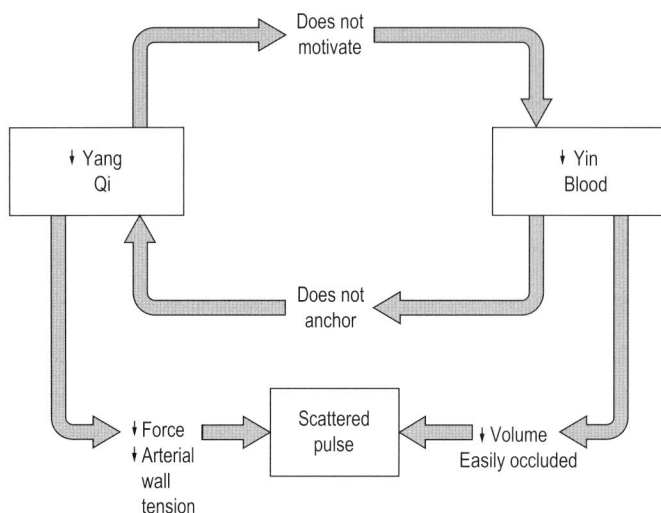

Figure 7.3
The development of the Scattered pulse.

- Width: The arterial width is increased, resulting in a wide pulse.
- Depth: The Scattered pulse is felt relatively strongest at the superficial level of depth.
- Pulse occlusion: The Scattered pulse is very easily occluded with pressure.

7.5.5.3 Clinical definition

The Scattered pulse is primarily characterised by its lack of arterial wall tension, presenting with an arterial wall that is virtually indistinguishable on palpation (Fig. 7.3). This marked reduction in the arterial wall tension results in difficultly clearly differentiating the boundaries between the arterial wall and the surrounding connective tissue. The Scattered pulse has a wide arterial diameter. Lacking force, it is palpated as an area of pulsating tissue. It is considered to be a pulsation without form and is easily occluded with finger pressure.

7.5.5.4 Comparison of definitions

While there is general agreement in the CM pulse literature regarding the main features of the Scattered pulse, its lack of arterial wall definition and general lack of force of pulsation, there are a number of other features that cannot be agreed on. The Scattered pulse is commonly described as a 'large' pulse, but this could be interpreted in a number of ways. It could be a reference to the overall forcefulness of the pulse (which is highly unlikely, as it is a vacuity-type pulse) or it could refer to the width of the arterial wall (most likely). Deng (1999), Flaws (1997), Li (Flaws trans) (1998) and Maciocia (2004) are some of the authors who refer to the appearance of the Scattered pulse at the superficial level of depth. In this respect it is considered to be 'without Root', being represented at the exterior but not present in the interior, and enabling it to be completely occluded with heavy pressure. All four authors have drawn from traditional pulse descriptions in the

Mai Jing, which could account for the similarities in their descriptions of the Scattered pulse.

A clear description of the Scattered pulse in the classical texts is difficult to find. In the *Mai Jing,* the term 'scattered' is used as a descriptor of other pulse qualities. For example, in the first chapter describing 24 separate pulse qualities, 'scattered' is used in both the description of the 'choppy' and 'dissipated' pulses (Wang, Yang (trans) 1997: p. 4). As noted by Hammer (2002: p. 62), there is no explanation of the term 'scattered' so we do not know exactly in what context it is being used. Although the 'scattered' pulse is not a designated pulse quality in the *Mai Jing,* the 'dissipated pulse' resembles the Scattered pulse described in other CM pulse literature.

However the Scattered pulse is also variously described as 'uncountable, uneven in rhythm, uneven in rhythm, showing no sign of pause' (Guangzhou College notes, 1991), 'large and irregular' (Amber & Babey-Brooke 1993) and 'feels as if it were "broken" into many tiny dots instead of flowing smoothly' (Maciocia 2004). These references to the irregularity of pulse rhythm appear to support the concept of extreme Qi and Blood vacuity affecting the heart's functional capacity to contract effectively, confirming the seriousness of the condition. One wonders why then is this pulse not included as a subdivision of the rhythm pulses? It would seem that the presence of arrhythmia is dependent on whether there is Heart involvement in the pattern, but is not an essential characteristic of the Scattered pulse quality. Rather, if irregularity of rhythm does occur then this indicates the extreme severity of the condition and would be identified as a change in an additional pulse parameter, rather than identifying it solely as the Scattered pulse.

Li (Flaws (trans) 1998: p. 110) has a number of descriptions for the Scattered pulse, including the phrase '*Or it may come many and depart few*' (our emphasis). This description could possibly refer to the manifestation of what is known in biomedicine as pulse deficit, which occurs when premature ventricular contractions (before the heart is properly filled) lead to a greatly decreased stroke volume so that the pulse wave cannot be felt at the radial artery. This results in a greater number of apical beats (as measured at the heart) compared to that felt in the radial pulse (Guyton & Hall 2006: p. 150).

The varying descriptions seem to imply that the Scattered pulse has possibly more than a single presentation, depending on the actual pattern of disharmony. This appears to be supported by Deng (1999: p. 105) who says 'Clinically, there ought to be close investigation of the changes in the disease circumstances.'

In fact, it is to be expected that the Scattered pulse will not be a commonly seen pulse in the average CM clinic, being usually seen in someone who is extremely sick. It must be remembered that many of these CM pulse qualities were originally developed hundreds of years ago, where the local acupuncturist or herbalist was the primary or sole provider of health care. Patients with a diverse spectrum of illnesses, ranging in chronicity and severity, would have been seen in their clinics. Correspondingly, a wide range of pulse qualities reflecting these differing health problems would have been observed. Today, in modern societies especially, the local general practitioner or hospital is the primary provider of healthcare, and some of the more extreme pulse qualities reflecting critical or severe illness are less likely to be seen in the CM clinic, and more likely to be encountered in a hospital ward or intensive care unit.

On the other hand, the increasing interest in 'alternative' or 'complementary' health services has also seen an increase in patients with more chronic or severe illnesses in CM clinics. Therefore the ability to recognise these CM pulse qualities and understand what they mean in terms of the effect of the disease process on Qi, Blood, Yin and Yang becomes ever more important.

7.5.5.5 Classical description from *Mai Jing* and *The Lakeside Master's Study of the Pulse*

> The dissipated pulse is a large yet scattered pulse. The dissipated pulse is an indication of Qi repletion but blood vacuity, presence (i.e., repletion) in the exterior but absence (i.e., vacuity) in the interior.
> *(Wang, Yang trans) 1997: p. 3).*

> Its edges are scattered and not restrained . . . Departs and comes without definitude
> *(Li, Flaws (trans) 1998: p. 111).*

7.5.5.6 CM indications

The Scattered pulse is considered to be a vacuity-type pulse, often associated with severe vacuity. Therefore, it can be seen in patterns such as:

- Severe vacuity of Qi and Blood
- Vacuity of Yuan Qi.

Severe vacuity of Qi and Blood

The Scattered pulse is a sign of severe disease, reflecting a severe vacuity of Qi, Blood, Yin and Yang. This may be due to chronic illness that, over time, consumes these substances, reflecting increasing vacuity of the organs involved in the transformation and transportation of Qi and blood, including the Spleen, Stomach, Lung, Kidney and Heart.

The Kidneys are considered to be the source of both Yin and Yang for the entire body, providing both the motive and nourishing aspects that support health. Therefore if Kidney function is affected, over time this can affect the functioning of all organs.

Severe vacuity of Yuan Qi or Kidney Qi

Yuan Qi provides the motive force for all the functional activity in the body. If this is exhausted, then Yang Qi will also be adversely affected. Yang Qi maintains the normal arterial wall tension. If Yang Qi is deficient then the arterial wall loses definition, blurring the boundaries between the artery and surrounding tissue.

- Clinical relevance: It is generally accepted that if the Scattered pulse is seen in a chronic or serious illness, this has a poor prognosis as it indicates a critical worsening of the condition.

  The Scattered pulse may also be seen in pregnant women, during the birthing process or as a sign of impending delivery (Deng 1999, Li, Flaws (trans) 1998, Lu 1996). While this is seen as a normal occurrence by some authors, with one interpretation being that it is a sign of the 'outgoing of Qi and blood in order to give birth' (Lu 1996: p. 118), Maciocia (2004) states that it may signify a prolonged and difficult labour. In addition its appearance during the course of pregnancy may also be pathological, associated with the risk of miscarriage (Li, Flaws (trans) 1998, Maciocia 2004).

7.5.5.7 Biomedical perspective

The Scattered pulse may occur as a result of neurogenic shock, a type of circulatory shock that occurs without any loss of blood volume. This can occur when there is a sudden loss of vasomotor tone throughout the body (Guyton & Hall 2006: p. 285). It is seen as the imbalance between parasympathetic and sympathetic stimulation of the smooth muscle in the blood vessels. As a result, extensive vasodilatation occurs, resulting in an increase in the vascular capacity so that the normal amount of circulating blood becomes inadequate to fill the circulatory system. This causes a decrease in the mean systemic filling pressure, which in turn leads to decreased venous return to the heart and resultant decreased cardiac output.

Neurogenic shock may occur as the result of trauma to the spinal cord, deprivation of oxygen to the medulla, depressant drugs, anaesthesia or severe emotional stress and pain (McCance & Huether 2006: p. 1629).

The vasodilatation and the lack of vasomotor tone are reflected in the distinct lack of tension in the radial arterial wall, and the lack of force is reflected in the decreased cardiac output.

As noted by Wiseman and Ellis (1996; p. 118), the appearance of the Scattered pulse 'indicates the dissipation of Qi and blood and the impending expiry of the essential Qi [essence] of the organs.' It is usually attended by other critical signs. From a biomedical perspective the Scattered pulse may be seen at the end stage of severe heart disease (Lu 1996: p. 110). This reflects the inability of the heart to contract effectively, leading to impaired circulation.

7.6 Pulse force

Pulse force is the most complex of all the pulse parameters because it depends on a range of variables such as the strength of cardiac contraction, blood volume and the tensile compliance of the arterial wall. It is how these variables interact at any given point in time that determines pulse force; a change in any one of these variables will cause a corresponding change in the overall pulse intensity and thus the perception of pulse force.

The parameter of pulse force is used to provide clinically useful information for both diagnostic and prognostic purposes and so is integral to further pattern differentiation, even when pulse force is not a requisite parameter for the CM pulse quality involved, or the pulse parameters do not form a recognisable CM pulse quality. A good example of this concept is using pulse force for differentiation of Yin vacuity Heat and an EPA Heat. Both patterns present with Heat signs and symptoms and so may have an accompanying increase in pulse rate, and so the Rapid pulse can form (>90 bpm). An increase in pulse rate or even the Rapid pulse provides information only in respect to the fact that Heat is present, but does not indicate whether the Heat is arising from a vacuity process (Yin vacuity) or a replete process (EPA Heat). Rather, accompanying changes in the pulse force should correspond with the process occurring; a forceful pulse usually indicates repletion (excess) while a forceless pulse generally indicates vacuity (deficiency), and so Yin vacuity Heat can be differentiated from an EPA Heat by assessing pulse force.

There are six CM pulse qualities that can be classified primarily according to the parameter of pulse force:

- Replete pulse (section 7.7.1)
- Firm pulse (section 7.7.2)
- Vacuous pulse (section 7.7.3)
- Faint pulse (section 7.7.4)
- Weak pulse (section 7.7.5)
- Soggy pulse (section 7.7.6).

These are complex pulse qualities, ranging from those that are abnormally forceful to those that have a decreased pulse force or can barely be perceived. They are differentiated further by changes in a number of other pulse parameters, but are most distinctly defined by the change in pulse force.

7.6.1 Differentiating between specific and descriptive terminology

Terminology such as 'replete', 'full', 'vacuous' 'empty' and 'weak' is often used interchangeably in the CM literature. The terms are used to describe changes in pulse force and used generically to identify the overall nature of an illness (or pattern), whether vacuous or replete. Unfortunately, these terms are also used to name specific CM pulse qualities. When used in this way the terms have a greater range of diagnostic meaning than when used as generic descriptors of illness and dysfunction. For example, a pulse that hits the finger with decreased intensity may be described as 'weak'. Thus it is inferred that a general vacuity pattern is occurring. This is not to be confused with the traditional CM pulse quality, the Weak pulse, which encompasses more than just a change in pulse intensity in its definition. That is, although the Weak pulse has a decrease in intensity (also inferring a vacuity pattern), it is also defined/noted as having changes in pulse width (it is thin) and is located at a specific level of depth (felt strongest at the deep level of depth and cannot be felt at the superficial level of depth). As such, the Weak pulse provides more specific information, not only about the nature of the disharmony (by the force), which is further specified by the pulse width, but also the location of the disharmony (via the level of depth).

This means that to avoid confusion and incorrect interpretation terms need to be distinguished or contextualised on whether they are being applied generically as descriptive terms, or specifically as diagnostic terms for specific CM pulse qualities. Clinically, this means that considered choices should be made to always use correct terminology always. This is paramount when there are several practitioners operating from the one clinic, or when several practitioners regularly confer, so terms are not misinterpreted or wrongly applied.

7.6.2 Pulse force and its assessment

The method for assessing pulse force requires evaluation of the intensity of the radial artery's pulsations hitting the palpating fingers. This is done by assessment of:

- Amplitude of the pulse wave
- Strength of cardiac contraction (and so the time taken for the pulse to reach maximum pulse amplitude)
- Contact area of artery being touched with the fingertips.

In assessing pulse force, the level(s) of depth where the pulse is most apparent need to be first identified. This is done by applying pressure simultaneously with all three fingers over the three pulse positions and varying the amount of pressure to examine each of the three levels of depth. This process is termed assessment of the *relative strength*, the level of depth where the pulse is felt most strongest, irrespective of whether the pulse is forceful, forceless or neither. (Sometimes two or all three levels of depth are similar in their level of strength.) Note should also be made of the presence or absence of the pulsation beyond Cun and beyond Chi pulse positions, as this can help in determining whether the pulse is forceful or not.

Once the level(s) of depth and positions are identified where the pulse is most apparent, then the assessment of the actual force of the pulse can be made. This is assessment of the *overall force*: the force reading which is used to identify several of the traditional CM pulse qualities. (Assessment of overall pulse force needs to be distinctly differentiated from assessment of *relative force*. Relative force refers to the 'subtle' comparative assess-

ment of differences in strength between positions, levels of depth or left and right arms. That is, irrespective of whether the pulse is forceful, forceless or neither, one side or position may be relatively stronger than the other (King et al 2002: p. 153). This concept and related application in different pulse assumption systems is discussed further in Chapter 9.)

There are two basic subdivisions of pulse force:

- Forceful
- Forceless.

Forceful

A forceful pulse is defined as having a large pulse pressure wave or amplitude, with the change in pressure occurring rapidly so that the pulse strikes the finger strongly and displaces a wide surface area on the fingertip (Fig. 7.4). It is defined as being forceful in at least two of the three traditional pulse positions and with the pulse likely to be apparent in the beyond Chi and/or beyond Cun pulse positions.

Forceless:

A pulse that is forceless is defined as either:

- A small pulse pressure wave (amplitude) striking the fingertip weakly with a small displacement of area on the fingertip; or
- A slow rate of change in the pressure pulse wave (amount of time required to reach maximum amplitude) and a wide displacement of surface area on the fingertip.

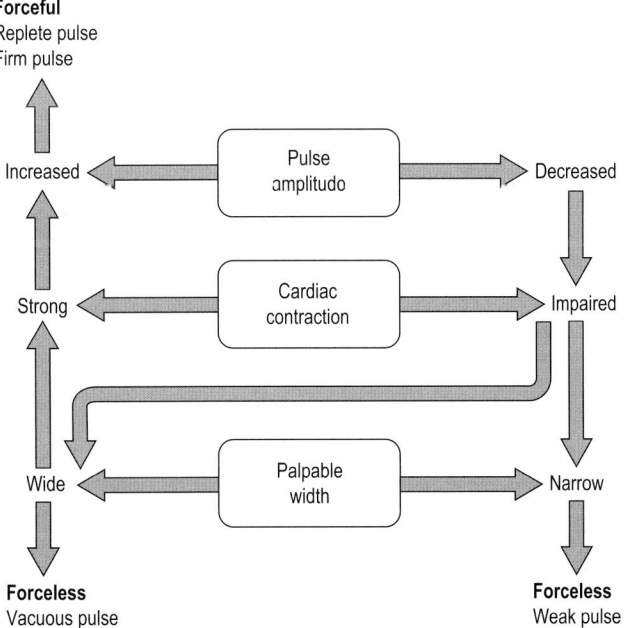

Forceful
Replete pulse
Firm pulse

Forceless
Vacuous pulse

Forceless
Weak pulse
Soggy pulse
Faint pulse

Figure 7.4
Factors affecting the formation of forceful and forceless pulses.

A forceless pulse may not be found in all three traditional positions and is unlikely to be found beyond the three positions. If it can be palpated beyond Chi, then it is usually difficult to detect.

7.6.2.1 Additional palpatory technique for assessing force

When evaluating pulse force the assessment of the pulse parameter 'ease of pulse occlusion' can provide useful information. Occlude the pulse and check whether the pulsation can still be felt at the proximal (body) side of your ring finger (positioned at the Chi position). This is not a failure to occlude the pulse but rather is due to the pulse waves hitting the barrier (your finger) that has blocked their normal pathway of progression along the radial artery. When a forceful pulse is present then a pulsation can still be apparent on that side of the finger.

When the pulse is very forceful, then pulse occlusion may be very difficult to achieve as well, especially at the Chi position.

7.6.2.2 A pulse that is neither forceless nor forceful

A pulse that presents as neither forceful nor forceless is often of no consequence in either the identification of some pathological CM pulse qualities or pulse assessment using the pulse parameters. Indeed, a pulse that is neither forceless nor forceful would usually be considered to be a 'normal' pulse presentation of this parameter.

The exception is when the 'neither' pulse force is either weaker or stronger than the individual's usual pulse force. If the individual's pulse is weaker than it usually is, then this may be seen as a sign of weakening Qi or Yang but does not necessarily mean that the Yang or Qi is definitively vacuous. Transient factors such as a poor night's sleep or hunger can often cause such temporary decreases in pulse force.

Similarly, if the pulse force for an individual has been forceless but starts to increase in intensity, then this can be viewed as a sign of improvement, a good prognostic sign (so long as it is not accompanied by adverse changes in other pulse parameters or other signs and symptoms).

7.6.2.3 Differences between left and right radial arteries

Assessment of the overall force of the pulse should be compared between the left and right arteries, either individually or with simultaneous bilateral palpation. If there is a significantly large discrepancy in force between the two sides (10–15 mmHg), the decreased pulsatile flow may be the result of arterial narrowing or occlusion (McCance & Huether 2006: p. 1069). (From a CM perspective more subtle differences relate to the Qi and blood balance and are discussed in Chapter 9.)

7.6.3 Regulation of pulse force: CM perspective

Pulse force is intrinsically linked with both Qi and Blood and their inter-relationship of function and form. Sufficient Qi is required to cause the blood to move in the vessels, longitudinally through the length of the arteries but also laterally, expanding the arterial wall. This relates to the heart's functional capacity to contract, thus Heart Qi, and the strength of that contraction, which is Yang force. For example, if Yang is vacuous then the heart contraction is weak and relatively slow and the pulse is felt without force. If Qi is weak then the heart's functional ability to contract at all is affected and so the rhythm becomes irregular. In this sense, Qi initiates function while Yang is the expression of the Qi's strength.

A pulse without force can also arises when the blood is vacuous. This is because blood is the medium for conducting the pulse force or Yang Qi throughout the body. When blood is vacuous, then Qi has nothing to act on and so Qi cannot interact physically with the pulse, and pulse force (Yang) is consequently felt diminished. As is often the case when blood levels fall, pulse pressure also falls and this is subsequently felt as a decrease in pulse amplitude and subsequently decreased pulse force. Conversely, when blood is abundant then the pulse will be felt forceful so long as the Qi and Yang are also abundant.

In this context, pulse force is affected when Qi and blood are affected. Changes in pulse force occur as a result of:

- External factors affecting the inter-relationship of Qi and blood; through consumption, damage, agitation or countering Qi and blood's intrinsic nature
- Internal factors affecting the inter-relationship of Qi and Blood; often involving dysfunction of the mechanisms associated with the production, movement, storage, function and maintenance of these.

7.6.4 Measures of pulse force: biomedical perspective

The force of the pulse refers to the impetus of the arterial pulsation striking the fingertip when the pulse is palpated. This is viewed as pulse amplitude.

7.6.4.1 Pulse amplitude as a measure of pulse force

From a biomedical perspective, the pulse amplitude is equated with pulse strength and pulse volume. The pulse amplitude is defined as the difference between the systolic and diastolic pressures (also known as the pulse

Box 7.9

Systole and diastole

Systolic pressure

- The pressure in the arteries as blood is pumped from the left ventricle into the aorta
- Affected by stroke volume, force of contraction and elasticity of arterial walls.

Diastolic pressure

- The pressure in the arteries as the heart relaxes and blood flows out of the main arteries and into the arterial system.
- Affected by the peripheral resistance, elasticity of blood vessels and blood viscosity (the higher the viscosity, the more resistance to flow) and also heart rate: the slower the heart rate, the more time there is for blood to flow out of the main arteries therefore decreasing diastolic pressure.

(Stables & Rankin 2005: p. 230)

Box 7.10

Objective measurements of pulse force

Walsh (2003) found that pulses recorded as being forceful using manual palpation in healthy subjects were associated with higher tonometry measurements showing a faster change in pressure with respect to time during systole. This means that maximum pulse amplitude or pulse height of the pulse wave, when achieved in a short period of time, often means more forceful pulses. For example, if the heart contracts strongly, the systolic peak is achieved more rapidly, resulting in a sharper incline to the peak. This causes a greater volume of blood to flow into the aorta at a given point in time. As a consequence, the pulse may feel 'full' or have increased pulse wave intensity. Alternatively, either a decrease in blood flow or ejection of the blood from the heart occurring over a longer period of time is associated with decreased arterial pressure and may be felt as either forceless or of 'normal' strength. In this situation, ventricular contraction determines the amount of force imparted into the blood forcing it to flow through the vessel.

Box 7.11

Factors affecting pulse pressure

Pulse pressure is affected by:

- Stroke volume (the amount of blood pumped from left ventricle into the aorta)
- Compliance of the arterial system (ability of arteries to accommodate blood flow from the heart)
- The nature of the ejection from the heart during systole.

This means the greater the stroke volume, the larger the amount of blood that needs to be accommodated in the arterial system, therefore the greater the pressure rise and fall: hence a larger pulse pressure (Guyton & Hall 2006: p 173).

size of the artery palpated . . . The amplitude of the pulse is thus the manifestation of force – of pressure multiplied by the area of the finger distorted by the pulse.

7.6.5 Regulation of pulse force: biomedical perspective

In general, the greater the difference in amplitude from normal (the larger the pulse pressure) the more forceful the pulse is felt under the finger, and the less divergence from normal, the weaker the pulse.

However, pulse force is also influenced by other factors such as arterial diameter, blood volume and the condition of the arterial walls (Box 7.11). Large amplitudes result in more distinct arterial pulsation because of the large differences in pressure – the larger the difference, the more noticeable any movement in the artery will be.

When viewed from a mechanical and flow wave perspective the manifestation of pulse force is likely to be due to a number of different pathways dependent on the illness and pathological processes (Box 7.12). The amplitude of the pressure pulse should not be solely mistaken for pulse force: large pulse amplitude does not necessarily mean a forceful pulse or small amplitude a forceless pulse. For example:

- Changes in the arterial wall tension affect the ability of the arteries to expand in response to the pulse wave, so affecting the perception of pulse force. Systolic pressure is raised if the arterial walls are stiff and are unable to expand easily. Consequently pulse force is raised.
- Increased pulse force can result from arterial narrowing or vasoconstriction. When arteries constrict there is less area for the pulse wave to act on, thereby proportionally increasing the pressure exerted from within the artery.

pressure) (Box 7.9). On average this is about 40 mmHg (assuming an average blood pressure of 120/80 mmHg) (Box 7.10). It was suggested by O'Rourke et al (1992: p. 19), that:

The amplitude of the palpable pulse depends on the amplitude of the pressure pulse and on the

Box 7.12

Biomedical conditions associated with changes in pulse pressure from the norm

Decreased pulse pressure may indicate:

- ↓ stroke volume due to cardiac tamponade, shock, tachycardia (decreased ventricular filling time)
- ↑ peripheral resistance due to cardiac or aortic dysfunction such as aortic stenosis, mitral valve problems, cardiac tamponade.

Increased pulse pressure may indicate:

- ↑ stroke volume due to aortic regurgitation (blood flowing back into left ventricle from the aorta after it has emptied)
- ↓ peripheral resistance and therefore ↑ peripheral vasodilation (therefore ↑ blood volume returning to the heart and ↑ cardiac output): fever, anaemia, hyperthyroidism, exercise, arteriovenous shunt (abnormal fistula between major artery and vein).

(Estes 2006: p. 263)

Box 7.13

Effects of the sympathetic and parasympathetic nervous system on cardiac function

Sympathetic stimulation

- ↑ strength of heart contraction and therefore stroke volume
- ↑ heart rate up to 180–200 bpm or more

This leads to an increase in cardiac output up to 2–3 times normal.

Parasympathetic stimulation

- ↓ heart rate to 20–40 bpm
- ↓ strength of cardiac contraction by 20–30%

The overall effect is to decrease cardiac output by 50%, a milder effect than the sympathetic response.

(Guyton & Hall 2006: pp. 112–113)

- How quickly the maximum amplitude is reached during heart contraction and the extent of the area of the finger being 'hit'. The quicker this occurs, the more likely the perception of the pulse is forceful.

7.6.5.1 Other factors affecting pulse force

Duration of systole and diastole

The perception of pulse force is also affected by the proportion of time the heart is in systole and diastole, which affects the volume of blood ejected into circulation by the heart (stroke volume). It is also affected by pressure indices affecting the end-systolic volume in the ventricles and so strength of heart contraction.

Autonomic nervous system

The activation of the sympathetic or parasympathetic nervous system affects the heart, leading to changes in cardiac output (see Box 7.13 for further information).

Body temperature and pulse force

Changes in body temperature due to either environmental conditions or disease can affect both the heart rate and, to a degree, the contractility of the heart. Changes in body temperature alter the rate of electrical discharge in the heart (Stables & Rankin 2005: p. 225).

A moderate increase in body temperature can increase the strength of cardiac contractility, therefore increasing the perceived force of the radial arterial pul-

sation. However, if this is prolonged it has an adverse effect on cardiac metabolic functioning resulting in eventual impaired cardiac function and therefore weaker contractions.

If the heart rate is greatly increased, both systole and diastole are shortened. Systole duration increases to the detriment of the diastolic duration. As a result, the left ventricle will not be filled sufficiently, adversely impacting on the cardiac output and also resulting in a weaker pulsation.

Ageing

Cardiac output is regulated in proportion to metabolic activity. Guyton & Hall (2006: p. 237) note that cardiac output declines with age, however they add that this is probably reflective of declining activity with age. This is associated with decreased skeletal muscle mass and therefore reduced oxygen and blood flow requirement reflected in a decreased cardiac output.

7.7 CM pulse qualities defined by pulse force

7.7.1 Replete pulse (Shí mài) 实脉

7.7.1.1 Alternative names

Full, Excess or Strong pulse.

7.7.1.2 Requisite parameters

Five pulse parameters are involved in the formation of the Replete pulse:

- Force: The Replete pulse has an increased pulse force that can be felt equally at all three levels of depth
- Depth: The Replete pulse can be felt equally strong at each level of depth
- Width: The arterial width is increased from that of normal, being termed 'wide'
- Length: Pulsations can be felt at all three traditional pulse positions of Cun, Guan and Chi and beyond Chi and/or beyond Cun
- Arterial wall tension: There is a slight increase in arterial wall tension which leads to a easily palpable arterial wall that retains its shape when moderate pressure is applied by the fingers.

7.7.1.3 Clinical definition

The Replete pulse is named for its strong arterial pulsations that hit the palpating fingers with an equally increased force at all three levels of depth and at the three traditional pulse positions Cun, Guan and Chi and beyond. The pulse force expands the artery both laterally and longitudinally so the pulse presents as wide under the fingers and long, extending beyond Chi and/or beyond Cun. There is a slight increase in arterial tension.

7.7.1.4 Identifying whether the Replete pulse is present

Step 1: When the fingers are placed over the radial artery pulsation with only the pressure of the resting fingers exerting pressure, the pulse may be easily palpated and is felt strongly under all three fingertips.

Step 2: With increasing finger pressure exerted over the radial pulsation, the pulse and artery resist deformation. With increasing finger pressure towards the radial bone the pulsation can be occluded with heavy pressure, but the pulse may still be felt against the proximal side of the ring finger at the Chi position. The finger pressure is then released slowly until the pulsation can be felt once more. At this deep level, the pulse can be felt as forcefully as it was at the superficial level of depth and at all three pulse positions.

Step 3: Once the superficial and depth levels of depth have been examined, the middle level of depth is assessed. The pulse can be felt equally strongly at this level of depth and at all three pulse positions. In this way, while pulse force is an important parameter in identifying this pulse, it also primarily depends on detecting the presence of pulse force at the three levels of depth and at the three pulse positions.

Step 4: This pulse will also present with an increased arterial width and a clearly defined arterial wall usually beyond the three traditional positions.

7.7.1.5 Classical description from *The Lakeside Master's Study of the Pulse*

The replete pulse is obtained both floating and sunken.
The pulse is large and also long,
Slightly bowstring.
It responds to the fingers driving, driving [description comes from the *Mai Jing*]
(Li, Flaws (trans) 1998: pp. 82–83).

7.7.1.6 CM indications

The Replete pulse usually indicates a pathological condition, always indicating the presence of a pathogenic factor, usually Heat or Fire. The one primary pattern associated with the Replete pulse is pathogenic Heat or Fire.

Replete pathogenic Heat or Fire
The Replete pulse indicates the presence of a strong pathogenic factor, usually Heat or Fire, generally resulting in the stagnation of Qi.

In the presence of pathogenic Heat, the appearance of the Replete pulse indicates that the antipathogenic Qi (Upright or Zheng Qi) is strong. The excessive force is a reflection of the struggle between the pathogen and the body's Zheng Qi as it attempts to overcome the pathogen. It would also be expected that the hyperactivity of Yang could also cause an increase in pulse rate, resulting in the appearance of the Rapid pulse.

The Replete pulse is formed as a result of the body's fight against the pathogenic factor, with blood and Qi overfilling the artery. Pulse force defines the Replete pulse and is determined by a combination of the strength of Yang Qi and the Yang nature of pathogenic Heat. Therefore the pulse has an increase in overall intensity, reflecting the summative accumulation of Yang Qi.

7.7.1.7 Clinical relevance

The Replete pulse can be seen in the pattern of Heat accumulating in the Triple Heater (Lu 1996: p. 86), where the Heat pathogen systemically affects the body, throughout the upper, middle and lower sections or Heaters of the body. This is also described in the *Bin Hu Mai Xue* (Li, Flaws (trans) 1998: p. 83) 'Heat brewing in the three burners produces strong fire. This is communicated to the intestines'.

Depending on what organs the Heat or Fire is affecting, the accompanying signs and symptoms will correspondingly vary. For example, the literature notes manic behaviour occurring when the Heart is affected by Heat, while in the middle Heater there may be vomiting as Heat causes the Stomach Qi to become 'rebellious'. Heat affecting the lower Jiao causes the fluids to dry, and constipation may dominate the clinical signs and symptoms.

7.7.1.8 Biomedical perspective

An extremely forceful pulse, such as the Replete pulse, may occur as a result of systemic bacterial infection. As described by Guyton and Hall (2006: p. 286) features include:

- Marked increased vasodilatation throughout body and especially in the infected tissue
- High metabolic rate caused by bacterial stimulation and high body temperature.
- High cardiac output (not in all patients).

It would be expected that there would be a resultant increase in pulse rate as well. As the severity of the bacterial infection progresses to septic shock, other processes start to occur. For example, red blood cells start to accumulate in the degenerating tissues, small blood clots begin to form throughout and, as a result of the clotting factors being consumed, haemorrhages occur in many tissues such as the intestinal tract (Guyton & Hall 2006: p. 286). This can be seen from a CM perspective as the heat injuring the fluids. If clinically significant, then the bleeding could eventually cause the pulse to form into the Vacuous pulse or Surging pulse.

7.7.1.9 'Replete' and relative strength

Many authors describe the occurrence of the Replete pulse in individual pulse positions. However, by definition, as explained in the 'Clinical definition' section above, it is impossible for the Replete pulse to occur in a *single* position, as part of the requisite changes in parameters is the appearance of the pulse in *all three* traditional pulse positions and beyond Chi and/or Cun.

Therefore, it is presumed that the term 'replete' in this case simply refers to a relative difference in strength (Box 7.13). As such, the 'replete' or increase in force occurring in a discrete position may not necessarily reflect pathogenic Heat (as the Replete pulse does) but may reflect another pathogenic mechanism such as obstruction or stasis.

7.7.1.10 Prognostic use

While the presence of the Replete pulse in a replete (excess) type pattern is seen as a positive indication that the signs reflect the pattern (Box 7.14), Deng asserts that its presence in a vacuity pattern signifies a critical condition and indicates that the pathogenic factor is strong and the Zheng Qi is weak (1999: p. 127).

7.7.2 Firm pulse (Láo mài) 牢脉

7.7.2.1 Alternative names

The Firm pulse is also known in CM literature as the Confined, Fixed or Prison pulse.

Wiseman & Ellis (1996) note in their revised translation of a Chinese medical teaching text that the term 'Firm pulse' is no longer used. Instead, such a pulse is described as 'stringlike and deep', a composite of two other CM pulse qualities. This does not seem to be the case in other modern CM pulse literature, where the Firm pulse is still included as a CM pulse quality.

7.7.2.2 Requisite parameters

The Firm pulse is a complex pulse quality and therefore has changes in five pulse parameters:

- Force: The overall intensity of the pulsation is increased
- Depth: The Firm pulse cannot be felt at the superficial level of depth and usually not at the middle level of depth. It is felt strongest at the deep level of depth
- Width: The arterial diameter is increased in the Firm pulse
- Length: Pulsations can be felt at all three traditional positions and beyond Chi and/or beyond Cun

- Arterial wall tension: The arterial wall can be easily palpated due to the increased arterial tension.

7.7.2.3 Clinical definition

The Firm pulse is a forceful pulse, felt strongest at the deep level of depth. It cannot be felt at the superficial level of depth. It has a wide diameter, and the arterial wall is distinct, so the artery is easily delineated from the surrounding tissue. It is perceived simultaneously by the three palpating fingers as a length of pulsating artery, extending beyond Chi and/or beyond Cun pulse positions. The Firm pulse probably develops from a 'drawing in' of the arterial structure so it sits deeper within the flesh.

7.7.2.4 Identifying whether the Firm pulse is present

Step 1: The pulse is best identified by firstly placing the fingers gently on the skin overlying the radial artery, with only the weight of the palpating fingers exerting downward pressure. At this superficial level of depth the radial pulsation cannot be felt.

Step 2: As finger pressure is exerted downwards the radial artery pulsation begins to be palpable, and with increasing finger pressure (pushing down towards the radial bone) the pulsation becomes more obvious. The arterial wall should be examined at this stage; it is distinctive and can be distinguished from the surrounding connective tissue. The arterial diameter can also be examined at this time; it should cause a broad area of the palpating finger to be indented, and is therefore classified as wide.

Step 3: Next, the deep level of the pulse is examined by increasing finger pressure so that the radial artery is occluded for a few seconds. The pulsation may still be felt at the proximal side of the ring finger, from the direction of the arterial blood flow, signifying a forcible pulsation. The finger pressure is then gently and slightly eased so that the pulsation can once again be felt. This is the deep level of depth and the pulsation will appear at its strongest at this level of depth. At this level of depth the pulsation hits the fingers forcefully. It can be felt under all three palpating fingers and beyond the Chi position.

Step 4: As finger pressure is released from the arterial pulsation, it decreases noticeably in force until it is imperceptible at the superficial level.

7.7.2.5 Classical description from *The Lakeside Master's Study of the Pulse*

The confined pulse is similar to sunken, similar to deep-lying.

[But it is] replete, large, and also long,
Slightly bowstring.
(Li, Flaws (trans) 1998: p. 104).

7.7.2.6 CM indications

The Firm pulse is a pathological pulse quality, occurring only in the presence of illness and dysfunction. There are two main patterns associated with the Firm pulse, both considered to be internal Replete type patterns:

- Replete pathogenic Cold in the interior of the body
- Internal obstruction due to Qi or Blood stasis

Replete pathogenic Cold in the interior of the body

This Firm pulse can be seen when pathogenic Cold enters the body and directly lodges in the interior. This may affect the internal organs such as the stomach, the intestines or the uterus, which are considered to be particularly vulnerable to an attack of external Cold directly passing to the interior of the body (Maciocia 2004). Alternatively, this may be due to consumption of excessively cold food (such as ice cream) or cold drinks. Cold in the stomach may present with abdominal pain and vomiting of clear fluids, Cold in the intestines usually presents with lower abdominal pain and diarrhoea, and Cold in the uterus may result in pain during menstruation.

Pathogenic Cold can also enter the meridian system. An example of this is an invasion of pathogenic Cold into the Liver channel, which may present clinically as a hernia.

Lu (1996) also notes that the Firm pulse may be seen in convulsions caused by Wind.

Internal obstruction due to Qi or Blood stasis

The Firm pulse may also arise as a result of the internal stagnation of Qi or blood so that neither Qi nor blood is able to reach the exterior. Stasis may be caused by retention of food, or may be due to pathogenic factors such as Cold or phlegm. Improper diet or emotional disturbance may adversely impact on the Liver and Spleen, leading to Qi stasis that, over time, results in the stasis of Blood.

The Firm pulse is commonly associated with abdominal masses due to either Qi or Blood stasis (Lu 1996). Qi stasis can result in the formation of masses of indefinite shape that can form or dissipate at irregular intervals, influenced by the state of Qi flow. The location of the pain is not fixed. Such masses are known as 'conglomerations' and are usually associated with disease in the Fu (Yang) organs and problems with Qi. 'Concretions' are also caused by stasis and have a definite form and fixed location, usually associated with problems of the Zang (Yin) organs and blood (Wiseman & Ye 1998: p. 92). Blood stasis type pain is usually fixed, stabbing and more severe in nature.

Mechanism of pulse formation

A deeply located pulse can indicate:

- The location of disease in the interior or
- The obstruction of Yang Qi in the interior so that Qi and blood cannot move outwards.

In the case of Qi stasis, the increased arterial tension indicates disturbance to the normal Qi flow, and a resulting hyperactivity of Yang that is unable to move outwards.

In the case of pathogenic Cold, the increased arterial tension is due to the contracting nature of Cold. It also reflects the obstruction of normal flow of Qi and blood by the Cold, which has a tendency to constrain Yang.

The increased force and wide arterial diameter seen in the Firm pulse imply the presence of a pathogenic factor and reflect the resulting obstruction of Qi and/or blood.

7.7.2.7 Clinical relevance

Pain is one of the most obvious symptoms that a patient will present with in cases of obstruction of Qi or blood. Pain is often accompanied by an increase in arterial wall tension in the pulse, reflecting the obstructed flow. The nature of the pain may differ according to its cause. Blood stasis will present as fixed and boring pain and abdominal masses associated with it will be hard. Qi stasis, on the other hand, has a more diffuse area of involvement, the pain tends to have a distending feel and may also change in location.

The pain can be quite severe in the case of the EPA of Cold entering directly into the interior, and will have an acute onset.

Interestingly, while Li (Flaws (trans) 1998) describes the pathogenesis relating to the presence of many of the other pathological CM pulse qualities in individual pulse positions, there is no discussion of the appearance of the Firm pulse (or Confined pulse, as it is known in *The Lakeside Master's Study of the Pulse*) in individual pulse positions. This may be because the Firm pulse usually arises due to pain due to the strong obstruction of Qi and/or blood, which will generally tend to have a systemic effect on the pulse, as occurs in all situations in which arterial tension is increased (Box 7.16).

7.7.3 Vacuous pulse (Xū mài)
虚脉

7.7.3.1 Alternative names

Empty, Deplete, Feeble, Deficiency or Weak pulse.

Box 7.16

The Firm pulse as a prognostic indicator

Both Li (trans. Flaws 1998) and Lu (1996) assert that the appearance of the Firm pulse in a patient who has suffered a severe blood loss denotes a poor prognosis. This is a situation in which the pulse is contradictory to the individual's actual state of health. That is, because blood is vacuous, the pulse should be easy to compress, and so the Firm pulse should not occur. Thus if the Firm pulse is occurring when blood is vacuous then this indicates that an EPA is residing in the vacuous space, falsely causing the pulse to present as strong. For an EPA to have done this indicates the Zheng Qi (Upright or antipathogenic Qi) is weak, implying that the pathogenic factor is strong.

7.7.3.2 Requisite parameters

The Vacuous pulse is a complex CM quality with changes in four pulse parameters:

- Force: The Vacuous pulse has a decreased pulse force. The perceived pulse force decreases with increasing finger pressure
- Depth: The Vacuous pulse is felt strongest at the superficial level of depth. (The pulsation actually disappears before we can palpate to the deep level of depth.)
- Width: The arterial width is increased from that of normal, resulting in a wide pulse
- Pulse occlusion: This pulse is easily occluded. There are also no perceived pulsations at the side of the finger when the pulse is occluded.

7.7.3.3 Clinical definition

The Vacuous pulse has a lack of intensity in the radial pulsation hitting the palpating fingers. The pulse is easily perceived with light pressure at the superficial level of depth and is also wide (due to vasodilation). However, although the arterial wall can be felt, this is due to a relative hyperactivity of Yang caused by an underlying vacuity and so the artery is easily occluded when finger strength is increased into the deeper levels of depth. Accordingly, the arterial wall loses its definition, becoming indistinct, and the pulsation is absent with heavy pressure (at the deep level of depth).

7.7.3.4 Identifying whether the Vacuous pulse is present

Step 1: The fingers are placed gently over the radial artery pulsation, with only the pressure of the resting fingers on the skin. The pulsation should be easily felt at this level of depth, although the overall strength is forceless. The arterial diameter is wider than would normally be expected. Moving the fingers side to side (medially and laterally) across the arterial wall may assist in identifying this pulse.

Step 2: With increasing finger pressure downwards towards the middle level there should be a noticeable decrease in overall force, with little resistance by the arterial wall to deformation.

Step 3: With an increasing amount of finger pressure the pulse will be easily occluded, before reaching the deep level of depth. No pulsation can be felt either under the palpating fingers or on the proximal side of the ring finger (positioned over the Chi position). The definition of the arterial wall decreases so that it cannot be felt.

7.7.3.5 Comparison of definitions

A number of pulse texts include the term 'slow' in their descriptions of the Vacuous pulse (Belluomini & Cheung 1982, Flaws 1997, Li (Flaws trans) 1998, Wang (Yang trans) 1997). Although mentioning the term 'slow' in the general description of the Vacuous pulse, Flaws (1997: p. 25), qualifies this by saying he does not include it in his personal definition, noting pulses that are 'floating, large and forceless' are commonly seen in his clinical practice.

In Huynh's 1981 translation of the *Bin Hu Mai Xue*, the Vacuous pulse (termed the Empty pulse) is described as having 'slow beats' but is *not* included in the section on the Slow pulse and its related types, nor is it accorded a number of beats per respiration. Deng (1999) includes the term 'arrives slowly' in his definition of the Vacuous pulse but also does *not* include the Vacuous pulse in the section on slow pulses, instead classifying it under pulses that are based on abnormal changes in strength.

A decreased rate (hence a Slow pulse) would suggest the presence of pathogenic Cold or a deficiency of Yang, accompanied by Cold signs and symptoms. However these patterns are not usually included in the indications for the Vacuous pulse. Rather than being an actual decrease in heart rate, the term 'slow' could possibly be interpreted as referring to the actual beat itself, the proportion of time that systole and diastole occur within each beat (see Chapter 2 for further information). That is, the actual pulse wave peak or time taken to full amplitude occurs over a relatively longer time, thus systole (which is perceived as the actual beat) is perceived as happening more slowly rather than a decrease in the pulse rate. As the intensity or strength of the pulse is also influenced by the both the force of the heart's contraction and how quickly this occurs, the pulse wave intensity will also feel less forceful than

it would if the contraction happened at a quicker rate. This, in conjunction with the wider than normal arterial diameter, further diluting pulse force. Overall, this means that the pulsation is perceived as forceless.

7.7.3.6 Classical description from the *Mai Jing*

> The vacuous pulse is a slow, large, and limp pulse, impotent when felt with pressure applied and giving the (feeling) fingers an impression of wide hollowness
> *(Wang, Yang (trans) 1997: p. 4).*

7.7.3.7 Specific definition versus descriptive terminology

It should be remembered that the term 'vacuous' is not only utilised as the name of a specific CM pulse quality but also as a generic term to describe any pulse that presents with a lack of force or is associated with a vacuity pattern. The terms 'vacuous' and 'weak' are often used interchangeably.

When the Vacuous pulse is used as a specific CM pulse quality, this refers to a pulse that is defined by changes in four pulse parameters, resulting in a pulse that is relatively strongest at the superficial level of depth, has a wide arterial diameter, hits the fingers without force and is easily occluded.

7.7.3.8 CM indications

The Vacuous pulse is, by nature and name, a vacuity-type pulse and therefore is the result of vacuity-type patterns, usually of both Qi and blood. Two patterns are associated with the formation of the Vacuous pulse:

- Vacuity patterns of Qi and blood
- EPA of summer heat.

Vacuity patterns of Qi and Blood
Blood and Qi have a mutual relationship; blood is considered to be the mother of Qi, and Qi engenders blood (Wiseman & Ye 1998). Blood vacuity is often accompanied by Qi vacuity signs, therefore the signs and symptoms accompanying the Vacuous pulse may include both blood and Qi vacuity signs: generally these include lethargy, shortness of breath, spontaneous sweating, pale complexion, low voice, dizziness, 'floaters' in eyes and pale tongue. Specific signs and symptoms will of course depend on the specific organs involved.

Mechanism of pulse formation
Qi, particularly the Yang aspect, works to maintain arterial wall tension; when Qi is vacuous the tension in the arterial wall is not maintained and the arterial diameter widens. Blood vacuity results in the decreased viscosity of the blood due to the decreased numbers of

Box 7.17

Signs and symptoms of heat exhaustion

- Fever
- Sweating
- Thirst
- Dizziness
- Hypotension
- Weakness
- Nausea
- Vomiting
- Tachycardia
- Decrease in urination

When severe, dehydration may lead to the cessation of sweating and if the core temperature continues to rise then changes in neurological status such as delirium, confusion or loss of consciousness may occur if the temperature is not decreased.

red blood cells. This results in decreased oxygen supply to the tissues and the resultant hypoxia causes the peripheral blood vessels to dilate in order to increase the blood flow through the tissues and back to the heart. This contributes to the increase in arterial diameter.

EPA of summer Heat

Clinically, the Vacuous pulse may be seen in heat exhaustion or heat stroke. This would be expected to have an acute onset and may occur during periods of extreme climatic heat. An EPA of summer Heat causes excessive heat in the body, consuming Qi and Yin fluids. This causes dehydration and causes the pulse to become forceless and easily occluded due to a decreased fluid volume in the arteries (decreased plasma volume). Li (Flaws trans 1998: pp. 81–82) describes the accompanying signs and symptoms as spontaneous sweating, very rapid pulse and fright palpitations (Box 7.17). He advises to 'nourish the constructive, boost the Qi', referring to the need to rehydrate, replenish fluids (an essential part of blood) and strengthen depleted Qi.

The elderly and very young are the most susceptible to this type of pattern, as both groups are prone to difficulties with thermoregulation.

Mechanism of pulse formation

Heat exhaustion/heat stroke is characterised by fluid and electrolyte loss, especially sodium, causing dehydration. There is a consequent reduction in arterial volume (loss of plasma) and a corresponding decrease in blood pressure.

From a CM perspective, the loss of Yin fluids deprives Yang of its stabilising anchor. As a result, Yang 'floats', moving upwards and outwards; the pulse becomes superficial, forceless and wide. The loss of both fluid and

Qi results in the lack of pulse force and its easy occlusion. The vacuous Yin means that Yang becomes relatively hyperactive and may also result in a Rapid pulse.

7.7.3.9 Differentiation of similar pulses

Both the Vacuous pulse and the Floating pulse are felt relatively strongest at the superficial level of depth. However, the Vacuous pulse is very easily occluded with minimal finger pressure whereas the Floating pulse may still be felt at other levels (although not as strong as the superficial level) with increased finger pressure.

Maciocia (2004: p. 474) prefers to use the term 'Empty pulse' to describe the Vacuous pulse and defines it as having:

> No strength and disappears with a light pressure, feeling empty; it is soft but also *relatively* big and distended at the superficial level.

There are differences in opinion about the severity of the Vacuous pulse. Maciocia (2004) describes it as indicating an early or middle stage of Qi vacuity, progressing in a more severe form to the Weak pulse (defined as deep, soft and without strength). Interestingly, he does not consider changes in arterial width to be an essential feature in his definitions of the Weak or Soggy pulses.

Lu (1996) also compares the Vacuous pulse (which Lu labels Deplete) and Weak pulse. However, while he agrees that they are both indicative of vacuity-type syndromes of Qi and blood, Lu considers the Vacuous pulse to reflect a more severe deficiency condition. This manifests in what he terms the 'more severe destruction of the mutual restriction of Yin and Yang or Qi and Blood', signified by the superficial location and increase in diameter. (See Chapter 8 for further discussion of the evolution of CM pulse qualities.)

Li (Flaws trans 1998) also identifies damage to essence and blood via 'bone-steaming'. This could be equated to Kidney Yin vacuity leading to consumption of Yin fluids and consequently Qi.

In spite of these difference there appears to be general consensus in the pulse literature about the pathogenesis leading to the development of the Vacuous pulse. A dual vacuity of Qi and Blood is hypothesised to be responsible for this pulse quality, and is usually associated with impaired organ functioning.

7.7.4 Faint pulse (Wēi mài) 微脉

7.7.4.1 Alternative names

Minute, Feeble, Minute, Indistinctive, Subtle, Diminutive or Evanescent pulse.

7.7.4.2 Requisite parameters

The Faint pulse is a complex CM pulse quality that has changes in four pulse parameters:

- Force: The Faint pulse has a greatly decreased intensity that further diminishes with increasing finger pressure; it is a difficult pulse to palpate because of the extreme lack of pulse force
- Width: The arterial width is greatly decreased, resulting in a very narrow arterial wall
- Pulse occlusion: This pulse is very easily occluded with slight finger pressure
- Arterial wall tension: The Faint pulse has a greatly decreased arterial wall tension.

The parameter of pulse depth is not specifically mentioned in traditional pulse literature concerning the Faint pulse. It is therefore assumed that depth does not play an important role in the formation of the Faint pulse and as such, it may be located at any level of depth depending on the pathogenesis. Of more importance is its extreme lack of force, extremely narrow width and its tendency to disappear with minimal finger pressure.

7.7.4.3 Clinical definition

The notable feature of the Faint pulse is the extreme presentation of changes in the pulse parameters, reflecting extreme vacuity. It is an extremely thin, forceless and easily occluded pulse. While easy occlusion and lack of force are descriptors of the Faint pulse, it is also defined in the literature as being a difficult pulse to locate due to its extreme lack of force. As such, the arterial pulsation may seem to 'fade' in and out of perception because of a small pulse amplitude.

Because of the lack of internal pressure force, the Faint pulse is easily obliterated by external finger pressure and so careful use of discrete pressure changes is required to locate the pulse. The arterial wall has little tensile force when finger pressure is applied so that it is perceived as having a lack of definition.

7.7.4.4 Identifying whether the Faint pulse is present

Step 1: Using the radial styloid process for guidance, the fingers are placed over the three traditional positions to locate the radial pulsation. The pulsation may be difficult to locate because of the greatly decreased force and lack of arterial tension.

Step 2: All levels of depth need to be examined in order to locate the pulsation. Once the pulsation is obtained, with slight finger pressure it should be easily occluded. The arterial width is very narrow, and it is also difficult to perceive because of the lack of vasomotor tone.

Step 3: If the arterial pulsation is very difficult to ascertain or seems to disappear then reappear, then this signifies the Faint pulse.

7.7.4.5 Classical description from the *Mai Jing*

> The faint pulse is a very fine, soft pulse possibly bordering on expiry, sometimes there and sometimes not [said in another version to be small; in still another to be quick under the fingers, in yet another to be floating and thin; in still another to come to almost an end when pressure is applied].
> *(Wang, Yang (trans) 1997: p. 4)*

7.7.4.6 CM indications

The Faint pulse is a pathological pulse quality representing an *extreme* vacuity of both Yang and Qi as well as blood. It always indicates a critical condition. Two main patterns are associated with the Faint pulse:

Severe Qi and Blood vacuity (chronic)

The severe vacuity of Qi and blood is usually due to chronic disease. This is known as 'vacuity desertion' (Wiseman & Ye 1998). The appearance of the Faint pulse denotes a critical worsening of a disease. Such severe vacuity usually indicates long-term hypofunctioning of the organs and may be caused by chronic lifestyle issues such as overexertion, insufficient sleep, poor diet and emotional disharmony.

Yang collapse or shock (acute)

From a CM perspective, this could refer to any acute situation where the separation of Yin and Yang occurs. This may be seen with high fever or massive blood and fluid loss such as haemorrhage, profuse sweating or severe vomiting and diarrhoea. The extreme and sudden loss of Yin means that Yang is no longer nourished and supported, leading to the collapse of Yang. (This is could be associated with hypovolemic shock.) This is reflected in signs and symptoms such as cold limbs, profuse beadlike sweating, no thirst, loose stools or incontinence of urine or stools, or unconsciousness.

7.7.4.7 Biomedical perspective

The Faint pulse is termed the 'weak and thready pulse' and can be seen in circulatory shock: that is, any condition where blood vessels are inadequately filled and blood is unable to circulate properly, such as heart failure. As a result of the decrease in circulating blood flow, initial compensatory mechanisms help to resolve the resulting decrease in blood pressure, such as vasoconstriction of peripheral blood vessels. This may occur in severe haemorrhage, profuse sweating or severe repeated vomiting. Acute trauma such as extensive burns can also contribute to loss of water and plasma, resulting in a reduced blood circulation (hypovolemic shock) and greatly increased blood viscosity (see section 7.4.2 for the stages of hypovolemic shock).

As noted earlier, shock generally progresses in three stages, with the third stage being irreversible and leading to death. The Faint pulse, as a critical pulse, may be equated with either the progressive or irreversible stage of circulatory shock. By this stage, positive feedback mechanisms have been initiated and perpetuate continuing damage to the heart and other tissues, further impairing cardiac output and leading to irreparable tissue and organ damage. As such, the Faint pulse is associated with severe exhaustion in critical conditions, and may be seen in dying patients.

The Faint pulse has a poor prognosis when it appears in chronic conditions, indicating further critical decline in homeostasis.

7.7.5 Weak pulse (Ruò mài) 弱脉

7.7.5.1 Alternative names

Frail, Infirm pulse.

7.7.5.2 Requisite parameters

The Weak pulse is a complex pulse quality characterised by changes in four pulse parameters:

- Force: The Weak pulse has a decreased overall intensity of pulsation
- Depth: It is found strongest at the deep level of depth and it cannot be felt at the superficial level
- Width: The arterial width is decreased from that of normal
- Ease of occlusion: With increasing finger pressure down to the deep level of depth, the pulse is easily occluded.

7.7.5.3 Clinical definition

The Weak pulse can only be palpated with medium to heavy pressure, being relatively strongest at the deep level of depth. Overall the pulsation is forceless, hitting the fingers with little intensity. It is easily occluded with increasing finger pressure and is unlikely to be still felt at the proximal side of the ring finger with pulse occlusion. It has a narrow but distinct pulse width (commonly described as 'threadlike').

7.7.5.4 Identifying whether the Weak pulse is present

Step 1: The fingers are placed gently over the radial artery pulsation, with only the pressure of the resting fingers on the skin. The pulsation should not be able to felt at this superficial level of depth.

Step 2: With increasing finger pressure downwards towards the middle level the pulsation may be able to be felt but with little intensity hitting the fingers.

Step 3: With an increasing amount of finger pressure, heading towards the deep level of depth, the pulsation should become apparent, although with a lack of overall intensity. The pulse has a narrow arterial width, displacing only a small area on the palpating finger. With heavier pressure, as the external pressure exerted on the arterial wall equals the internal pressure, the pulsation ceases so that no pulsation can be felt either under the palpating fingers or on the proximal side of the ring finger (positioned over the Chi position). Simultaneously, the definition of the arterial wall decreases so that it cannot be felt.

7.7.5.5 Classical description from the *Mai Jing*

The weak pulse is a very soft, deep, and fine pulse bordering on expiry under the (feeling) fingers when pressure is applied [said in another version to be impalpable unless pressure is applied and absent when pressure is released] *(Wang, Yang (trans) 1997: p. 4).*

7.7.5.6 CM indications

The Weak pulse occurs in vacuity patterns and is generally seen as a pathological pulse quality. The occurrence of the Weak pulse at the deep level of depth indicates the inability of Yang to circulate Qi to the exterior of the body. It also specifies that the problem is located in the interior of the body, involving organ involvement. The Weak pulse can occurs as the result of vacuity of both Qi and Blood, particularly Yang. The circumstances in which the pulse manifests include:

- Pathology
- Age-related changes.

The diagnostic meaning of the pulse is further differentiated on the basis of:

- Constitutional health and age of the patient
- Presence or absence of other illnesses.

Vacuity of both Qi and Blood, particularly Yang Qi

While the Weak pulse reflects a dual vacuity of Qi and blood, Yang Qi vacuity is the predominating feature. Yang Qi vacuity signifies hypoactivity of physiological functioning, exhibiting signs and symptoms that reflect the damage to the warming and moving aspects of Yang Qi. Cold signs and symptoms accompany the Weak pulse, such as aversion to cold, cold extremities, pale complexion, lethargy, loose stools, a desire for warm drinks, increased urinary output and spontaneous sweating.

- Mechanism of pulse formation: Vacuous Yang Qi cannot propel blood with sufficient strength, therefore the pulsation is felt forceless and at the deep level of depth. Deficient blood fails to expand the pulse resulting in a narrow pulse, and provides an inadequate medium for Qi movement.

Constitutional health

If the Weak pulse occurs in someone who is young, Lu (1996) considers this to be a sign of a weak constitution, inherited from parents. This constitutional weakness may predispose the individual to increased attack by EPAs. In this case, the pulse may not present as the Floating pulse in response to the presence of an EPA because of the body's already depleted Qi. Pre-Heavenly Essence or Jing represents the inherited energy from each parent at the time of conception and cannot be replenished.

Long-term illness

Chronic illness causes the consumption of both Yin and Yang over time. The appearance of the Weak pulse is seen as a natural reflection of this underlying vacuity. This may be the result of organ hypofunction and can be seen in vacuity patterns of the Kidney (sore knees, tinnitus, aching bones) and Spleen (digestive problems, tiredness, muscle weakness).

Age-related changes

Qi and blood are traditionally considered to diminish with the natural progression of age, and the Weak pulse is said to appear in older people as a reflection of this decline. However, a vacuity of Qi and blood is considered to be pathological, whether age related or not, and it would be expected that there would be accompanying abnormal signs and symptoms associated with Qi and blood, depending on which predominates.

7.7.5.7 Biomedical perspective

From a biomedical perspective, the Weak pulse may indicate problems with the heart affecting the cardiac output and resulting in decreased pulse amplitude. Clinically, the Weak pulse can be seen in prolonged chronic illness.

7.7.5.8 Comparison of similar CM pulse qualities

The Weak pulse and Soggy pulse both have decreased pulse force and pulse width. They are differentiated by the level of depth at which the arterial pulsation can be felt relatively strongest. The Weak pulse is felt relatively strongest at the deep level of depth, while the Soggy pulse is felt relatively strongest at the superficial level of depth. As such, these are in fact similar pulse types, albeit found at different levels of depth. Accordingly, the underlying pathogenesis of each pulse quality reflects both the similarities and differences between them.

Both the Weak and Soggy pulses are considered to be indicative of Qi and blood vacuity, reflected in the overall lack of intensity in pulsation and the decrease in arterial width. However, it is the level of depth that further differentiates the causal background, with the Weak pulse reflecting the predominance of Yang Qi vacuity. The Soggy pulse, on the other hand, is mainly indicative of either Yin vacuity or an EPA of Damp. Therefore, the Soggy pulse is felt relatively strongest at the superficial level of depth, which reflects involvement at the exterior of the body. The vacuity of Yin means that the Soggy pulse cannot be felt at the deep (or organ/Yin) level of depth.

7.7.6 Soggy pulse (Rú mài) 濡脉

7.7.6.1 Alternative names

Soft, Weak, Floating or Frail pulse.

7.7.6.2 Requisite parameters

The Soggy pulse has changes in four pulse parameters:

- Force: The Soggy pulse has a decreased pulsatile force
- Depth: This pulse is relatively strongest at the superficial level of depth, decreasing in force with increasing finger pressure
- Width: The arterial width is decreased, resulting in a narrow pulse
- Ease of occlusion: The Soggy pulse is easily occluded with increasing finger pressure.

7.7.6.3 Clinical definition

The Soggy pulse lacks force in the arterial pulse pressure wave, hitting the finger with little intensity. It has a thin but distinct arterial diameter (often described as thread-like), felt strongest at the superficial level of depth and easily occluded when further pressure is applied (before the deep level of depth can be reached).

7.7.6.4 Identifying whether the Soggy pulse is present

Step 1: The fingers are placed gently over the radial artery pulsation, with only the pressure of the resting fingers on the skin. The pulsation should be easily felt at this level of depth, although the overall strength is forceless. The arterial wall is defined so that the arterial width can be described as thin, displacing a narrow area of skin on the palpating fingertips.

Step 2: With increasing finger pressure downwards towards the middle level there should be a noticeable decrease in overall force, with little resistance by the arterial wall to deformation. As finger pressure is increased the arterial pulsation is easily occluded so that no pulsation can be felt either under the palpating fingers or on the proximal side of the ring finger (positioned over the Chi position).

The pulse cannot be felt at the deep level of depth, as it is occluded well before reaching this level of depth.

7.7.6.5 Classical description from the *Mai Jing*

> The soft pulse is a very soft pulse as well as floating and thin [said in another version to be absent when pressure is applied but potent when pressure is released; in still another to be small and soft; soggy instead of weak in yet another, where the soggy pulse is said to be like the clothes in water which are reachable only to a gentle hand.]
>
> *(Wang, Yang (trans) 1997: p. 4).*

7.7.6.6 CM indications

The Soggy pulse is a pathological CM pulse quality and is associated with vacuity-type patterns. The Soggy pulse usually indicates vacuity of Qi and blood or Yin; however, an EPA of Damp may complicate this pattern. Two main patterns associated are with the Soggy pulse:

- Vacuity of Qi and blood or Yin
- Vacuity of Qi and blood complicated by an EPA of Damp

Vacuity of Qi and Blood or Yin

The Soggy pulse may arise due to vacuity of Qi and the concurrent vacuity of either blood or Yin. Blood vacuity may arise due to loss of blood through abnormal bleeding from the nose, stomach or throat known as 'flooding invertedly' (Li, Flaws (trans) 1998: p.107). Alternatively, Yin vacuity signs such night sweating and 'steaming of the bones' (tidal fever, restless sleep and agitation) may occur, a sign that the body's nourishing and cooling abilities have been compromised.

- Mechanism of pulse formation: The inadequate expansion of blood vessels due to deficient Yin (fluid) or blood inadequately filling the vessel, the pulse is consequently forceless, decreased in width and easily occluded. As Yin is depleted, Yang is no longer anchored and so moves upward, resulting in a superficially located artery.

Vacuity of Qi and Blood complicated by an EPA of Damp

Exogenous damp can enter the body through the pores of the skin, settling in the flesh. As Clavey (1995: p.124) notes:

Even just locally, however, in the surface tissues, the pathogenic damp can interrupt normal fluid movement and cause edema.

The Damp EPA enters the body whose physiological processes are already impaired by Qi and blood vacuity. Qi vacuity compromises the body's ability to defend itself from external attack and may also enhance the effect of the pathogen. If the Spleen is affected this may impact on the body's ability to further transform and move fluids throughout the body.

The Dampness trapped in the tissue both impairs and consumes Yang Qi, leading to a forceless pulse. It compresses the pulse, resulting in an arterial diameter that is narrow, already depleted by Qi and blood vacuity.

Other authors mention that the Soggy pulse is indicative of chronic Dampness such as 'postviral fatigue syndrome' (Maciocia 2004: p. 481).

7.7.6.7 Body types and the Soggy pulse

It is noted in some pulse texts that the Soggy pulse is the pulse most likely to be felt in thin individuals. This appears to come from the *Mai Jing* (Wang, Yang (trans) 1997: p. 10) which claimed that 'The pulses in females are inclined to be more soggy and weaker than in males' and 'if the person is small, a female, or thin, the pulse is (accordingly) small and limp.' However this is contradicted in a modern CM text that notes 'Obese people tend to have fine and deep pulses, while thin people have large pulses' (Wiseman & Ellis 1996: p. 118).

Because of the contradictory nature of the information pertaining to body and pulse width and in the absence of demographic information, instead of generalising about this relationship, it is necessary to evaluate the pulse width within the context of the other presenting signs and symptoms, as well as the changes in other pulse parameters.

7.7.6.8 Comparison of similar CM pulse qualities

The Weak pulse and Soggy pulse are similar in their presentation, differentiated by the level of depth they are located (Table 7.2). The Weak pulse is strongest at the deep level of depth, while the Soggy pulse is strongest at the superficial level of depth. This is symbolic of their pathogenesis, with the Weak pulse generally indicating Yang vacuity and therefore being vacuous at the Yang level, and the Soggy pulse indicating Yin vacuity and therefore not found at the deep level of depth (which represents Yin).

7.7.6.9 Clinical relevance

The Soggy pulse is often seen in Yin vacuity patterns, the exact signs and symptoms of which may depend on the organ(s) affected (Fig. 7.5). The Soggy pulse is commonly noted as the CM pulse quality seen in Damp

Table 7.2 ● Comparison of CM pulse qualities defined primarily by pulse force

	Replete pulse	Firm pulse	Vacuous pulse	Weak pulse	Soggy pulse	Faint pulse
Pulse force	↑↑ force	↑↑ force	↓ force	↓ force	↓ force	↓↓ force Difficult to feel
Pulse occlusion	Retains form with increasing finger pressure due to increased internal resistance within artery. With significant pressure, pulse is occluded. May still pulsate at side of finger while occluding pulse.	Retains form with increasing finger pressure due to increased internal resistance within artery. With significant pressure, pulse is occluded. May still pulsate at side of finger while occluding pulse.	Easily occluded before reaching the deep level of depth.	Easily occluded due to the lack of internal resistance (decreased volume and force)	Easily occluded due to the lack of internal resistance (decreased volume and force)	Very easily occluded due to the lack of internal resistance (decreased volume and force)
Pulse depth	Felt at all levels of depth	Deep level of depth. Cannot be felt at the superficial level	Superficial level of depth	Deep level of depth. Cannot be felt at the superficial level	Superficial level of depth Cannot be felt at deep level of depth	May be seen at any level, depending on underlying pattern
Arterial width	↑ width	↑ width	↑ width	↓ width	↓ width	↓↓ width
Pulse length	Long	Long	–	–	–	–
Arterial wall tension	Slight ↑ tension	↑ tension	↓ tension, the arterial wall is easily deformed with finger pressure	–	–	Significantly ↓↓ tension. Difficult to feel arterial pulsation.

– not a requisite pulse parameter for this CM pulse quality.

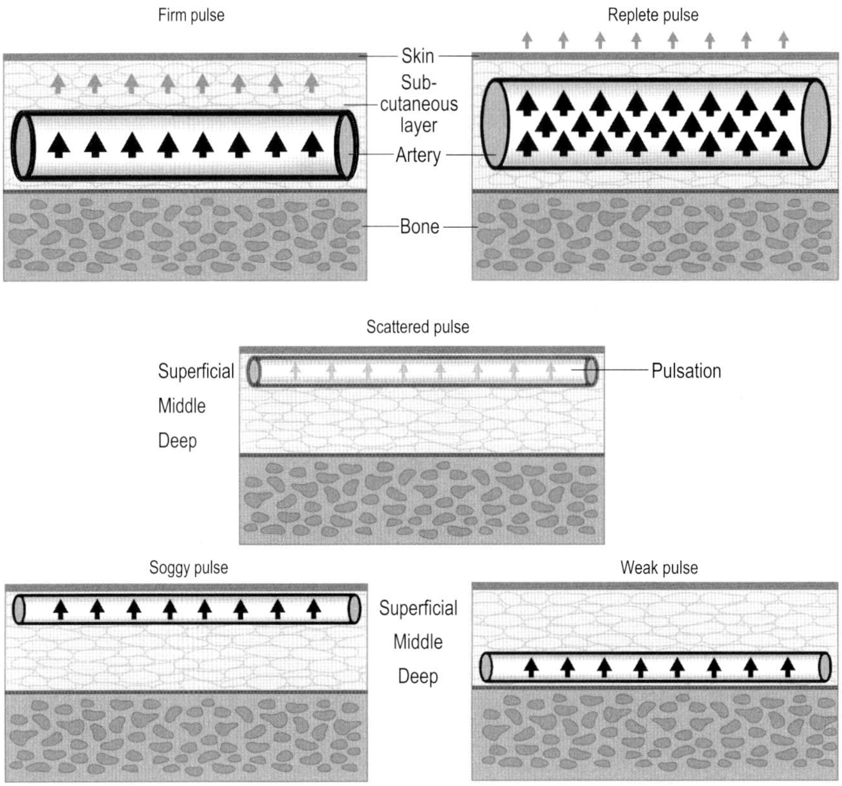

Figure 7.5
Schematic representations of the Replete, Firm, Soggy, Weak and Scattered pulses.

patterns, particularly associated with underlying Spleen Qi vacuity and digestive dysfunction (Kaptchuk 2000, Maciocia 2004, Wiseman & Ellis 1996).

Lu (1996) asserts that the Soggy pulse can be seen in postpartum women, signifying both Qi and blood vacuity.

7.8 Pulse contour and flow wave

The final parameter of pulse contour and flow wave primarily encompass the actual longitudinal movement of blood flow through the radial artery and its interaction with the arterial wall. Together these contribute to the formation of the contour or shape of the pulse.

7.8.1 Classifying CM pulse qualities according to pulse contour

There are four specific CM pulse qualities that are defined by the shape of the pulse contour and flow

wave. The contour pulses include one of the most commonly diagnosed pulses in clinical practice, the Slippery pulse, and one that is rarely seen, the Stirred (or Spinning Bean) pulse. They are:

• Slippery pulse (section 7.9.1)
• Rough pulse (section 7.9.2)
• Surging pulse (section 7.9.3)
• Stirred (Spinning Bean) pulse (section 7.9.4).

7.8.2 Definition of pulse contour and flow wave

The contour of the pulse refers to the shape of the pulsation that can be felt by the palpating fingers. It is formed by the pressure wave as it moves through the artery, deforming the arterial wall and propagating the longitudinal forward movement of blood (the flow wave). The pulse contour and the flow wave are influenced by a number of interacting factors including:

• Flexibility of the arterial walls and their relative tension
• Volume of blood/fluids within the circulatory system

- Amplitude or strength of the pulse
- Blood viscosity (flow varies inversely with the viscosity of the blood; McCance & Huether 2006)
- Condition of the lumen of the arterial wall, which influences the nature of the movement of the flow wave through the artery.

7.8.3 Assessment of pulse contour and flow wave

The assessment of pulse contour and flow wave involves two aspects:

- Evaluation of the consistency of the blood flow
- Evaluation of the pressure and flow wave and their impact on the arterial wall.

7.8.3.1 Evaluation of the tactile sensation of the flow wave contour

This involves assessing the nature or texture of the movement of blood as it passes through the radial artery underneath the fingers. There are number of questions that must be addressed when assessing this parameter:

- Does the blood flow feel smooth or turbulent? Is the blood flow consistent?
- Are there changes in the intensity of pulse force? This may make the pulsation appear stronger or weaker at times.
- Is the contour formed by each pulsation distinctly uniform or does it seem to change in shape?

7.8.3.2 Evaluation of the interaction of the pressure wave and flow wave on the arterial wall

We need to assess how the pulse wave feels:

- On arrival at the fingers
- As it passes underneath the fingers
- As it moves away from the fingers

This relates to the upward rise of the pressure pulsation, the peak and then the receding pressure (preceding the arrival of the next pulsation) and its interaction with the arterial wall. Different segments of the pulse wave may be more distinctive than others. For example, the arrival of the pulsation may be more distinctive than its departure. Alternatively, both the arrival and departure of the pulsation may be clearly felt.

7.8.4 Regulation of pulse contour and flow wave: CM perspective

The smooth flow of Qi and blood depends on four important factors. Lu (1996) notes that if any of these factors are compromised, pathological changes in the pulse contour may occur. These factors are:

- The presence of sufficient Qi and Yang
- The quantity and quality of Yin fluids
- The internal condition of the arterial wall (the tunica intima): a smooth arterial lumen ensures unimpeded laminar blood flow
- The external environment surrounding the arteries (connective tissue, organs, peritoneum, etc.): compression of arteries may adversely affect the distensibility of the artery.

7.8.4.1 Presence of sufficient Qi and Yang

Qi is the commander of the blood (Fig. 7.6). In this capacity, it produces, moves and keeps the blood within the blood vessels (specifically a function of Spleen Qi). Therefore Qi vacuity may affect the normal flow of blood, ultimately leading to sluggish flow or even stagnation of blood. In particular, Yang Qi is important to provide the Heart with the sufficient control over the blood and the vessels so that blood has the momentum to be propelled through the arterial system. Therefore Heart Yang has an important role in the circulation of Qi and blood not only in the chest but also throughout the body. If sufficient blood cannot reach the vital organs, then this can lead to functional problems with the transformation and transportation of Qi, blood and body fluids. This in turn may perpetuate or exacerbate the vacuity of Qi and blood. If Spleen Qi is vacuous, this may affect the production and consequently quantity of both Qi and blood.

7.8.4.2 Quantity and quality of Yin fluids

Blood is the mother of Qi, nourishing Qi and enabling its functional activity throughout the body (Wiseman & Ye 1998). Because of this close relationship between Qi and blood, the volume of blood or Yin fluids in any of its forms may impact on the tangible manifestation of Qi on blood flow, affecting pulse contour, pulse force, pulse width and the depth at which the pulse is most readily located. Therefore the quantity and quality of Yin fluids, encompassing blood, body fluids and Essence, also influences how blood moves through the arterial system (Fig. 7.7).

The pulse is affected by increases and decreases in blood/fluid volume in the following ways:

Increased volume

An increase in the volume of body fluids can affect the flow wave and pulse contour, depending on where the increase in volume occurs in the arterial system or in the connective tissue.

Increased fluid volume can develop as a result of abnormal fluid transformation and transportation

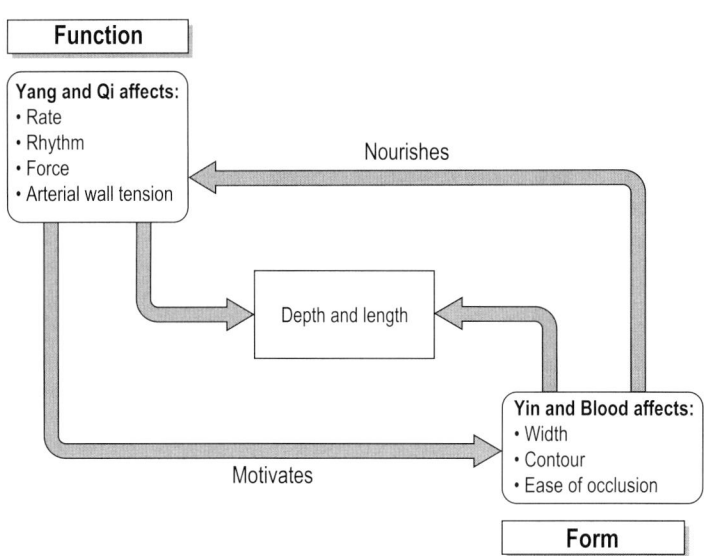

Figure 7.6
The mutual relationship between Qi and Blood.

involving the Spleen, Lung and Kidney and the Triple Heater. Fluid retention can occur due to normal water loss being inhibited, for example the inhibition of sweating or urination, and this can result in excess fluid moving into the blood vessels, leading to increased blood volume. Alternatively, fluid can accumulate in the limbs as oedema, in the lungs as phlegm or in the abdomen causing distension.

Clavey (1995: p. 134) notes that the close relationship between blood and fluids means that accumulated fluids can also interrupt normal blood flow, impacting on other bodily functions. For example the Shui Fen (water separation) syndrome illustrates what happens when oedema disperses menstrual blood 'separating it pathologically into water and Qi so that blood cannot flow into the uterine vessels, thus causing amenorrhoea'.

Conversely, increased production of fluids may not necessarily be pathological but may happen routinely as the result of normal increased metabolic demands, such as those occurring during pregnancy.

Decreased volume
Decreased fluid volume may occur as the result of the damage or loss of blood, body fluids, Yin or Essence. This can influence the radial arterial pulsation in the following ways:

- Insufficient filling of the artery so that it feels 'hollow' and is therefore very easily occluded
- The artery fails to be expanded and therefore the arterial diameter is narrower than it should be
- Insufficient fluids may lead to turbulent flow through the arteries, causing changes in both the pulse contour (shape) and pulse force

- Decreased Yin may lead to the relative hyperactivity and outward movement of Yang, due to the loss of the anchoring effect of Yin.

7.8.4.3 Internal environment of arteries

The smooth flow of Qi and blood requires unimpeded access to arteries that have smooth walls to encourage the laminar flow of blood. Obstruction of the flow of Qi, blood or both through the arteries leads to irregular changes in the pulse contour, as blood moves turbulently through the arteries (for example, the Rough pulse). The aetiology behind the obstruction to Qi and blood flow may be varied, encompassing both replete and vacuity patterns. For example, the presence of pathogenic factors may adversely affect Yang Qi and its ability to move blood. Damp has a congealing, sticky effect, resulting in the sluggish flow of Qi and blood. Heat or Fire, on the other hand, can dry up body fluids causing them to congeal over time, leading to the formation of Phlegm, and consequently the impaired flow of blood and Qi.

7.8.4.4 External environment surrounding the arterial system

The arterial system is extensive, with the arteries passing through connective tissue, muscles, organs, the gastrointestinal system and numerous other tissues to supply oxygen and nutrients throughout the body. The arteries may be partially compressed by the tissues through which they pass, so that blood flow through part of the arterial system is compromised. This may result in blood flow varying in intensity as it makes its way through the affected tissue.

Possible causes of arterial compression include:

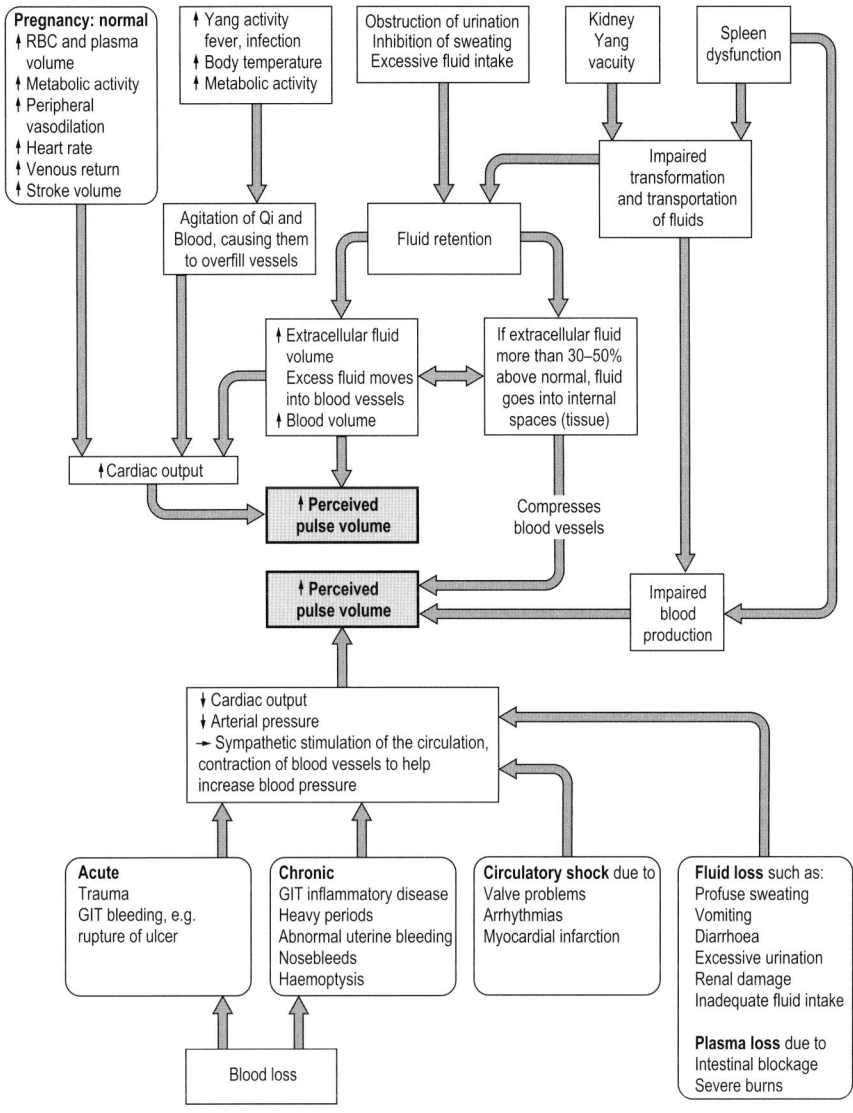

Figure 7.7
Factors affecting pulse volume.

- Food retention: Undigested food trapped in the stomach may cause abdominal distension or discomfort. The accumulated food may result in compression of the blood vessels, adversely affecting the flow of both Qi and blood in the area.
- Oedema: Fluids accumulating in the connective tissue and flesh may also compress blood vessels, so that normal expansion and contraction of the artery walls in response to the pulse and flow wave from the heart is inhibited.
- Trauma: Physical trauma may also result in disruption to blood flow through tissues.

7.8.5 Regulation of pulse contour and flow wave: biomedical perspective

There are numerous factors that can affect the pulse contour and flow wave. These are integrally related to the factors that affect pulse force and pulse width such as blood volume. As with the CM perspective, it is the interaction of these following factors that form the pulse contour and flow wave:

- Volume of blood/fluids in the circulatory system
- Cardiac output, in particular stroke volume (the amount of blood expelled from the left ventricle into the aorta during systole) and resulting pulse amplitude
- Blood viscosity; flow varies inversely with the viscosity of the blood (McCance & Huether 2006, Tortora & Grabowski 2000)
- Compliance of the arterial walls and their relative tension
- The condition of the lumen of the arterial wall, which influences the nature of the blood flow.

7.8.5.1 Smooth versus turbulent flow

The pulse contour and flow wave can be interpreted in terms of the smoothness of the blood flow and its relative state of turbulence. McCance & Huether (2002: p. 962) note that 'Where flow is obstructed, or the vessel turns, or blood flows over rough surfaces, it becomes turbulent . . . Resistance increases with turbulence'.

The condition of the lining of the arteries influences the fluidity of the blood flow. A rough lumen encourages turbulent flow. Atherosclerotic plaques inside the arteries may also impede flow, decreasing the arterial diameter and also causing disruption to the smooth surface lining the inner surfaces of the arterial wall.

7.8.5.2 Blood viscosity

Viscosity may also impact on blood flow. The viscosity of blood depends on the ratio of plasma volume and the number of circulating red blood cells. The more viscous the blood, the more sluggish the blood flow. Conversely, the lower the blood viscosity the faster and more turbulent the blood flow (Fig. 7.8).

Factors affecting blood viscosity include anaemia (decreased viscosity due to decreased size or numbers of red blood cells), dehydration (increased viscosity due to loss of body fluids through severe sweating, diarrhoea or vomiting) and plasma loss (increased viscosity due to loss of blood volume but not red blood cells).

7.8.5.3 Pregnancy

A number of changes in the cardiovascular system occur very early during pregnancy, one being a decrease in peripheral vascular resistance. It is hypothesised that this provides the stimulus for the activation of the renin–angitensin–aldosterone axis, responsible for the increase in plasma volume and cardiac output (Chapman et al 1998, cited in Poston & Williams 2002). These changes are apparent at about 5 weeks after conception. During normal pregnancy the increase in blood volume (on average about 1.5 litres) is due to both an increase in red blood cells (by 15–18%) and plasma volume (about 40–50%). This results in physiological anaemia and represents hypervolaemia or haemodilution, which is deemed a necessary adaptation of pregnancy in order to accommodate for cardiovascular changes and expected loss of blood at delivery (Coad & Dunstall 2005). The increased plasma/blood volume also provides increased systemic oxygen supply, increased renal filtration and helps to disperse increased heat production due to increased metabolic activity (Estes 2006).

7.9 CM pulses defined by pulse contour

7.9.1 Slippery pulse (Huá mài) 滑脉

The Slippery pulse is defined by changes occurring in a single pulse parameter. However, despite its seeming simplicity, the parameter of pulse contour encompasses a number of diverse variables associated with blood flow and the arterial wall structure. It should be noted that although the indications of the Slippery pulse all point towards repletion patterns and therefore by association, increased pulse force, this is not a requisite pulse parameter.

7.9.1.1 Alternative names

Although the name 'Slippery pulse' is most commonly used, it is also known in CM literature as the Smooth or Rolling pulse, which also aptly describe the shape of the pulse contour and how the flow wave moves under the palpating fingers.

7.9.1.2 Requisite parameters

- Pulse contour and flow wave: The Slippery pulse has a rounded shape or contour to the palpating

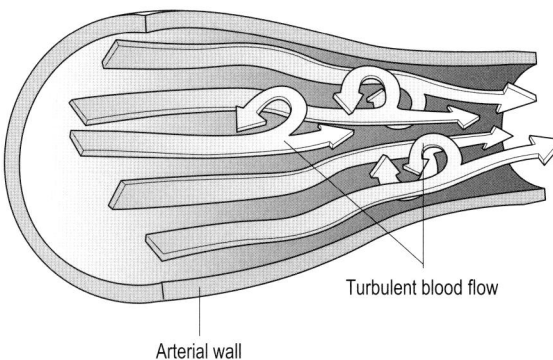

Figure 7.8
Turbulent blood flow. (Adapted from Part B of Figure 29.33 of McCance & Huether 2006, with permission of Elsevier Mosby.)

Turbulent blood flow

Arterial wall

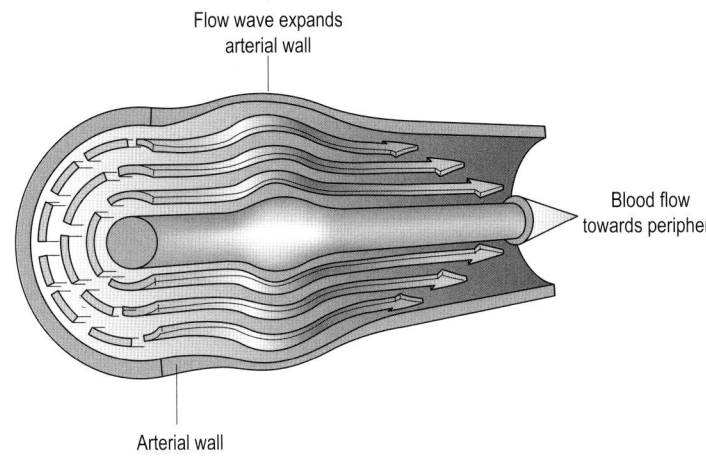

Flow wave expands
arterial wall

Blood flow
towards periphery

Arterial wall

Figure 7.9
Schematic representation of the flow wave and contour contributing to the formation of the Slippery pulse. (Adapted from Part A of Figure 29.33 of McCance & Huether 2006, with permission of Elsevier Mosby.)

finger. As the pressure wave travels along the radial artery, the arterial wall expands and contracts with ease as blood is pushed through the artery (the flow wave).

7.9.1.3 Clinical definition

The Slippery pulse is characterized by the smooth fluidity of blood flow under the palpating finger. The pulsation can be clearly felt expanding the arterial wall: the flow wave hitting and passing under the palpating finger, resulting in a distinct dilatation and contraction of the arterial wall so that a relatively large surface area of the artery is affected. The arterial wall returns to a normal resting state once the pressure wave departs, until the next wave arrives. This sensation is often described as giving the impression of 'smoothness' or a 'rolling' type of action and is characterised by a lack of friction between the flow wave and the palpating fingers. The pulse relates primarily to the longitudinal flow of blood and its interaction with the arterial wall (Fig. 7.9).

7.9.1.4 Classical description from *The Lakeside Master's Study of the Pulse*

A slippery pulse goes and comes, advances and retreats
Flowingly, uninhibitedly, unfurled, revolving
It responds to the fingers like a pearl (or bead)
[*Mai Jing*]
(Li, Flaws (trans) 1998: p. 76).

7.9.1.5 CM indications

The Slippery pulse can represent health, or may be considered to be a pathological pulse quality, depending on the accompanying signs and symptoms. There are five main conditions that can result in the Slippery pulse:

- Health
- Pregnancy

- Presence of pathogenic factors such as Phlegm, Damp or Heat
- Food retention
- Menstrual cycle: Occurs at certain times during the cycle

Health

The Slippery pulse can be an indication of good health, signifying abundant Qi and blood filling out the blood vessels. This signifies that Yin and Yang are well balanced and harmonious. The *Mai Jing* notes (Wang, Yang (trans) 1997: p. 21):

(A pulse) emerging swiftly followed by falling is called slippery. What does this imply?
The master answers:
Falling is pure Yin, while emerging is righteous Yang. When Yin and Yang are in harmony and cooperate, the pulse is slippery.

Pregnancy

The Slippery pulse is traditionally associated with a healthy pregnancy. It reflects the normal production of the extra blood and Qi that is required to supply the developing fetus with sufficient nutrients to grow and develop. This pulse is said to occur in the first trimester and is considered to be a healthy sign of a normally progressing pregnancy.

The Slippery pulse is also considered to be a diagnostic indicator of pregnancy. If the pulse is identified as Slippery and there is amenorrhoea (no periods) in someone whose periods are usually regular (Li, Flaws (trans) 1998: p. 76), then this may be a sign of pregnancy. In addition to the overall Slippery quality, an increased force in both Chi positions and the left Cun position is also deemed necessary by Maciocia (1998: p. 76). However, this theory in general should be used with some degree of caution, as the Slippery pulse can also occur in someone who is not pregnant, as the

159

Box 7.18

Underlying causes of Phlegm production

- EPA of Wind
- Dysfunction of Spleen, Lung or Kidney's transformation and transportation functions
- San Jiao dysfunction of Qi transformation and fluid movement
- Stress or emotional imbalance leading to Liver Qi stagnation
- Constitutional Yin vacuity
- Dietary: consumption of cold/ raw foods or overeating
- Lung Yin deficiency
- Kidney Yang deficiency: due to ageing or excessive sexual activity.

(Clavey 1995: Ch. 7)

Box 7.19

Signs and symptoms commonly associated with Damp

- Feeling of heaviness
- Lethargy
- Loose stools
- Nausea
- Abdominal distension
- Chest distension
- No appetite or thirst
- White greasy tongue coat.

result of a pathological process such as pathogenic Damp, Phlegm or Heat.

Pathogenic factors such as Phlegm, Damp or Heat

The Slippery pulse is commonly associated with pathogenic Phlegm, Damp or Heat. These pathogens may occur individually or in varying combinations.

- Phlegm: This has a varied aetiology due to either external pathogens or endogenous causes, often involving vacuity (see Box 7.18). Many of these factors ultimately result in stasis or obstruction that congeals fluids. Phlegm may also arise due to the prolonged retention of Damp in the body, as a further progression of Damp. The presence of Heat may lead to the congealing of fluids or Damp, producing Phlegm.

  Because Phlegm has multiple causes and pathogenic mechanisms, this may be reflected in the varying changes in pulse parameters. In other words, Phlegm may manifest in differing pulse qualities, not necessarily only the Slippery pulse. As noted previously in section 7.3, phlegm may also result in the Stringlike (Wiry) pulse, which would tend to reflect the underlying stagnation of Liver Qi as the causal factor. There may also be changes in rate or the level of depth at which the pulse can be found depending on the nature of the Phlegm.

- Endogenous (internal) Damp: Internal Damp may be the result of Spleen or Kidney dysfunction, leading to impaired transformation and transportation of fluids. Alternatively Damp may

arise due to dietary indiscretions such as the overconsumption of Damp-forming foods such as dairy (cheese, ice cream, milk) cold, raw food, citrus fruits and oily, fried or greasy foods. This can impact on the function of the Spleen and stomach, impairing transformation of food and drink and the distribution of fluids. Damp is greasy or sticky in nature and associated with the presence of excess fluids in the circulatory system or fluids trapped in the tissue. (See Box 7.19 for common Damp signs and symptoms.)

- Exogenous (external) Damp: Alternatively, the Slippery pulse may be caused by external pathogenic Damp due to climatic, environmental or living conditions 'If one is affected by the dampness Qi of the earth, then this harms the skin, the flesh, the sinews, and the vessels' (Unschuld 2003: p. 197). This would be seen as a replete-type pulse. However, the Moderate pulse and Soggy pulse are also associated with an EPA of Damp. The Soggy pulse may arise instead of the Slippery pulse if the individual has an underlying deficiency that may predispose them to external attack. The pathological Moderate pulse, with its slow rate, may be associated with pathogenic Cold Damp.

- Heat: The Slippery pulse may arise due to pathogenic Heat causing hyperactivity of both Qi and Blood, leading to excessive filling of arteries. Heat may have the additional effect of causing fluids to congeal, leading to the formation of Damp or Phlegm.

Food retention

Retained food may be caused by the regular consumption of Damp-inducing foods and alcohol which impact adversely on the Spleen and Stomach. This leads to impaired digestive function, and the retained food may transform into phlegm. As noted by Clavey (1995: p. 184), this is termed 'food phlegm' and is linked to Phlegm-Damp.

Menstrual cycle

The Slippery pulse may be seen at different times during the menstrual cycle. Maciocia (1998: p. 77) describes the normal pulse during menstruation as 'somewhat Slippery, Big and slightly rapid'.

It may be expected that at other times during the menstrual cycle the building up of blood and Yin in expectation of potential fertilisation (around mid-cycle, approximately days 11–15) may be reflected in the Slippery pulse. At this time of the cycle Yin is described as being 'at the peak of its cycle, the Chong vessel is full of Blood' (Lyttleton 2004: p. 36). From a physiological perspective, oestrogen is at its peak. There appears to be some limited initial biomedical support for this, with research showing increased radial artery distensibility (related to the ability of the artery to expand and contract and peripheral vasodilatation) occurring around ovulation (days 13–15) (see Box 7.20 for more information).

7.9.1.6 Biomedical perspective

Recent research has shown possible support for the manifestation of the Slippery pulse during pregnancy, revealing differences in radial arterial blood flow in pregnant women compared to non-pregnant women (Chen & Clarke 2001) (Fig. 7.10). However, while it is hypothesised that this may be reflected in changes leading to the possible formation of the Slippery pulse (Fig. 7.11), unfortunately a manual palpation component to identify possible CM pulse maladies was not included in the study to allow for correlation of objective pulse changes with manually assessed CM pulse qualities (see Box 7.21).

7.9.1.7 Comparison of the Slippery pulse with other CM pulse qualities

The Slippery pulse should not be confused with a Rapid pulse, which is defined as having an increase in heart rate. While the Slippery pulse may appear to be rapid due to the ease with which it slips beneath the finger, when the actual rate is calculated, the rate should fall within the normal range of 60–90 bpm. If the Slippery pulse is caused by Heat, then the pulse rate may be rapid as well.

The Slippery pulse is also commonly mistaken for the Stringlike (Wiry) pulse, even though their respective descriptions are quite different (see Box 7.22). The Stringlike and Slippery pulses are probably some of the most commonly seen pulse qualities in clinical practice.

Often in CM case studies, the pulse will be explained as being both Slippery and Stringlike (Wiry). As these are quite different pulse qualities in terms of the pulse parameters involved, how are these two pulse qualities seen in combination? If we examine what the main focus of each pulse is, we can see that they are actually

---

Box 7.20

The menstrual cycle and possible hormonal effects on radial artery distensibility

In a study undertaken to look at radial artery distensibility during the menstrual cycle, it was found that fluctuations did indeed occur during different phases of the menstrual cycle. Giannattasio, Failla, Grappiolo et al (1999) found that radial artery distensibility was increased markedly in the ovulatory phase (days 13–15) compared with the luteal phase (days 21–29) and follicular phase (days 3–5), which were decreased. Blood hormonal measurements showed that during the ovulatory phase oestradiol (oestrogen) was at its highest level, along with luteinising hormone (LH) and follicle-stimulating hormone (FSH). During the luteal phase, progesterone and antidiuretic hormone (ADH) were at their peak.

It is suggested that the variation in radial artery distensibility appears to be at least partially dependent on the sex hormones. The authors suggest that previous studies showing the existence of oestrogen receptors in vascular smooth muscle cells and the vasodilatory effects of oestrogen administration in animals, and the effects of increased oestrogen during pregnancy leading to an increase in arterial distensibility in both animals and humans, all point towards increased oestrogen levels in the ovulatory stage causing arterial distensibility.

The arterial stiffness of the luteal phase is due to an increase in the contraction of vascular smooth muscle in the arterial wall. While this may be due to a decrease in oestrogen levels during the luteal phase, it is likely to include other factors such the effects of increased progesterone and ADH levels that may reinforce the effect of decreased oestrogen levels or potentially have additional effects on the distensibility of the vascular wall.

161

---

concerned with different aspects of the pulse (see Box 7.23). The Stringlike (Wiry) pulse is mainly focused on the physical characteristics of the arterial wall (external aspect), while the Slippery pulse is primarily concerned with the flow wave and the forward longitudinal movement of blood (internal aspect). The Slippery pulse may sometimes be accompanied by increased arterial wall tension, but this would be seen as a relative increase, as the rounded contour of the pulse still dominates the pulse. As such, the tension would not be retained on increased finger pressure, indicating that the increased arterial wall tension is not the definitive Stringlike (Wiry) pulse. For example, this may be seen in conditions where Liver Qi encroaches on the Spleen and Stomach, leading to digestive disturbances. If we understand that increased arterial tension usually

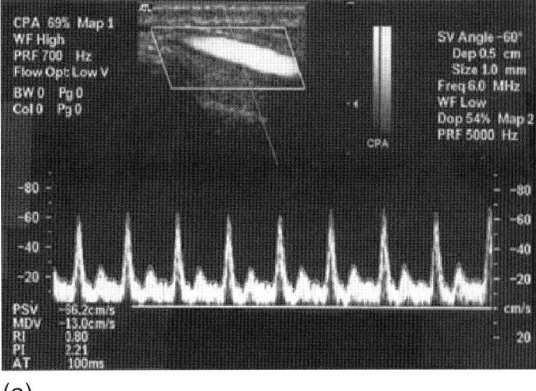 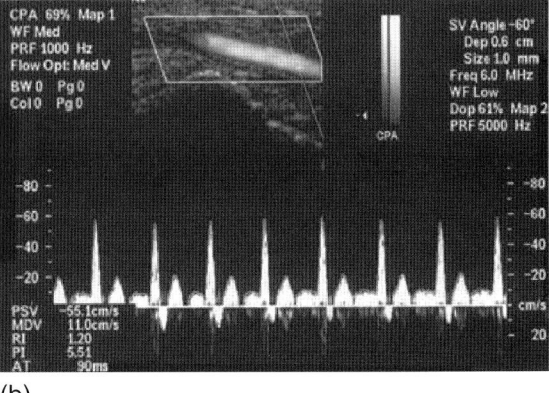

(a)　　　　　　　　　　　　　　　　　　(b)

Figure 7.10
Typical Doppler wave forms in the radial artery of (a) pregnant and (b) non-pregnant women. (From Chen & Clark 2001, with permission of Blackwell Publishing.)

Box 7.21

Pregnancy and changes in radial arterial blood flow

A research study has found that 'the physical properties of the blood flow pattern in the radial artery are different between pregnant and non pregnant women' (Chen & Clarke, 2001). It is hypothesized that oestrogen plays a role in the peripheral vasodilatation in two ways: inhibiting movement of calcium ions into vascular smooth muscle cells and stimulating nitric oxide, both of which cause relaxation of the smooth muscle.

This study also showed that blood flow pattern in pregnant women is believed to be less pulsatile than in non-pregnant women, 'throughout the entire cardiac cycle, whereas reversal flow and an absence of flow were detected in the non-pregnant women' (Chen & Clarke, 2001). They surmised that the decreased fluctuation of blood flow impact on the radial artery wall may contribute to the presentation of the CM 'smooth' pulse, described as feeling like 'a group of small glass balls running underneath the fingertips'. This is a reference to the Slippery pulse.

This is mirrored in CM thought, which has traditionally believed that pregnancy may be recognised, even at early stages, by the changes in certain characteristics such as the pulse contour in the radial artery pulse that occur during pregnancy (Maciocia 1998).

Box 7.22

Slippery pulse versus Stringlike pulse

- Slippery pulse: Blood flow forms the artery around itself: blood flow dominates arterial structure
- Stringlike (Wiry) pulse: The arterial wall is constricting blood flow: arterial structure dominates the contour of blood flow

the Slippery pulse. It can reflect health, as a sign of abundant Qi or blood, or as a pathological pulse quality it often occurs as a result of impaired Spleen Qi, particularly of Yang. Therefore the Moderate pulse may perhaps be considered to be a vacuity version of the Slippery pulse, with the Yang Qi vacuity affecting not only Spleen function but also slowing down metabolic activity generally, hence the decreased pulse rate. The accompanying signs and symptoms will also help to further differentiate the pattern. It must be remembered that pulse diagnosis is only one of the four examination procedures and that the other diagnostic indicators are also essential when formulating a diagnosis.

7.9.2 Rough pulse (Sè mài) 涩脉

The Rough pulse is a complex pulse quality that is primarily concerned with the nature of the blood flow through the radial artery and the effect that this has on the pulse contour. It is often contrasted with the Slippery pulse, described as its opposite in terms of the fluidity of the blood flow through the radial artery.

means obstruction, this may give us a clearer understanding of the underlying aetiology behind the pulse or alternatively, the extent of the pathogenesis.

The Moderate pulse, although known for its change in pulse rate (it is defined as slow), is also commonly described as having a rounded pulse contour similar to

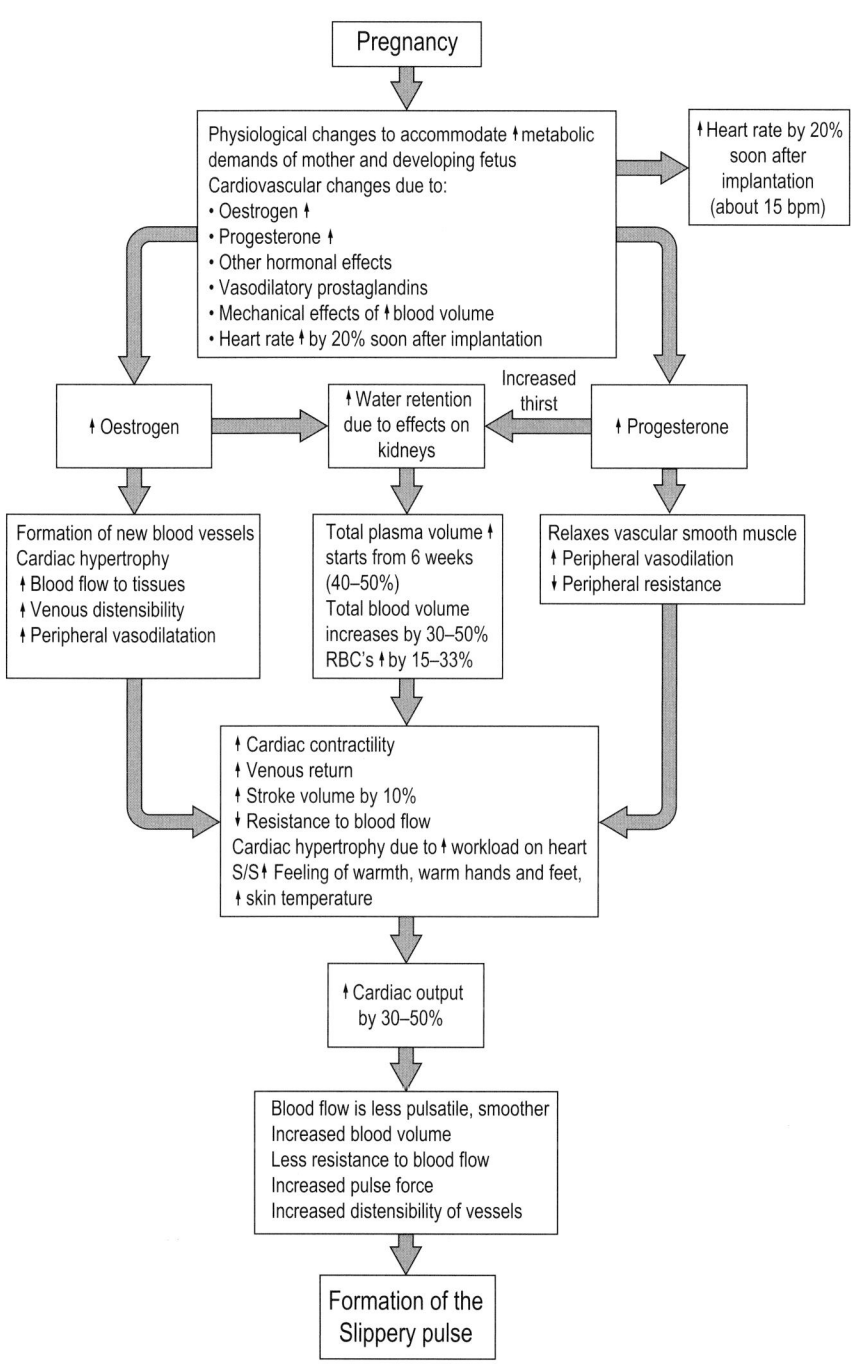

Pregnancy

Physiological changes to accommodate ↑ metabolic demands of mother and developing fetus
Cardiovascular changes due to:
• Oestrogen ↑
• Progesterone ↑
• Other hormonal effects
• Vasodilatory prostaglandins
• Mechanical effects of ↑ blood volume
• Heart rate ↑ by 20% soon after implantation

↑ Heart rate by 20% soon after implantation (about 15 bpm)

↑ Oestrogen

↑ Water retention due to effects on kidneys

Increased thirst

↑ Progesterone

Formation of new blood vessels
Cardiac hypertrophy
↑ Blood flow to tissues
↑ Venous distensibility
↑ Peripheral vasodilatation

Total plasma volume ↑ starts from 6 weeks (40–50%)
Total blood volume increases by 30–50%
RBC's ↑ by 15–33%

Relaxes vascular smooth muscle
↑ Peripheral vasodilation
↓ Peripheral resistance

↑ Cardiac contractility
↑ Venous return
↑ Stroke volume by 10%
↓ Resistance to blood flow
Cardiac hypertrophy due to ↑ workload on heart
S/S↑ Feeling of warmth, warm hands and feet,
↑ skin temperature

↑ Cardiac output by 30–50%

Blood flow is less pulsatile, smoother
Increased blood volume
Less resistance to blood flow
Increased pulse force
Increased distensibility of vessels

Formation of the Slippery pulse

163

Figure 7.11
Likely effects of pregnancy on the cardiovascular system and the development of the Slippery pulse.

Box 7.23

Pulse terminology

Unschuld (2003: p. 262) talks about the possibility of the terms such as 'rough' or 'smooth' being perhaps 'remnants of a time when the condition of the skin above the vessels, rather than the movement in the vessels below the skin, was considered a valuable parameter'. In this context, the term 'smooth' would reflect that the skin has been moistened and nourished, a sign of that there is sufficient Blood and body fluids. Conversely, skin that feels overly moistened or 'waterlogged' (oedema) may reflect fluid pathology. Similarly 'rough' may refer to the skin's lack of nourishment or moistening, reflecting a vacuity of blood or fluids. The interpretation of this terminology continues to resonate with the current indications of the both the Slippery and Rough pulses as defined today.

Box 7.24

The Three Five pulse: a subcategory of the Rough pulse

The Three Five pulse is a subcategory of the Choppy pulse that is mentioned in a number of modern CM texts (Kaptchuk 2000, Maciocia 2004, Townsend & De Donna 1990). It refers to the frequently changing rate of the pulsation so that sometimes it beats three times per respiration and sometimes five times per respiration (it does involve misted beats). Townsend & De Donna (1990) note its link to Heart or circulatory disease, but the other authors do not elaborate on its meaning.

This should be distinguished from normal sinus arrhythmia that is noted for its increased pulse rate during inspiration and decreased pulse rate on expiration and may be seen in healthy young adults, particularly men (see section 6.6 for more information.)

7.9.2.1 Alternative names

The Rough pulse is also known throughout the CM literature such as the Choppy, Dry, Hesitant, Uneven, Grating or Difficult pulse. The differing interpretations of the various terms used to name the Rough pulse may be responsible for the diverse range of descriptions for this pulse quality between CM texts and even within individual pulse definitions (see Box 7.24).

7.9.2.2 Requisite parameters

The Rough pulse is a complex pulse quality with changes in two pulse parameters:

- Pulse contour: This has an irregular shape to the palpating finger, lacking a feeling of fluidity of flow
- Pulse force: This may vary in intensity and the timing of systole and diastole.

7.9.2.3 Clinical definition

The Rough pulse is marked by variations in pulse force and, accordingly, pulse contour. The pulse wave appears to change in intensity, resulting in a pulse that sometimes feels forceful and at other times seems to decrease in force. This impacts on the palpating fingers as a change in pulse amplitude so that, with an even amount of pressure exerted on the artery, the pulse sometimes is felt forcefully and at other times it presents as forceless.

The term 'irregular' is often used to describe the Rough pulse. However, the irregularity described is associated with the changing intensity of pulse force. This may be caused by a change in the duration of systole and diastole or an inconsistency in blood flow, resulting in intra-arterial turbulence and poor propagation of the pulse pressure wave. This is perceived as an 'unevenness' by the palpating fingers.

The Rough pulse does not have missed beats, has a regular rhythm and is within the normal rate parameters.

7.9.2.4 Classical description from *The Lakeside Master's Study of the Pulse*

> Fine and slow, going and coming difficult, short and scattered. Possibly one stop and again comes (*Mai Jing*).
> Uneven, not regular (*Su Wen*).
> Like a light knife scraping bamboo (*Mai Jue: Pulse Knacks*).
> Like rain wetting sand.
> Like a diseased silkworm eating a leaf (*Li, Flaws (trans) 1998: p. 78*).

7.9.2.5 CM indications

> A slippery pulse shows abundant blood but scanty Qi. A choppy pulse shows scanty blood but abundant Qi. A large pulse shows abundance of both blood and Qi.
> (*From the Mai Jing (Wang, Yang (trans) 1997: p. 24*).

The Rough pulse is associated with two main patterns, vacuity and repletion, further differentiated by manual palpation using the parameter of pulse force:

- Vacuity of Yin fluids such as body fluids, blood or Essence
- Repletion causing stasis or obstruction of blood.

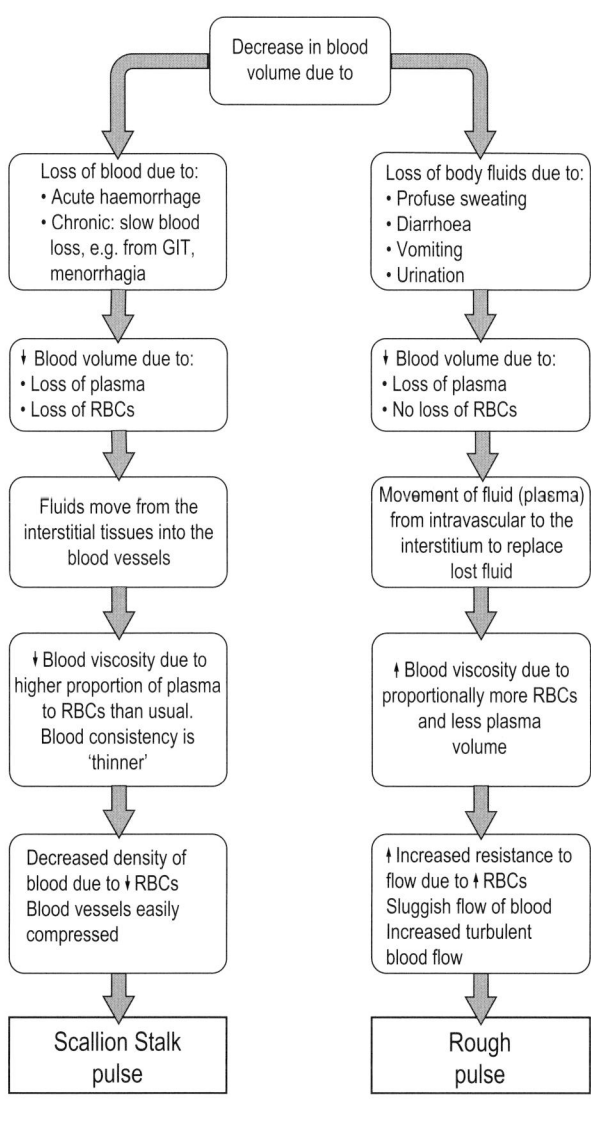

Figure 7.12
Fluid loss versus blood loss and the effects on the pulse.

165

Vacuity of Yin fluids such as body fluids, Blood or Essence

The Rough pulse may be seen in body fluid loss, blood vacuity or the consumption of Kidney Essence (Fig. 7.12). Vacuity of Yin fluids leads to impaired blood flow through the arteries, resulting in an unsmooth flow of blood.

- Yin fluid loss: Fluid loss may occur due to profuse sweating or severe vomiting, leading to dehydration. Acute trauma such as severe burns or tissue damage may also result in loss of plasma volume. Intestinal obstruction may also result in large loss of plasma into the intestinal lumen (Guyton & Hall 2006: p. 285). If fluid loss is severe, plasma may move from the circulatory system to replace the severely depleted fluid. This

results in increased blood viscosity, which can lead to the sluggish flow of blood and increased turbulence, hence the appearance of the Rough pulse (see Boxes 7.6 and 7.7).

- Vacuity of blood or Kidney Essence in pregnancy: From a CM perspective, the appearance of the Rough pulse in pregnancy is always pathological. At the beginning of pregnancy the Rough pulse indicates possible miscarriage and towards the end of pregnancy it may indicate an increased risk of eclampsia (Maciocia 1998).

During pregnancy various cardiovascular changes occur naturally, accounting for the increased force and 'slipperiness' of the pulse, including dramatic increases to blood volume, particularly plasma volume. The increase in plasma volume correlates positively with both birth weight and placental weight. An unusually low increase in plasma volume is associated with low birth weight, stillbirth and recurrent miscarriages (Coad & Dunstall 2005: p. 263). This correlates with the CM perspective of the appearance of the Rough pulse, in its vacuous form, which implies that the normal increase to blood volume has been impaired, resulting in insufficient blood to nourish and support the rapidly growing fetus. As Lyttleton (2004: p. 319) notes, if there is dual vacuity of blood and Qi then this may result in decreased fetal growth.

Lu (1996) states that Kidney impairment may lead to the Kidney Essence (also an important component in the production of blood) being consumed and this may also lead to infertility or in the case of pregnancy, miscarriage.

- Obstruction with underlying vacuity: Li (Flaws (trans) 1998: p. 80) also links the Rough pulse with an invasion of cold dampness into the 'constructive', an aspect of the blood, causing 'blood impediment'. Wiseman & Ye (1998: p. 32) define this as a *bi* (blockage) pattern occurring in patients with underlying Qi and blood vacuity, resulting in numbness and painful limbs. While the pulse is described as 'faint, rough', other changes such as 'fine and tight at the cubit' are also mentioned. 'Tight' may refer to the increased tension that arises due to the obstruction (signified by pain) while 'fine' may reflect the underlying vacuity, although this is difficult to know without further clarification by the author.

Replete patterns associated with stasis of Qi and Blood

The Rough pulse is also related to the stasis of normal Qi and blood flow. Some authors consider this pulse quality to be a sign of unhealthy lifestyle, seen in physically unfit people with an erratic lifestyle and diet, leading to stagnant Liver Qi with Damp (Townsend & De Donna 1990). As a result, Qi stasis eventually leads to the sluggish flow of the blood. However, other types of blood stasis may occur as the result of obstruction due to pathogenic factors or retained food.

- Cold Damp: The Rough pulse may occur with pathogenic Cold Damp, as the Cold contracts the vessels while Damp also causes stasis leading to obstruction of blood. In the Mai Jing, a discussion of the various causes of the 'internal binding (of evils)' giving rise to masses in the lower abdomen notes that 'If the pulse arrives choppy, it points to the disease of cold dampness' (Wang, Yang (trans) 1997: p. 23). This pattern is also described by Lu (1996: p 71).
- Retained food: Food retention may result in a Rough pulse because of its physical compression of

the blood vessels due to the accumulation of undigested food in the stomach. However, the undigested food may exacerbate the pathogenesis by the transformation of the retained food into Damp and eventually Phlegm, which further impacts on Qi and blood flow.

- Blood stasis affecting fertility and pregnancy: The Rough pulse may occur in patterns of blood stasis associated with the menstrual cycle, impacting on both the ability to become pregnant and also the viability of the pregnancy. Blood stagnation may impact on the endometrium and also the Chong Mai (also called the 'Sea of Blood'), one of the Eight Extra meridians associated with the menstrual cycle and fertility.

Endometriosis is a condition where endometrial tissue is found outside the uterus in the pelvic cavity. This can range from tiny spots to masses that distort the pelvic organs and can be found on or inside the ovaries, tubes, bladder or bowel (Lyttleton 2004: p. 167). For some women this may be non-symptomatic, but for others it may be the source of pain, menstrual problems and infertility. During pregnancy, the damage to the endometrium from endometriosis may affect the blood supply to the placenta, affecting its development and therefore increasing the risk of miscarriage (Lyttleton 2004).

Endometriosis is commonly associated with Blood stasis in terms of signs and symptoms such as stabbing pain, clotted menstrual blood and abdominal masses. It should be noted that if the pain associated with the blood stagnation is strong, then the overriding pulse quality that may be felt is the Tight pulse (Lyttleton 2004: p. 95). Lyttleton notes that endometriosis is also associated with Phlegm Damp and Kidney Yang vacuity, with the production of mucus secretions that obstruct to normal functioning of the reproductive system. All of these patterns may result in the obstruction of normal flow of Qi and thus Blood, reflected in the appearance of the Rough pulse.

7.9.2.6 Biomedical perspective

From a biomedical perspective, irregularities in pulse force may indicate a lack of smooth muscle tone in the arteries or changes in the force of the cardiac contraction (Tortora & Grabowski 1996: p. 631). Therefore cardiovascular dysfunction may potentially also result in the Rough pulse.

Conditions such as polycythemia vera, a genetically based disease that results in the overproduction of red blood cells and blood volume (sometimes twice as much as normal), may result in very sluggish blood flow due to the greatly increased viscosity of the blood (Guyton

& Hall 2006: p. 428). This may cause increased turbulence of blood flow.

7.9.2.7 Comparison of definitions

There is a wide divergence of descriptions and indications for the Rough or Choppy pulse. It is traditionally described as 'fine and slow' (Li, Flaws (trans) 1998, Wang, Yang (trans) 1997) in the classical texts. Within these definitions, there are references to the pulse 'coming and going with difficulty' as well as terms such as 'short' and 'scattered'. There are also references to an irregularity of rhythm 'possibly one stop and again comes' or 'with an interruption but the ability to recover'.

When examining the individual parameters of the pulse the following points can be noted:

- Pulse rate: When authors do include 'slow' in their definitions of the Rough pulse, it is often then categorized with other pulses associated with a decrease in pulse rate, for example Li Shi zhen (Huynh (trans) (1985) and Deng (1999)). However, many modern CM definitions do not include change of rate in their interpretations of the Rough pulse. The term 'slow' could possibly be interpreted as a decrease in the rate at which systole and diastole occur within a cardiac cycle, which may also account for the phrase 'coming and going with difficulty' or the indication that the pulse feels 'hesitant' rather than slow (Lu 1996: p. 71).

- Pulse rhythm: The reference to the interruption of pulse rhythm is not expanded on in the traditional definitions; therefore it is difficult to be sure of their nature or the context in which they occurred. An interpretation of its use may have been to signify the severity of the underlying pathological process of blood vacuity or stasis, as was commonly attributed to the Rough pulse; in particular, the use of 'possibly' may imply that this was not the normal occurrence. As the presence of rhythm irregularities often indicate heart organ involvement, the appearance of dysrhythmias, in conjunction with the other changes in parameters that signify the Rough pulse, would seem to indicate the progressive severity of the condition. Modern CM texts do not usually include the parameter of pulse rhythm in their definitions of the Rough pulse. Rather, the focus is on the texture of the blood flow and the changing pulse intensity.

- Pulse width: The term 'fine' continues to be used in modern definitions of the Rough pulse but is usually used in the context of the vacuity patterns only, particularly of blood or Essence (Jing). Therefore, it is not considered an essential part of the CM pulse definition.

Other pulse terms used to describe the Rough pulse

The terms 'short' and 'scattered' are sometimes utilised in the description of the Rough pulse. It is described as short by Maciocia (2004: p. 477) who notes that the pulse lacks 'continuous movement between the three positions and does not feel like a wave'. However, this description is not a common component of other definitions for the Rough pulse.

'Scattered' is used in the traditional pulse definitions of the Rough pulse in the *Mai Jing* and *The Lakeside Master's Study of the Pulse*. However it is poorly defined, if at all, and the possible interpretations of 'scattered' are too varied for this term to be of clinical use.

Hammer discusses the Choppy pulse as having 'small 'hills' and 'valleys' as one rolls one's finger along the pulse' and 'the varying heights are static' (2002: p. 63). He further describes it as 'like rubbing it [the finger] across a washboard'. Although these descriptions imply a variation in pulse wave height, he notes that the Choppy quality is 'relatively stable and fixed in terms of the vertical movement and has little of the restive wave activity associated with Changing Intensity and Amplitude [a specific and separate pulse quality as defined by Hammer and his colleague, Dr Shen]'.

A common interpretation of the Rough pulse encompasses varying pulse force. However, Hammer identifies a distinctly separate pulse quality defined as a pulse having a change in intensity and amplitude (see above), and says that the Choppy pulse is not this type of pulse. It is therefore unclear whether the 'hills' and 'valleys' Hammer is referring to are a result of the actual arterial pulsation or alternatively, perhaps part of the physical structure of the artery wall, possibly referring to a tortuous arterial wall that is not smooth.

There are distinctive pulse qualities in biomedicine that could possibly be equated with the Rough pulse. For example, pulsus alternans is defined by pulse beats that alternate in strength. This can palpated as alternating increase and decrease in amplitude, hence a distinctive change in pulse amplitude despite having a regular rhythm. This is due to the alternating force of left ventricular contraction and is commonly indicative of severe impairment of left ventricular function. It can also occur during or after paroxysmal tachycardia (sudden increase in heart that may last from a few seconds to a number of hours). However, pulsus alternans can also be seen in individuals without heart disease for several beats following a premature or ectopic beat (a heart contraction that occurs before the normal contraction is expected (O'Rourke & Braunwald 2001: p. 1256). See section 6.6 for more information about ectopic beats and tachycardia.

It is possible that the Rough pulse was used to describe a number of pulses that exist but do not fit easily into any of the other standard CM pulse quality definitions. For example, a forceless pulse that has a slow rate of pressure increase, leading to a delayed systolic peak and subsequent slow collapse, correlates well with the description of the pulse as slow and going and coming with difficulty. This will also result in a forceless pulse due to the low volume (small pulse pressure), further fulfilling the descriptions of its decreased width. From a biomedical perspective, this is recognised as the pulsus parvus et tardus which often occurs with discrete obstruction to left ventricular output, for example occurring in aortic valve stenosis (O'Rourke et al 1992: p. 74).

7.9.3 Surging pulse (Hóng mài) 洪脉

7.9.3.1 Alternative names

Flooding, Overflowing, Full, Tidal or Vast pulse.

7.9.3.2 Requisite parameters

The Surging pulse is a complex pulse quality with changes in three pulse parameters:

- Pulse contour and flow wave: The Surging pulse has a distinctive flow pattern, hitting the fingers distinctly but then pulse pressure decreases slowly.
- Pulse width: The arterial diameter is increased, resulting in a wide pulse.
- Force: There is an increase in pulse force

7.9.3.3 Clinical definition

The Surging pulse is a wide pulse. The initial part of the pulse wave pushes strongly against the side of the finger (in contrast to the Replete pulse, which pushes strongly upwards displacing the fingers vertically) but this is not sustained for the duration of the pulsation, continuing underneath the fingers with relatively diminished intensity. The most noticeable aspect of the pulsation is the initial forceful longitudinal movement of the pressure and flow wave, resulting in an expansion of the arterial wall.

7.9.3.4 Classical description from the *Nei Jing* and the *Mai Jing*

> The surging pulse is a very large pulse [floating and large in another version] under the fingers. *(Wang,Yang (trans) 1997: p. 3).*

> When the pulse comes with much strength but goes completely weak, this is called the flooding pulse. *(Ni trans 1995: p. 32).*

7.9.3.5 CM indications

The Surging pulse is now considered a pathological CM pulse quality associated with febrile disease, but it was traditionally described as the normal pulse for summer in the *Nei Jing*.

As a pathological pulse quality, the Surging pulse may be caused by either a replete external pathogen (Cold or Heat) or vacuity Heat pattern. These patterns include:

- Yang Ming stage of Six Division channel pattern identification
- Qi level of the Four Levels pattern identification
- Deficiency of Yin with hyperactivity of Yang.

Yangming stage of Six Division channel pattern identification

This theory deals with externally contracted febrile disease. The Yangming stage is the second stage and is associated with the progression of an external Cold pathogen into the interior of the body, transforming into extreme Heat. This pattern is usually accompanied by severe thirst and agitation, high fever, profuse sweating and the Surging pulse.

The Six Division pattern identification was initially mentioned in the *Nei Jing* but was described in greater detail in the *Shan Han Lun*, the classic text on externally contracted febrile disease.

From a CM perspective, high fever is a sign of that the body's Zheng Qi is strong and fighting off a very strong pathogen. Subsidence of the fever is a sign that the Zheng Qi is overcoming the pathogenic factor (Wiseman & Ellis 1996: p. 226).

The Surging pulse reflects the transformation of the Cold pathogen into Heat, the subsequent increase in Yang and the struggle with the Zheng Qi. It also reflects the damage to fluids by the strong heat. This may be the cause of the pulsation's tendency to hit the fingers strongly at first (increased Yang Qi) but then drop off gradually, as the fluids have been damaged and cannot sustain support for the Yang Qi (Yang is exuberant but Yin is weak).

Qi level of the Four Levels pattern identification

This theory also deals with externally contracted febrile diseases but is concerned with Heat pathogens and the effect of their progression into the interior of the body. In this particular pattern, an EPA of Heat transforms into severe heat and is very similar to the Yangming pattern described above. Signs and symptoms include high fever, severe thirst, agitation and profuse sweating. However, the Heat pathogen is able to transform into more severe heat much more rapidly than the previous pattern (Wiseman & Ellis 1996: p. 239).

As in the previous pattern, the Surging pulse is the result of the struggle between the Heat pathogen and the body's Zheng Qi (Upright Qi).

Deficiency of Yin with hyperactivity of Yang

This is a severe vacuity-type pattern that results from the consumption of Yin and the resulting hyperactivity of Yang. This version of the Surging pulse is usually found in patients with very weak constitution due to chronic illness (leading to consumption of Yin) or complicated by severe loss of blood (Lu 1996: p. 104). In such circumstances the appearance of the Surging pulse signifies a bad prognosis.

Townsend & De Donna (1990) ascribe ageing, poor diet and excessive consumption of alcohol or drugs as possible factors responsible for diminished Yin and the manifestation of the Surging pulse. The severe vacuity of Yin can no longer control the Yang, which becomes hyperactive.

7.9.3.6 Biomedical perspective

Febrile disease has systemic effects on the circulation, increasing metabolic activity, regardless of the cause. Fever also causes certain mechanisms to place in order to reduce the body temperature. These include:

- Sweating
- Vasodilatation, which transfers heat to the skin to be dispersed.

Sweating increases greatly when the body's core temperature rises above 37°C. A further increase of 1°C in temperature causes 'enough sweating to remove 10 times the basal rate of body heat production' (Guyton & Hall 2006: p. 895).

The vasodilatation may account for the increased width of the Surging pulse, and the increased metabolism may account for the perceived increase in pulse force. However, as noted in the clinical definition, this perceived force increase is not maintained for the duration of the pulsation. This may be the result of the injured fluids, depleted because of the increased fluid loss through compensatory sweating.

7.9.3.7 Comparison of similar CM pulse qualities

The Replete pulse is a pulse that is long and associated with either abundant Qi and blood (health) or Heat which agitates Qi and blood. Although both the Replete and Surging pulses are associated with Heat, the Surging pulse also signifies damage to fluids, which may occur concomitantly or may be pre-existing.

7.9.4 Stirred pulse (Spinning Bean pulse) (Dòng mài) 动脉

The Stirred pulse is not commonly seen. In some CM texts it is included as one of the ten 'Unusual' or 'Death' pulses and is generally considered to be associated with critical illness.

7.9.4.1 Alternative names

Spinning Bean, Stirring or Tremulous Pulse.

7.9.4.2 Requisite parameters

The Stirred pulse is a complex pulse quality that has changes in four pulse parameters:

- Pulse contour and flow wave: The pulse contour is rounded. It has a tendency to vibrate in its position, with a lack of smooth motion.
- Length: The Stirred pulse is a short pulse, occupying only one position, usually the Guan position.
- Rate: The pulse rate is rapid, >90 bpm.
- Force: There is an increase in pulse force.

7.9.4.3 Clinical definition

The Stirred pulse is rapid (>90 bpm) and short (occurring only in one position, usually the Guan position) and forceful, hitting the finger with intensity. It is noted for its quick succession of pulse pressure waves ('vibrating': rapid heart rate), with the pulse amplitude causing the arterial wall to be palpated by the finger as a 'curved' surface.

7.9.4.4 Classical description from the *Mai Jing*

> The Shan Han Lun (Treatise on Cold Damage) says 'Contention between Yin and Yang is called stirring . . . A rapid pulse that is perceptible only in the Guan with no ends in the upper or lower position. (i.e., the Cun or Chi) and which is large as a bean stirring and rotating in a small way is called a stirring pulse' *(Wang, Yang (trans) 1997: p. 5)*.

7.9.4.5 CM indications

The Stirred pulse usually occurs in an acute context, resulting from severe heat, trauma, pain, severe fright or cardiac-related dysfunction.

The Stirred pulse is associated with the severe disruption to the normal flow of Qi and blood and is considered to be the result of 'Yin and Yang wrestling' (Li, Flaws (trans) 1998: p. 116). The idea of two opposing yet interactive forces in dynamic motion has been an integral part of the philosophical theory underlying Chinese medicine, reflected by information in the *Book of Changes (Yi Jing)* which stated that 'It is because hard and soft push each other that changes and transformations occur' (Unschuld 2003: p. 85). Therefore the Stirred pulse may occur in sudden fright due to adverse flow of Qi and blood, whereas in physical trauma there may be severe obstruction of Qi and blood in the local area causing severe pain.

7.9.4.6 Clinical relevance

The Spinning Bean pulse is said to occur in reaction to sudden and extreme shock, fright, pain or physical trauma. It may be seen in severe fevers, myocardial infarction (heart attack), and shock (disturbance to normal circulation). Modern CM practitioners do not expect to see this pulse often in clinical practice, as these situations are more likely to be dealt with in an intensive care unit or other hospital settings.

7.9.4.7 Biomedical perspective

When the heart's ability to pump blood becomes impaired, for example from myocardial infarction (decreased blood flow to heart muscle), circulatory reflexes are activated to restore cardiac output. This involves stimulation of the sympathetic nervous system and inhibition of the parasympathetic nervous system. Strong sympathetic stimulation has the dual effect of increasing the myocardial contraction and increasing the ability of blood to flow back to the heart. This greatly increases cardiac output. Heart activity also increases, increasing heart rate.

Circulatory shock similarly activates sympathetic reflexes to in an attempt to restore cardiac output, which may account for the increase in pulse rate and increased force.

7.10 Revision of the 27 CM pulse qualities

See Tables 7.3 and 7.4.

7.11 Using the pulse parameter system

Although much is made of the complexity of the pulse taking process, some CM authors believe that it should not be a difficult skill to learn, if both the theories and standard textbook definitions of each pulse quality are learnt and memorised (Porkert 1983, Flaws 1997). As discussed extensively in Chapter 4, the difficulties experienced in pursuit of this goal are usually due to the wide range of varying definitions that exist for the CM pulse qualities. The main aim of the pulse parameter system of pulse assessment is to limit the subjectivity of the process by providing a consistent methodology and concrete pulse definitions. As such, the integral components of the pulse parameter system are:

- Learning and memorising which pulse parameters are involved in the formation of each CM pulse quality and the nature of the changes occurring
- Understanding the theory and mechanisms underlying each of the pulse parameters
- Following a consistent methodology for examining the pulse, collecting and interpreting the pulse information.

Table 7.3 ● Revision of the simple pulse parameters and the simple CM pulse qualities associated with them

Defining pulse parameter	CM pulse quality	Specific pulse parameters involved	Changes in pulse parameters present
Rate	Slow pulse (Chí mài)	Rate	Decreased ≤60 bpm
	Rapid pulse (Shuò mài)	Rate	Increased ≥90 bpm
	Moderate pulse (Huǎn mài)	Rate	60 bpm
Depth	Floating pulse (Fú mài)	Depth	Strongest at the superficial level
	Sinking pulse (Chén mài)	Depth	Strongest at deep level
	Hidden pulse (Fú mài)	Depth	Strongest at deep level, deeper than Sinking pulse
Length	Long pulse (Cháng mài)	Length	Extends beyond Cun, Guan and Chi
	Short pulse (Duǎn mài)	Length	Cannot be felt in all three pulse positions
Width	Fine pulse (Xì mài)	Width	Decreased width: narrow diameter
Rhythm	Skipping pulse (Cò mài)	Rhythm	Irregular interval between beats at irregular intervals
		Rate	Increased ≥90 bpm
	Bound pulse (Jié mài)	Rhythm	Irregular interval between beats at irregular intervals
		Rate	Decreased ≤60 bpm
	Intermittent pulse (Dài mài)	Rhythm	Regularly irregular: consistently misses a beat in a distinctive pattern. No rate change

Table 7.4 ● Revision of the complex pulse parameters and the complex CM pulse qualities associated with them

Defining pulse parameter	CM pulse quality	Specific pulse parameters involved	Changes in pulse parameters present
Arterial wall tension	Stringlike pulse (Xián mài)	Arterial wall tension Pulse occlusion Length	Increased arterial tension Retains form with increasing finger pressure Increased length: long
	Tight pulse (Jǐn mài)	Arterial wall tension Force Width Length	Increased arterial tension Increased force Increased diameter: wide Increased length: long
	Scallion stalk pulse (Kōu mài)	Arterial wall tension Force Width Depth Pulse occlusion	Increased arterial tension Decreased force Increased diameter: wide Strongest at the superficial level Easily occluded
	Drumskin pulse (Gé mài)	Arterial wall tension Force Width Depth Pulse occlusion	Increased arterial tension Decreased force Increased diameter: wide Strongest at the superficial level Easily occluded
	Scattered pulse (Sàn mài)	Arterial wall tension Force Width Depth Pulse occlusion	Greatly reduced arterial tension-little definition of arterial wall Decreased force Increase in diameter: wide Relatively strongest at the superficial level Very easily occluded
Force	Replete pulse (Shí mài)	Force Depth Width Length Arterial wall tension	Increased force Felt equally at all three levels of depth Increased diameter: wide Extends beyond Cun, Guan and Chi Increased arterial tension
	Firm pulse (Láo mài)	Force Depth Width Length Arterial wall tension	Increased force Strongest at the deep level Increased diameter: wide Extends beyond Cun, Guan and Chi Increased arterial tension
	Vacuous pulse (Xū mài)	Force Depth Width Pulse occlusion	Decreased force Strongest at the superficial level Increased diameter: wide Very easily occluded
	Faint pulse (Wēi mài)	Force Width Pulse occlusion	Extreme lack of force Very narrow Very easily occluded
	Weak pulse (Ruò mài)	Force Depth Width Pulse occlusion	Decreased force Strongest at the deep level Decreased diameter: narrow Easily occluded
	Soggy pulse (Rú mài)	Force Depth Width Pulse occlusion	Decreased force Strongest at the superficial level Decreased diameter: narrow Easily occluded

Table 7.4 ● Revision of the complex pulse parameters and the complex CM pulse qualities associated with them—cont'd

Defining pulse parameter	CM pulse quality	Specific pulse parameters involved	Changes in pulse parameters present
Pulse contour and flow wave	Slippery pulse (Huá Mài)	Pulse contour and flow wave	Smooth and rounded contour with a distinct expansion and contraction of arterial walls, conforming to flow wave. Can feel the pulse both arrive and depart smoothly.
	Rough pulse (Sè mài)	Pulse contour and flow wave Force	Contour feels irregular or has uneven texture to the palpating fingers Irregular: changes in intensity
	Surging pulse (Hóng mài)	Pulse contour and flow wave Width Force	The flow wave has a distinct arrival under the finger and an indistinct departure. Increased diameter: wide Increased force
	Stirred (Spinning bean) pulse (Dòng mài)	Pulse contour Flow wave Length Rate Force	Rounded Vibrating due to quick succession of beats Usually felt in only one position Increased: ≥90 bpm Increased force

A comprehensive knowledge of the clinical definitions and specific changes to pulse parameters for each of the 27 CM pulse qualities will enhance your ability to recognise them when they manifest themselves.

7.11.1 The appearance of multiple CM pulse qualities

As often noted in various CM pulse texts, it is not unusual for CM pulse qualities to appear in combination. However, in Chapters 6 and 7, an examination of the pulse parameter profiles reveals that there are some CM pulse qualities that simply cannot coexist. The Floating pulse and Sinking pulse cannot, by definition, appear simultaneously, likewise with the rate-related pulses. Another example of this was presented in Chapter 4 in the discussion of two complex pulse qualities, the Stringlike (wiry) pulse and Slippery pulse, which are primarily defined by two distinct pulse parameters. In this case, while a pulse may present with degrees of changes in both of these pulse parameters, neither is definitive enough to allow the pulse to be designated as either traditional CM pulse quality. To do so would lose valuable pulse information.

Pathogenic factors can often trigger changes in multiple pulse parameters that do not normally appear

together as a particular CM pulse quality profile. For example, pathogenic Heat results in hyperactivity of Yang. This has the effect of agitating Qi and blood, resulting in an expansive movement of blood flow so that it can be felt in the radial artery as a length of pulsation, hence termed 'long'. If the Heat is enough to elevate the body temperature then this results in an increased pulse rate. Therefore the pulse may be identified equally as both the Long and Rapid pulses. However, a Rapid pulse may occur without the Long pulse and vice versa.

Although changes in simple pulse parameters do occur together, it is usually a combination of these that lead to the identification of a specific CM pulse quality. For example, for a pulse that is found at the deep level of depth and cannot be felt at the superficial level, and is forceless and narrow, instead of identifying it as a forceless Sinking and Fine pulse, we would identify this as the Weak pulse.

Common combinations of CM pulse qualities often include a simple and a complex pulse quality. For example, assessment of the pulse during the onset of a cold or flu following exposure to cold climatic conditions may reveal pulse parameter profiles for both the Floating and Tight pulses, which may appear simultaneously in an EPA of Wind Cold. This would be described as a pulse that is forceful, has increased tension in the arterial wall that leads to a slight sideways movement and is found to be strongest a the superficial level of depth. The appearance of the pulse strongest at the superficial level of depth can be an indication that the exterior of the body is the focus of pathogenesis. In this particular case, the EPA has activated the Zheng Qi of the body so that Qi and blood rush to the surface as a defensive mechanism. The over-forceful nature of the pulsation indicates an excess within the body and signifies that both the Zheng Qi and pathogenic factor are strong, while the increased arterial tension reflects the effect of the Cold causing contraction of the muscles and blood vessels.

As such, these changes in the pulse parameters represent the pathological processes currently taking place in the body and signify specific changes in pulse parameters that are not normally linked together in any of the single traditional CM pulse qualities. Therefore, more than one CM pulse quality may be present.

Sometimes a pathogenic factor triggers changes in normal function (reflected in changes in pulse parameters) that, over time, can lead to changes in other pulse parameters and the transition of one CM specific pulse quality into another. Using the example above, the invasion of Wind Cold into the body presents with a Floating and Tight pulse. As the body's defensive Qi struggles with the pathogen, this causes Heat, which agitates Qi and blood; but as the struggle progresses the Heat increases and this causes fluids to be depleted. This results in a progression of the pulse into the Surging pulse, still forceful but starting to slightly reflect the damage to Yin fluids. The increased arterial tension in the pulse has receded due to the transformation of the Cold pathogen into Heat. The concept of progression of illness and its effect on the pulse is explored further in Chapter 8.

7.11.2 Practical application of the pulse parameter system

In terms of applying this system to diagnostic practice, we need to ensure that we examine the pulse in a methodical way, looking at each one of the parameters. Table 7.5 outlines the aspects of the pulse that need to be examined each time. This is the first step in identifying any changes in pulse parameters.

With a clear understanding of the mechanisms that result in changes to individual pulse parameters, the appearance of CM pulse qualities in certain disease states or ill health may be better understood. This is important because often the presenting pulse does not fit any of the criteria of the 27 CM pulse qualities (Box 7.25). This does not necessarily mean that the pulse information cannot be used, as the changes in individual pulse parameters can be used to shed light on the pathogenic process that is taking place. For

---

full details of the pulse taking procedure, see section 5.11.3.

The general pulse assessment process is outlined in Figure 7.13. It is recommended that you make use of the checklist for the CM pulse qualities (Table 7.6) and the summary of the CM pulse qualities in Tables 7.3 and 7.4 when you are initially starting to learn the pulse parameter system. These will help you to familiarise yourself with the terminology, pulse parameters and definitions for each of the CM pulse qualities, simplifying the identification process from the pulse information you have collected in Table 7.5. These tables are included for convenience but are not meant to be limiting, so include more information if you feel it is necessary.

7.11.3 Using the CM theory underlying the pulse parameters

Having identified the pulse parameters involved, use the checklist (Table 7.3) to note whether your parameter profile correlates with any of the 27 CM pulse qualities. You may find more than one CM pulse quality, as it is common for them to occur in conjunction with one another. For example, if the pulse rate is 95 bpm and equally strong at all three levels of depth, hits the fingers forcefully, is felt beyond Chi and is wide with a well-defined arterial wall, we would identify both the Rapid and Replete pulses.

However, what do you do if, having evaluated the pulse, you find that the pulse profile does not fit any of the specific CM pulse qualities? Rather than trying to fit any changes in pulse parameters into a specific pulse quality profile, and risk losing valuable pulse information, another way of utilising the information obtained from radial pulse palpation is to relate the changes occurring in the pulse and accompanying signs and symptoms, to the effect on the different substances,

Table 7.5 ● Pulse parameter assessment form

Pulse parameter	Factors to consider	Pulse assessment findings: Change in the pulse parameters Relevant diagnostic information
Rate	Beats per minute (bpm)	
	Extraneous factors: exercise levels, medication, stress, caffeine intake, prior exertion (for example, exercise or hurrying)?	
Rhythm	Is the rhythm regular (even intervals between each beat)?	
	If there are irregularities, do these occur erratically or regularly?	
	How often? When? Accompanied by stress?	
	Does the person suffer from palpitations?	
Depth	At what level of depth is the pulse the strongest?	
	Can it be felt at all levels of depth?	
	Does the strength vary between levels?	
Width	Is the pulse narrow or wide?	
	Neither? Appropriate width?	
Length	Can you feel the pulse at Cun,	
	Guan and Chi?	
	Can you feel it beyond Cun?	
	Can you feel it beyond Chi?	
	Does the artery wall have a continuous feel beneath the three fingers? That is, like a length of artery rather than having to feel the pulsation at each individual position?	
Arterial wall tension	Can you feel the arterial wall clearly?	
	Is there increased tension in the artery? Does the arterial wall feel hard?	
	Is it difficult to feel the arterial wall?	
Force	Does the pulse strike the finger:	
	Forcefully;	
	Without force;	
	With moderate force?	
Ease of occlusion	Does the pulse occlude easily with little pressure?	
	Does it feel 'empty' or lacking substance?	
	Does the artery feel solid, as though it is full?	
	Can you still the arterial distinctly wall even though the pulsation has been occluded?	

Table 7.5 ● Pulse parameter assessment form—cont'd

Pulse parameter	Factors to consider	Pulse assessment findings: Change in the pulse parameters Relevant diagnostic information
Pulse contour and flow wave	Can you feel the both the ascending and descending change in pressure?	
	Are they even in strength?	
	Can you feel the expansion and contraction of the artery walls?	
	Does the artery move side to side laterally?	
	Does the pulse move smoothly or unevenly under the finger? Does it have a particular shape?	
	Rounded, or does it vary in shape?	

Table 7.6 ● Specific CM pulse quality checklist

TCM pulse quality	Rate	Rhythm	Depth	Length	Width	Arterial tension	Pulse contour and flow wave	Pulse occlusion	Force
Slow pulse (Chí mài)	✓								
Rapid pulse (Shuò mài)	✓								
Moderate pulse (Hǔan mài)	✓						✓		
Racing pulse (Jí mài)	✓								
Floating pulse (Fú mài)			✓						
Sinking pulse (Chén mài)			✓						
Hidden pulse (Fú mài)			✓						
Long pulse (Cháng mài)				✓					
Short pulse (Duǎn mài)				✓					
Fine pulse (Xì mài)					✓				
Skipping pulse (Cò mài)	✓	✓							

Table 7.6 ● Specific CM pulse quality checklist—cont'd

TCM pulse quality	Rate	Rhythm	Depth	Length	Width	Arterial tension	Pulse contour and flow wave	Pulse occlusion	Force
Bound pulse (Jié mài)	✓	✓							
Intermittent pulse (Dài mài)		✓							
Stringlike (Wiry) pulse (Xián mài)				✓		✓		✓	
Tight pulse (Jǐn mài)				✓	✓	✓			✓
Scallion Stalk pulse (Kōu mài)			✓	✓	✓	✓		✓	✓
Drumskin pulse (Gé mài)			✓	✓	✓	✓		✓	
Scattered pulse (Sàn mài)			✓		✓	✓		✓	
Replete pulse (Shí mài)			✓	✓	✓	✓			✓
Firm pulse (Láo mài)			✓	✓	✓	✓			✓
Vacuous pulse (Xū mài)			✓		✓			✓	✓
Weak pulse (Ruò mài)			✓		✓			✓	✓
Faint pulse (Wēi mài)			✓		✓			✓	✓
Soggy pulse (Rú mài)			✓		✓			✓	✓
Slippery pulse (Huá mài)							✓		
Rough pulse (Sè mài)							✓		✓
Surging pulse (Hóng mài)					✓		✓		✓
Stirred (Spinning Bean) pulse (Dòng mài)	✓			✓			✓		✓

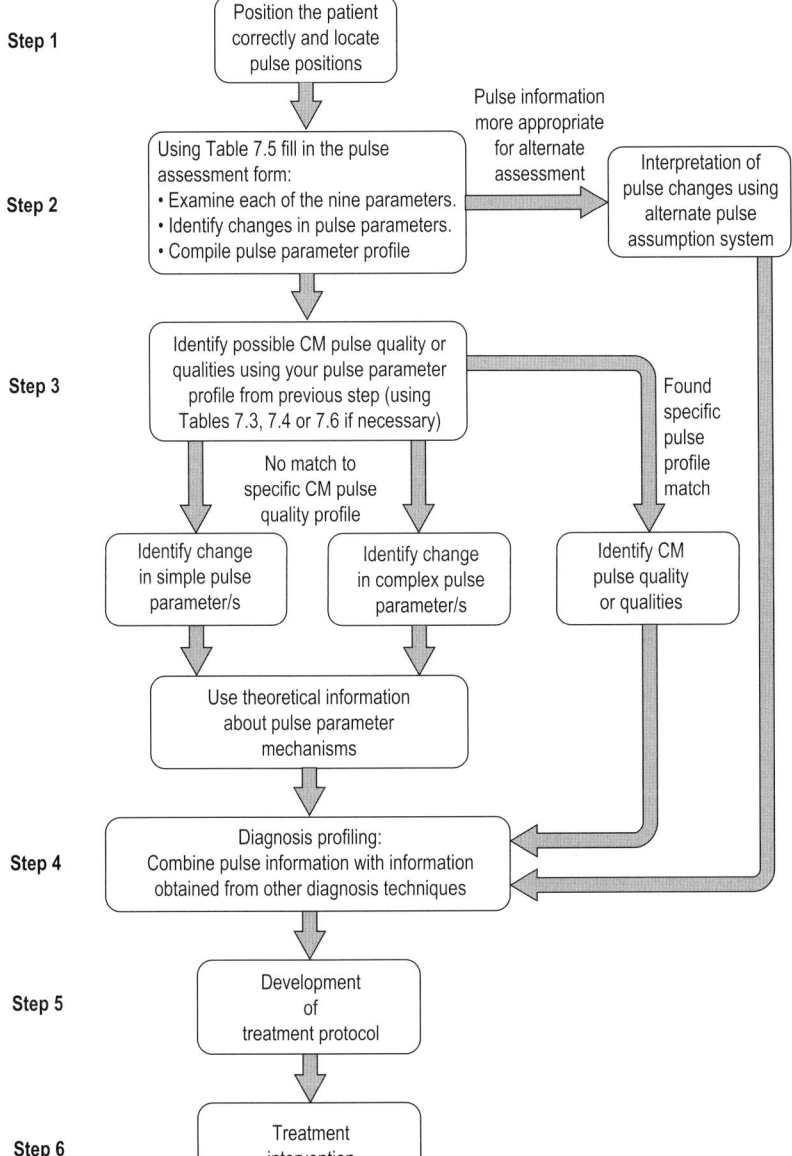

Figure 7.13
Pulse parameter assessment process.

such as Qi, Yang, Yin, and Blood, involved in the formation of the pulse. The mechanisms behind the pulse parameters have been discussed in detail throughout Chapters 6 and 7, in the accounts of the specific CM pulse qualities. Tables 7.3 and 7.4 briefly summarise this information, noting the effect on the pulse parameters. Note that this is a theoretical construct, so although this information may generally apply in most cases, occasionally there may be some contradictory findings. Remember that pulse diagnosis is only part of the holistic diagnostic procedure employed in order to gain a complete understanding of the patient's presenting problems and, as such, was not intended as a solitary diagnostic technique.

This concludes our account of the pulse parameter assessment system. The next chapter explores the connections that exist between many of the CM pulse qualities in terms of their shared pathological mechanisms and progression of disease.

References

Amber R, Babey-Brooke A 1993 Pulse diagnosis: detailed interpretations for eastern and western holistic treatments. Aurora Press, Santa Fe, NM

Chen D, Clarke J 2001 Analysis of a clinical sign in traditional Chinese medicine using Doppler ultrasound. Australasian Radiology 45:452–456

Chen S, Lin Y, Meng Q et al 1996 Comparative study on the mechanism of formation of pulse manifestations in coronary heart disease and hematopathic patients. Journal of Traditional Chinese Medicine June 16(2):143–146

Cockcroft J R, Wilkinson I B, Webb D J 1997 Age, arterial stiffness and the endothelium. Age and Aging 26-S4: 53–60

Clavey S 1995 Fluid physiology and pathology in traditional Chinese medicine. Churchill Livingstone, South Melbourne

Coad J, Dunstall M 2005 Anatomy and physiology for midwives, 2nd edn. Elsevier, Edinburgh

Deng T 1999 Practical diagnosis in traditional Chinese medicine. Churchill Livingstone, Edinburgh

Estes M E 2006 Health assessment and physical examination, 3rd edn. Thomson Delmar Learning, Southbank, Vic

Flaws B 1997 The secret of Chinese pulse diagnosis, 2nd edn. Blue Poppy Press, Boulder, CO

Giannattasio C, Failla M, Grappiolo A et al 1999 Fluctuations of radial artery distensibility throughout the menstrual cycle. Arteriosclerosis, Thrombosis & Vascular Biology 19: 1925–1929

Guyton A, Hall J 2006 Textbook of medical physiology, 11th edn. Elsevier Saunders, Philadelphia

Guangzhou Chinese Medicine College April, 1991 Inspection of the tongue and pulse taking. April. Guangzhou, China

Hammer, L (2002) Workshop: tradition and revision. Clinical Acupuncture and Oriental Medicine 3: 59–71

Kaptchuk T J 2000 Chinese medicine: the web that has no weaver. Random House, London

Kelly B A, Chowienczyk P 2002 Vascular compliance. In: Hunt B J, Poston L, Schachter M, Halliday A W (eds) An introduction to vascular biology: from basic science to clinical practice, 2nd edn. Cambridge University Press, Cambridge

King E, Cobbin D, Walsh S et al 2002 The reliable measurement of radial pulse characteristics. Acupuncture in Medicine 20(4):150–159

Li S Z, Flaws B (translator) 1998 The lakeside master's study of the pulse. Blue Poppy Press, Boulder, CO

Li S Z, Huynh HK (translator), Seifert GM (editor) 1985 Pulse diagnosis by Li Shi Zhen. Paradigm, Brookline, MA

Lu Y 1996 Pulse diagnosis. Science and Technology Press, Jinan

Lyttleton J 2004 Treatment of infertility with Chinese medicine. Churchill Livingstone, Edinburgh

McCance K L and Huether S E 2006 Pathophysiology: the biologic basis for disease in adults and children. Elsevier Mosby, St Louis

Maciocia G 1989 The foundations of Chinese medicine. Churchill Livingstone, Edinburgh

Maciocia G 1998 Obstetrics and gynaecology in Chinese medicine. Churchill Livingstone, Edinburgh

Maciocia G 2004 Diagnosis in Chinese medicine: a comprehensive guide. Churchill Livingstone, Edinburgh

Ni M (translator) 1995 The Yellow Emperor's classic of medicine: a new translation of the neijing suwen with commentary. Shambala, Boston

O'Rourke M F, Kelly R P, Avolio A P 1992 The arterial pulse. Lea & Febiger, Philadelphia

O'Rourke R, Braunwald E 2001 Physical examination of the cardiovascular system. In: Braunwald E, Fauci A, Kaspar D et al (eds) Harrison's principles of internal medicine, Volume 1, 15th edn. McGraw-Hill, New York, Ch 225

Porkert, M 1983 The essentials of Chinese diagnostics. Acta Medicinae Sinensis Chinese Medicine Publications, Zurich

Poston L, Williams, D 2002 Vascular function in normal pregnancy and preeclampsia. In: Hunt B J, Poston L, Schachter M, Halliday A W (eds) An introduction to vascular biology: from basic science to clinical practice, 2nd edn. Cambridge University Press, Cambridge

Rogers C 2000 The five keys: an introduction to the study of traditional Chinese medicine, 3rd edn revised. Acupuncture Colleges Publishing, Sydney

Stables D, Rankin J (editors) 2006 Physiology in childbearing with anatomy and related biosciences. Elsevier, Edinburgh

Tortora G J, Grabowski S R 2000 Principles of anatomy and physiology, 9th edn. John Wiley & Sons, Inc., New York

Townsend G & De Donna Y 1990 Pulses and impulses. Thorsons, Wellingborough

Unschuld P 2003 Huang di nei jing su wen. University of California Press, Berkerley

Walsh S 2003 The radial pulse: correlation of traditional Chinese medicine pulse characteristics with objective tonometric measures [PhD]. University of Technology, Sydney

Wang S H, Yang S (translator) 1997 The pulse classic: a translation of the mai jing. Blue Poppy Press, Boulder, CO

Wiseman N, Ellis A (translators and editors) 1996 Fundamentals of Chinese medicine, revised edn. Paradigm, Brookline, MA

Wiseman N, Ye F 1998 A practical dictionary of Chinese medicine 2nd edn. Paradigm, Brookline, MA

Genesis of pulse qualities

8

Chapter contents

8.1 Same disease different pulse; different pulse same disease 179

8.2 External pathogenic attack versus internal dysfunction 179

8.3 Blood 188

8.4 Qi 196

8.5 Yin vacuity 198

8.6 Yang vacuity 198

8.7 Health 199

8.8 The Unusual or Death pulses 200

8.1 Same disease different pulse; different pulse same disease

A clinical complication for the use of pulse diagnosis is that there can be a range of quite distinctly different pulse qualities that form in response to apparently the same illness or dysfunction. Blood vacuity or anaemia is an apt example of this. Blood vacuity pulses can present with both increased and decreased changes in the arterial width. With this in mind, there is still a further complication with the similarity of some pulses; while they are similar, diagnostically they reflect different pathological processes and the general health of the patient. This situation is aptly described in the Chinese medical axiom:

> Tong bing yi zhi,
> Yi bing tong zhi,
> Different disease, one treatment
> Same disease, different treatments

For this reason the traditional CM pulse qualities presents in Chapters 6 and 7 will be discussed in a comparative manner in this chapter with respect to the pathologies, dysfunction or health states that they reflect.

8.2 External pathogenic attack versus internal dysfunction

External pathogenic attack (EPA) refers to pathogenic agents external to the body that give rise to illness and can cause dysfunction. From a biomedical perspective this can broadly relate to common colds and influenzas and encompass other viral, fungal and bacterial agents. In a CM context, categorisation of illness due to pathogenic agents is based on the resultant signs and symptoms, the body's response to the pathogenic agent. In this sense, pathogenic agents causing fever are broadly classified as *Heat*; pathogenic agents causing swelling and oedema are classified as *Damp*. There are also *Cold*, *Dry* and *Wind* pathogenic agents in addition to Heat and Damp. Pathogenic agents can also combine to form complex conditions such as Damp Heat as seen in viral infections such as varicella (chickenpox).

A traditional assumption associated with the pulse when EPA attacks the body is the movement of the body's defensive Qi to accumulate or move outwards to the superficial regions of the body. The pulse correspondingly becomes relatively stronger at the superficial levels of depth. EPAs are a perverse version of Qi, certainly pathogenic, but still Qi. In this sense, when a pathogen attacks the body then there is extra Qi, additional to the normal levels of Qi in the body. The addition of the Qi makes the overall force of the pulse increase. This occurs in addition to the increasing defensive Qi levels at the external parts of the body to counter the EPA and reflected in the pulse as being strongest at the superficial level of depth.

When the pulse is distinctly stronger at the superficial level of depth, and consequently less strong at the middle and deep levels of depth, then this is termed a Floating pulse reflecting the movement of defensive Qi to counter the pathogen.

The Floating pulse also occurs with internal dysfunction causing conditions of hyperactivity such as seen in states of anxiety or stress. This is termed *Yin vacuity (Yin deficiency)*. This occurs when the body's ability to control Yang is compromised, causing increased activity of Yang. The Floating pulse occurs as Yang moves upwards and outwards, which is seen as pulling the Qi and blood with it. Another useful way of looking at this is via the control mechanisms of the autonomic nervous system; the parasympathetic nervous system's counter control to the sympathetic nervous system, and the related feedback systems are no longer able to keep activity in check.

The Floating pulse can therefore occur in the presence of EPA but also with internal dysfunction. As there are two quite distinct aetiologies, the Floating pulse can be further differentiated by the related changes in other accompanying pulse parameters. In this case the Floating pulse due to an EPA is accompanied by an increase in pulse force, reflecting the increased metabolic demands of the body to combat the pathogen. The Floating pulse resulting from Yin vacuity will have a decrease in pulse force reflecting the empty-type hyperactivity occurring.

There are a range of pulse qualities that occur with external attack by pathogenic agents. Although most of these pulse qualities are strongest at the superficial level of depth, they will by no means all present as a Floating pulse. Depending on the changes in other pulse parameters, usually in regard to the type of pathogenic agent, several other traditional pulse qualities can develop. There are specific differences in the parameters of these pulses that differentiate them from the Floating pulse, as there are specific differences in the parameters of the Floating pulse to further differentiate it from other superficially occurring pulses. Additionally, not all acute pathogenic attacks will result in a superficially strong pulse, because sometimes the pathogen goes directly into the interior and affects organ function. The pathogen can also mutate, so one pulse quality occurs initially and as the pathogen mutates so the pulse quality also changes. The Tight pulse in response to Cold EPA moving to the Replete pulse occurs as the Cold EPA becomes warmed by the body's heat. (Fig. 8.1)

Following is a discussion on the pulses formed with different pathogenic agents. Additionally, some of these pulse qualities can also occur via mechanisms reflecting internal dysfunction of the body's homeostasis or balance and are not necessarily due to an EPA; the discussion focuses on these differences and hence appropriate classification methods.

8.2.1 Pulse qualities reflecting Damp

The term 'damp' is used both descriptively and diagnostically. Descriptively it is used to describe any accumulation of fluids or moisture. This can be apparent as with the retention of fluid clearly seen with swelling of the ankles or face, overproduction of mucous, runny nose or coughing mucous from the lungs (Box 8.1). When the term 'damp' is applied diagnostically, it is used to describe the pathogenesis or cause of the illness as arising from Damp. In this sense, it is used to describe the symptomatic manifestation of Damp signs and symptoms. The term also loosely encompasses phlegm, which occurs when fluids congeal.

Damp illness can arise from internal and external causes. As an internal cause, Spleen Yang Qi vacuity or digestive weakness often gives rise to Damp accumulation as the distribution and transformation function of moving fluids and nutrients around the body is compromised and so fluid accumulates producing Damp. Diet-related causes are also common when particular food groups causing Damp are eaten in excess or are unable to be appropriately digested. For example, dairy products, raw foods, cold foods, oils and uncooked foods can be causes of Damp accumulation, often affecting the Spleen Qi and/or Yang. Damp formation also arises from external causes. For example, external pathogenic agents such as Cold have a congealing affect on the fluid in the body producing dampness, or Damp can arise from Damp pathogenic agents as well.

From a pulse diagnosis perspective, four of the traditional pulse types are associated with Damp:

- Slippery pulse (section 7.9.1)
- Soggy pulse (section 7.7.6)
- Moderate pulse (section 6.4.3)
- Fine pulse (section 6.12.1).

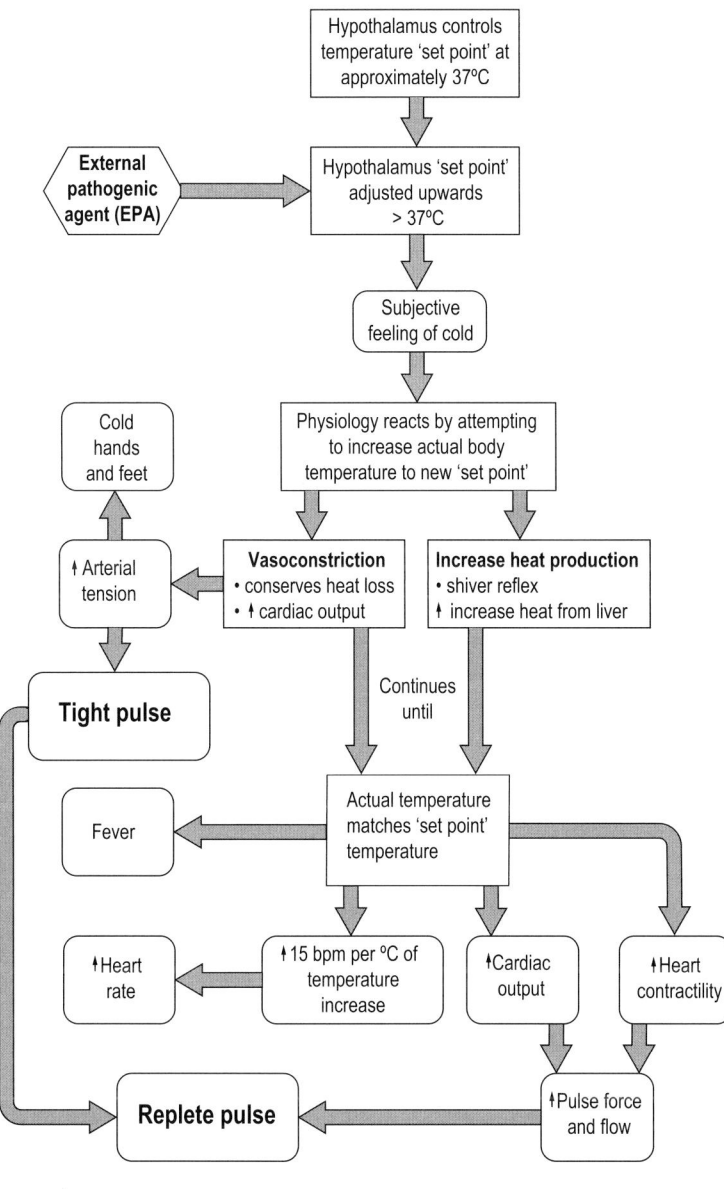

Figure 8.1
The likely transformation of an EPA of Cold to Heat and the formation of the Tight pulse and consequent formation of the Replete pulse. (Developed from information in Dinarello & Gelfand 2001).

Damp signs and symptoms

- Feelings of heaviness/fullness
- Lethargy
- Nausea/bloating
- Oedmea/fluid retention
- Copious urination
- Readily combines with pathogens of Cold and Heat

One other pulse quality can be categorised with Damp, and is associated with the formation of phlegm in particular:

- Stringlike (Wiry) pulse (section 7.5.1).

The first four pulses associated with Damp can be divided into two categories based on the parameters of their formation. The first grouping is that of Fine pulse and Soggy pulse, similar in width. The second grouping is the Moderate pulse and Slippery pulse, similar in contour. The two groupings are quite distinctly different. The first is a change in the physical characteristic of the artery, that of width, while for the second grouping it is a noticeable change in the pulse wave contour. Each is discussed in further detail below.

8.2.1.1 Fine pulse and Soggy pulse

The Fine and Soggy pulses are similar in their presentation, presenting with a reduction in arterial width and are forceless. In fact, as the Fine pulse is often used as a general descriptor of all superficial narrow pulses, the Soggy pulse and Fine pulse, in this instance, are one and the same for the presentation of damp. The Soggy pulse is a narrow pulse, an extension of the Fine pulse, because it has changes in other parameters which the Fine pulse does not.

The pathogenesis of the formation of these pulses arises from damp due to internal vacuity, or where damp has caused internal vacuity of Yang.

The Soggy pulse generally reflects vacuity of Qi and Yin/Blood but also presents with a further decreased force when damp is present. In this situation there is no distinct change in the contour of the pulse wave, as seen with the Slippery pulse and Moderate pulse. The forceless nature of the pulse which occurs in the Soggy pulse arises from the damp impairing the ability of the pulse wave or Yang to expand. Damp pathogenesis from an EPA is additionally reflected in the presentation of the Soggy pulse, felt strongest at the superficial level of depth where the body's defensive Qi rises to fight the pathogen.

8.2.1.2 Slippery pulse and Moderate pulse

The Slippery and Moderate pulses are very similar in their presentation, both presenting with distinct contour changes in the accompanying pulse wave. They are differentiated by the parameter of pulse rate and also by the strength and speed of cardiac contraction. The Slippery pulse is described as occurring in the presence of heat and so the pulse rate is likely raised. There would additionally be an increase in the strength and speed of cardiac contraction so the pulse is also felt strong and distinct. The Moderate pulse has a pulse rate of 60 bpm – reflecting a relative cold pathogen. As such, both pulse qualities can represent damp but are differentiated by the nature of the damp, whether hot or cold. There are probably additional differences in the

underlying mechanisms of pathogenesis which further differentiate the two pulses. For the Moderate pulse, the damp is seen as having a constraining affect on the body's activity (Yang). This suggests that the constitutional strength of the individual has a distinctive role in whether the Slippery or Moderate pulse will occur. (The difference between the Moderate pulse and Soggy pulse in this instance is that there is sufficient arterial volume with the Moderate pulse, while with the Soggy pulse, blood is vacuous or of not good quality.)

The contour changes associated with the Slippery and Moderate pulses can be explained by the appropriate physiological strength of the Qi and blood, in spite of the presence of a pathogenic agent. The pulse can then be seen to represent relatively new illness. (For the Soggy pulse the Qi and blood have been affected or were already depleted when the Damp pathogen arose.)

When Qi and blood are abundant, and there are no apparent signs of illness, then a similar pulse presentation of the Slippery pulse and Moderate pulse can occur as a sign of health. In this instance, the Slippery pulse is differentiated from the Moderate pulse by the parameter of pulse rate. The Moderate pulse has a pulse rate of 60 bpm.

Possible parameter changes associated with Damp (Table 8.1)

- Arterial width narrows: The Soggy pulse and Fine pulse form because blood is already depleted so Damp compresses the pulse.
- Pulse contour and flow wave changes: The Moderate pulse and Slippery pulse form only when blood is abundant or arterial volume is full (whether from blood or fluid accumulation).

8.2.1.3 Stringlike (Wiry) pulse (Xián mài)

The Stringlike (Wiry) pulse can reflect the consequences of a particular form of damp termed *phlegm*. Phlegm

Table 8.1 ● Comparison of pulse parameters and the traditional CM pulse qualities associated with Damp

	Slippery	Moderate	Wiry	Fine	Soggy
Rate		✓			
Tension			✓		
Contour	✓	✓			
Force					✓
Depth					✓
Length			✓		
Width				✓	✓

occurs as a result of congealed fluids due to pathogenic factors such as heat or fire, or from the poor circulation of fluids causing these to collect and congeal. The Spleen and Lungs are often linked to internal causes of phlegm formation because of their functional relationship with circulating and transforming fluids.

Phlegm is an obstructive substance impeding the normal flow of Qi and blood through the tissue and organs, placing stress on the system. Phlegm causes obstructions, obstructions cause pain. An increase in arterial tension is therefore not an unexpected response. (Note that phlegm is divided into further complex patterns dependent on other signs and symptoms. Relevant texts should be consulted for further information.)

8.2.1.4 Clinical application of the damp pulses

Clavey (2003) notes that diagnosis of damp or phlegm conditions should not depend solely on on the pulse. He notes that a lack of a 'damp pulse' does not preclude the presence of damp (p. 296). The reason for this is that damp is often a symptomatic consequence of dysfunction. For example, when the body's Yang warming function is impaired, moisture accumulates and congeals producing damp. In this situation, damp is secondary to the primary Yang vacuous condition. Lyttleton (2004) describes a scenario of infertility in a patient due to blockage of the reproductive organs due to Phlegm-Damp in which the damp pathology does not manifest on the pulse:

> . . . if the accumulation of Phlegm-Damp is isolated in a discrete location (e.g. one fallopian tube) then it may not register on the pulse. If Kidney Yang deficiency or Liver Qi stagnation are contributing causes of the Phlegm-Damp, their characteristics may be felt on the pulse instead (p. 96).

8.2.2 Pulse qualities that reflect Cold EPA

Cold by nature contracts and obstructs, it congeals fluids and counters the warming nature of Yang. Heat produced from metabolism is an expression of the body's Yang-related functions and so when a pathogen of Cold invades then the body's physiological functions are affected. This can arise in signs and symptoms such as chills and aversion to cold (Box 8.2). Cold invasion affects the pulse in three ways:

- Pulse rate: Qi is seen as a motive force, giving rise to and ensuring the regularity of the heart contraction and movement of blood in the vessels. Pulse rate is a reflection of the functional activity

---

Box 8.2

Cold signs and symptoms

- Aversion to cold
- Chills
- Preference for warmth and warm drinks
- Clear coloured urine
- Combines with pathogens of Wind and Damp
- Pulse parameters:
  - Slow rate
  - Increased arterial tension

---

of Yang to speed up or slow the heart rate. As Cold counters the Yang then the pulse rate slows (but importantly, heart rhythm is not interrupted as the heart Qi remains functional).

- Arterial tension: Cold has a contracting action on the flesh, and arterial tension increases as the Cold contracts the flesh. An increase in tension can also be viewed in this respect as the body's attempt to maintain internal warmth, conserve the Yang, by reducing the area of the artery and Qi and blood exposed to the pathogenic Cold: a defensive mechanism to prevent internal invasion of Cold. Control of temperature regulation from a biomedical perspective is associated with the hypothalamus, which increases the body's 'normal' temperature to a higher set point, and so the physiological response is an attempt to conserve body heat in order to raise body temperature to the new set point (see Fig. 8.1) From a CM perspective, an increase in arterial tension can also refer to the obstructive action of Cold on the normal flow of Qi and blood. Obstruction is associated with pain, and pain causes an increase in sympathetic nervous system activity further affecting arterial wall tension.

- Level of depth and strength: The level of depth at which the pulse is felt strongest with Cold pathogens is variable and depends on the body's immune function and the intensity of the Cold pathogen. This is because acute Cold pathogens are known to affect the internal organs almost immediately, while other types follow a progressive movement from the exterior to the interior over time. In the former case the pulse is felt strongest at the deep level of depth and in the latter, at the superficial level of depth.

Five traditional pulse qualities are associated with Cold invasion or are attributable to the presence of a Cold EPA:

- Slow pulse (section 6.5.1)
- Drumskin pulse (section 7.5.4)
- Tight pulse (section 7.5.2)
- Firm pulse (section 7.7.2)
- Hidden pulse (section 6.9.3).

Of these five traditional pulse qualities, the Slow pulse is the simplest to recognise and will nearly always be accompanied by signs and symptoms that reflect Cold. It is likely to combine with the other four pulse qualities when Cold pathogens are present. For example, the Tight pulse due to Cold will have increased arterial tension and a decrease in pulse rate.

The remaining four pulses range from those that form when there is an acute EPA Cold attack affecting the external regions of the body through to serious and chronic internal attack by Cold EPA. Of these the Tight pulse, Firm pulse and Hidden pulse can be arranged sequentially to reflect the continuation of a Cold EPA from the external regions of the body into the interior. (In addition to Cold EPA all three pulses also occur when there is stagnation of food, indicating a relationship/pathway between the pathology and their formation; see Fig. 8.2.)

8.2.2.1 Slow pulse

A decrease in pulse rate is a generic change in the parameter of rate that occurs when Yang is affected causing pulse rate to slow. If the pulse rate falls to

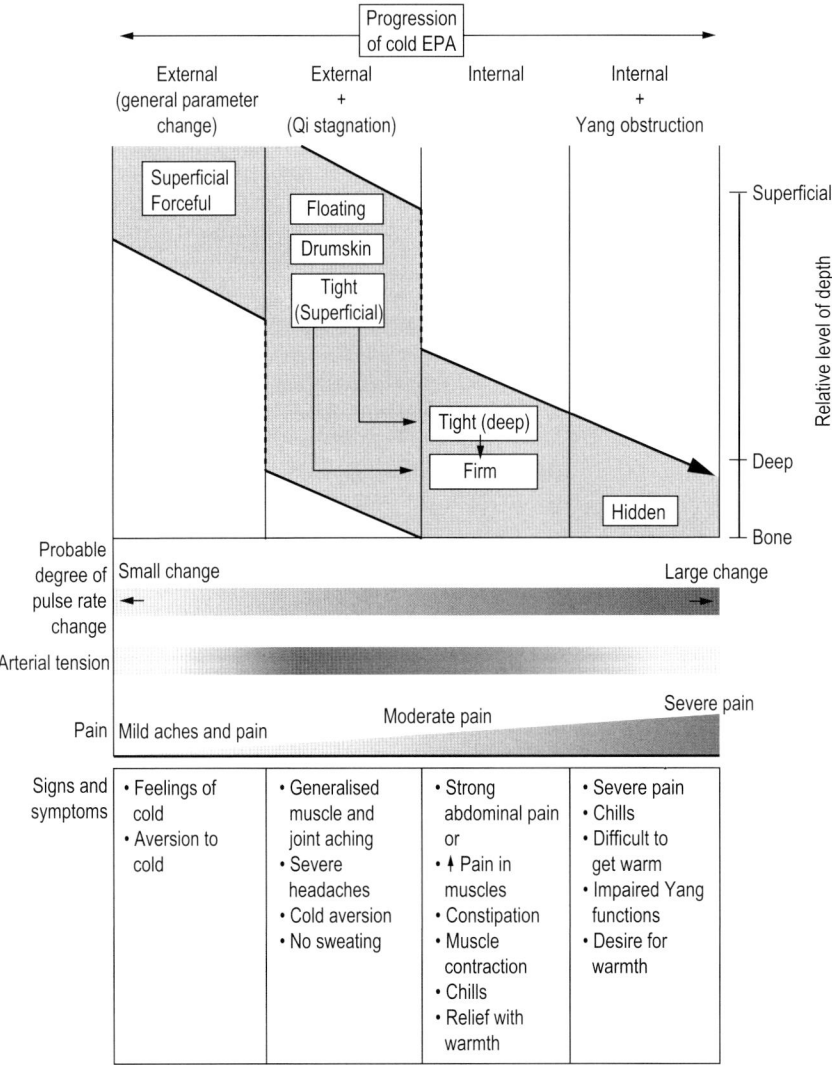

Figure 8.2
Progression of Cold EPA from the exterior to the interior and consequent formation of likely pulse qualities.

60 bpm or less then this is the Slow pulse. A decrease in pulse rate is likely to occur in combination with the other pulse qualities listed above, when caused by a Cold EPA aetiology.

The Slow pulse is the simplest of the five traditional pulse qualities to recognise associated with a Cold EPA. Yet, a decrease in the pulse rate with Cold need not be so great as to cause the rate to fall to 60 bpm or less, the range ascribed for categorising the pulse rate as the Slow pulse. The Slow pulse can also occur from internal Yang problems which slows the pulse. This is termed Yang vacuity (or Yang deficiency). (Yang vacuous pulses are discussed elsewhere.) In this sense the Slow pulse alone is not diagnostically specific enough to differentiate between a Cold EPA and Yang vacuity. It is necessary to assess the presentation of other pulse parameters to do this. Pulse force is an important additional parameter for this purpose: an increased force occurring with a decrease in pulse rate would likely indicate an EPA of Cold, whereas a decrease in both pulse force and pulse rate indicates dysfunction arising internally from Yang vacuity. When Yang is deficient the pulse sinks, being felt at a deeper level of depth than is normally felt for the affected individual.

Progression of Cold in the body

There are situations in which the body's immune system is weak and so an EPA of Cold quickly goes internally and affects the organs directly. The digestive organs of the Stomach and intestines are prone to this occurring. In this situation, Cold continues to have its contracting affect, obstructing the free flow of Qi and blood. Fixed abdominal pain is symptomatic of this scenario. The formation of the Firm pulse or Tight pulse may result. The Firm pulse is a natural continuum of the Tight pulse when the Cold pathogen is either chronic or is causing severe pain.

The presence of Cold internally will counter the associated organ's Qi or functional capacity, and eventually the body's Yang. Eventually, a Yang vacuous condition will arise over time in spite of the initial problem having arisen from an 'excessive' Cold EPA. In time, the pulse continuum progresses from a pulse with strength to one without strength.

8.2.2.2 Tight pulse and Drumskin pulse

The two other Cold-related pulses are the Tight pulse and the Drumskin pulse. These are both complex pulse qualities, developing from changes in several pulse parameters. Both are distinctive pulses with their associated increase in arterial tension.

The Tight pulse can occur with general internal obstructive disorders associated with poor digestion, so needs to be carefully differentiated from its Cold causation with assessment of other signs and symptoms as well. Using the pulse parameters, a Tight pulse caused by Cold and the Tight pulse caused by obstruction (not necessarily Cold related) can be differentiated by changes in pulse rate. The Tight pulse will probably occur with a generic decrease in pulse rate when due to a Cold EPA. When food obstruction is due to Cold, which occurs in a situation where a Cold EPA goes internally and causes obstruction, then the Tight and Slow pulse will also manifest.

The Drumskin pulse can also occur in the presence of a Cold EPA, as is apparent in the increase in arterial tension due to vasoconstriction, but its formation is primarily due to tensile stress in other layers of the arterial wall due to underlying blood vacuity. When the blood and fluid levels are normal and a Cold EPA invades, then the Drumskin pulse will not occur (Box 8.5).

8.2.3 Pulse qualities that reflect Heat

Heat by nature is expansive and supplements the normal functional activity of Yang in the body. Feeling hot, fever, sweating, flushed face are signs of pathogenic illness arising from Heat (Fig. 8.3). Heat additionally agitates blood and Qi, thus affecting the pulse.

Heat affects the pulse in three ways.

- Pulse rate: Pulse rate is a reflection of the functional activity of Yang. As Heat adversely supplements the Yang, then pulse rate increases. From a biomedical perspective this is an increased activity of the cardiac cells in response to an increased metabolic rate affecting core body temperature.
- Pulse length: Heat adversely affects the normal flow of Qi and blood via its expansive heating quality. This is sometimes described as heat agitating the blood and Qi. The result is a pulse which extends beyond the Cun, Guan and Chi pulse positions. That is, the pulse becomes more apparent with palpation along its entire length and not just at these three pulse positions at the wrist.
- Pulse contour: Heat produces a variation in the pulse contour with a more distinctive pulse wave. Heat causes cardiac cells to contract more quickly and strongly, resulting in a more forceful pulse. From a CM perspective the change in the pulse from Heat EPA reflects the agitating affect of heat on Qi and Blood as core body temperature increases.
- Pulse force: Pulse force increases and is a direct reflection of the increased strength of contraction of the cardiac cells and subsequent increased stroke volume.
- Arterial width: By increasing the surface area of the artery the body attempts to lose more heat to

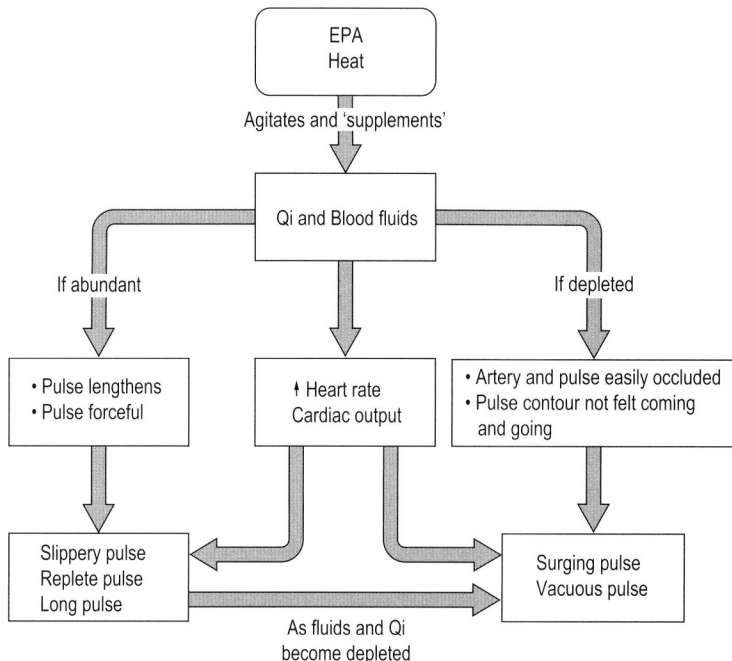

Figure 8.3
Affect of an EPA Heat on pulse parameters and the formation of traditional pulse qualities with consideration to the relative strength of Qi and Blood (fluids).

the environment: a defensive mechanism to prevent heat from damaging the body's Yin. Heat has an expansive action on the flesh and blood flow so the pulse wave contour comes to dominate the pulse quality and is felt wide.

- Level of depth: As a Heat pathogen invades the body so the body's Qi responds by rising to meet the invading EPA. The pulse becomes relatively stronger at the superficial levels of depth. With Heat pathogens, the pulse is likely to be felt with strength at the other levels of depth as well.

There are five traditional pulse qualities attributable to the presence of a Heat EPA:

- Rapid pulse (section 6.5.2)
- Slippery pulse (section 7.9.1)
- Replete pulse (section 7.7.1)
- Vacuous pulse (section 7.7.3)
- Surging pulse (section 7.9.3).

Of the five traditional pulse qualities, the Rapid pulse is the simplest to recognise and will always reflect Heat. It is likely to combine with the other four pulse qualities when Heat pathogens are present. For example, the Slippery pulse due to Heat will have an increase in pulse rate, when this is >90 bpm, then the pulse is Slippery and Rapid.

The remaining four pulse qualities can be subdivided into two further categories. The first category includes pulse qualities in which the underlying Qi and blood are agitated but remain abundant:

- Slippery pulse (section 7.9.1)
- Replete pulse (section 7.7.1).

The second category contains pulses that are also associated with Heat pathology but have injury to the Qi and blood from the Heat pathogen:

- Vacuous pulse (section 7.7.3)
- Surging pulse (section 7.9.3).

8.2.3.1 Vacuous pulse and Surging pulse

The formation of the Vacuous pulse and Surging pulse is described in the classical literature as occurring as a result of Heat agitation of the Qi and blood but differs from the Slippery pulse and Replete pulse as Heat has also caused injury to the Qi and blood. This is reflected in the Vacuous pulse parameter of arterial occlusion, in which the pulse is easy to occlude. When pulses are easily occluded this indicates that the arterial or pulse volume (blood and fluids) is impaired. Impaired arterial volume causes decreased blood pressure, so that the resistance of the artery to finger pressure is also lessened. This is additionally noted by the lack of increased arterial tension that usually accompanies blood vacuity, indicating that the Qi is equally injured.

For the Surging pulse, the injured state of the Qi and blood caused by Heat pathogen is reflected in the diastolic segment of the pulse wave contour and in the parameter of pulse length. Unlike the Replete pulse and Slippery pulse, the Surging pulse is not felt beyond the Cun or the Chi pulse positions. That is, although heat

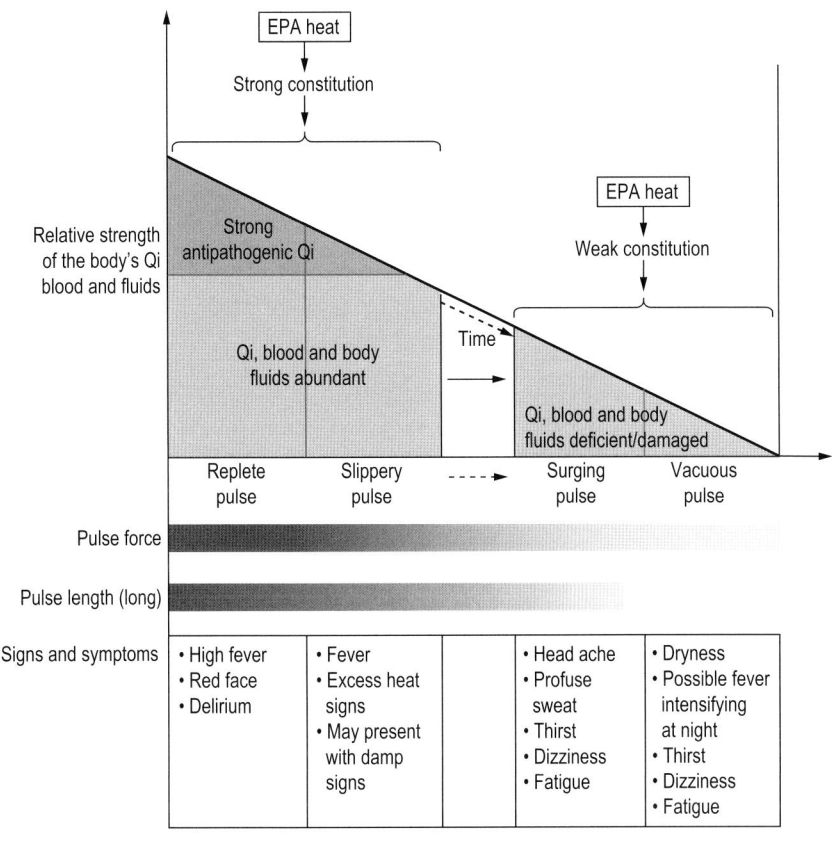

Figure 8.4
Temporal progression of a Heat EPA and consequent formation of likely pulse qualities with respect to the relative strength of Qi and Blood (fluids).

187

is agitating the Qi and blood, these substances are not abundant enough to lengthen the palpable pulse beyond the three pulse positions.

The diastolic segment of the Surging pulse wave is described traditionally as 'debilitated', giving the sense that cardiac contraction should be strong causing a distinct sudden rise in the pulse wave hitting the fingers during systole, but because the blood and fluids are injured, no substance is present for the pulse force to continuing moulding the pulse contour during diastole, and so the pulse wave is not apparent.

The Surging pulse is sometimes described as felt 'coming but not going'. This could also be interpreted as the pulse wave being felt hitting the proximal (body side) of the finger when palpating the pulse, but not felt going under the finger to the distal side (finger side).

An additional perspective on the formation of the Vacuous pulse and Surging pulse is that rather than Qi and Blood being damaged as a consequence of the heat Pathogen, the Qi and blood were already deficient before contraction of the Heat pathogen. As with the formation of the Drumskin pulse, it is the underlying

vacuity of Qi and blood that may give rise to the Vacuous pulse and Surging pulse when Heat EPA occurs. When Qi and blood are abundant, then the Replete pulse and Slippery pulses are likely to occur instead.

Also, the Vacuous pulse and Surging pulse can indicate a prognostic and temporal progression of a Heat EPA. For example, if Qi and blood are abundant, then the Replete/Slippery pulse will form. As the heat injures these, then the Surging pulse and Vacuous pulse may arise.

As a continuum, the Vacuous pulse and Surging pulse can arise from the Slippery pulse and Replete pulse when the heat begins to injure the blood, fluids and Qi. From this perspective there are prognostic guides that can be derived from these pulse groupings. For the Slippery pulse and Replete pulse, the Qi and blood remain uninjured so the patient will recover back to normal health and function once the pathogen is resolved. In contrast, the Surging pulse and Vacuous pulse represent an injury to the Qi and blood so recovery will be slower (Fig. 8.4).

8.2.3.2 Slippery pulse and Replete pulse

Both the Slippery pulse and the Replete pulse form in the presence of Heat via the agitation of Qi and blood. Although the Qi and Blood are agitated by Heat, the formation of the pulses indicates that the Qi and blood remain strong and prognosis is good.

Both pulses are similar in the filling of the vessel, but the Slippery pulse has a distinct change in the pulse contour and is strong whereas the Replete pulse is felt equally strong at all three levels of depth. Characteristics of the two pulses may combine to form a unique pulse quality not adequately defined by either the Slippery pulse or Replete pulse definition.

8.2.3.3 Rapid pulse

The Rapid pulse is the simplest of these five pulse qualities, defined simply by an increase in the pulse rate parameter. The Rapid pulse can also occur from internal Yin problems; that is, dysfunction within the organs can lead to impaired Yin function causing a hyperactivity of the Yang and increasing the pulse rate. This is termed Yin vacuity (Yin deficiency). In this sense, increased pulse rate alone is not sufficiently diagnostic to differentiate between a Heat EPA and Yin vacuity and it is necessary to assess the presentation of other pulse parameters to do this. Pulse force is an important additional parameter for this purpose: an increase in force occurring with an increase in pulse rate is likely to indicate an EPA of Heat, whereas a decrease in pulse force occurring with an increase in pulse rate indicates dysfunction arising internally from Yin vacuity. Furthermore, the increase in pulse rate is pronounced for an EPA Heat, whereas for Yin vacuity the rate may increase but not substantially so.

8.2.4 Pulse qualities that reflect Wind

Only one pulse quality occurs with an EPA Wind attack, and even then, it is a generic pulse quality that can form in the presence of any EPA attack. This is the Floating pulse.

According to CM theory, Wind as a pathogenic agent often combines with other aetiology factors producing combinations of EPAs. For example, Wind can combine with Cold, Heat or Damp producing EPAs of Wind-Cold, Wind-Heat and Wind-Damp. In this scenario, a likely response of the pulse is to form pulses that reflect the other accompanying EPAs. This is a likely explanation for the paucity of Wind-specific pulses.

From a pulse parameter perspective, the parameter of arterial tension is related to Wind and could be used to identify Wind EPA. The parameter often presents as an increase in arterial tension. The Stringlike (Wiry) pulse, or variations of this in which there is an increase in arterial tension, were traditionally associated with Wind according to the classical writings of the *Nei Jing*. Sometimes, the Stringlike (Wiry) pulse was classically viewed as a healthy pulse when occurring in the season of spring (Unschuld 2003).

In contemporary times an increase in arterial tension is nearly always viewed as a pathological indicator of underlying tension and stress involving the liver. The increase in tension associated with liver dysfunction is still associated with the concept of Wind, but Wind arising internally. Wind can obstruct the free flow of Qi and blood. Conditions relating to internal Wind include stroke (transient ischaemic attack or cardiovascular accident) Parkinsonism, epilepsy and similarly related neurological conditions. Internal Wind is the result of chronic pathological processes affecting the blood and circulation of Qi. Stress and tension are readily linked to the concept as well. An increase in arterial tension relates to an increase in sympathetic nervous system activity and is a common response to pain.

8.3 Blood

In CM, blood is described primarily as having a nourishing or nutritive function, nourishing the skin, tissue and bones. A healthy quantity and quality of blood is required for maintaining concentration, emotional stability (poor blood can give rise to stress, tension, anxiety affecting the Shen) and is important in the restorative outcomes of sleep. Blood is also seen as the physical or denser aspect of Qi, yet it is inherently Yin because of the density and moisturising function that accompanies its nutritive capacity (Maciocia 2004). When Blood quality is compromised or its quantity depleted then the nourishing and moisturising aspect is also impaired, and this is reflected in the pulse.

The pulse is intrinsically linked with the flow of blood in the arteries. It is not surprising to realise that nearly one third of the traditional pulse qualities either relate directly to or have an association to the diagnosis of blood pathologies or conditions that impact on the blood.

Blood pathologies fall into three broad categories:

- Blood vacuity (deficiency)
- Blood stagnation
- Blood heat.

8.3.1 Blood vacuity

Blood is thought of as the internal volume of the artery that gives the vessel form. It would be natural to consider that the pulse width would decrease concurrently with Blood vacuity. However, the traditional pulse qualities commonly mentioned in relation to Blood vacuity differ considerably in their presentation. Some pulse qualities manifest with a narrow arterial diameter, as would be expected if the blood is 'vacuous', yet there are other pulse qualities which manifest with a wide arterial diameter in the presence of Blood vacuity. It is this contradiction that commonly causes confusion and difficulty when applying pulse findings within a diagnostic framework.

Blood vacuity in CM is defined by a specific grouping of signs and symptoms that occur in individuals in whom the blood quality and/or quantity is reduced or compromised, and the blood's nutritive and moistening function is similarly impaired (Box 8.3). Additionally, when blood is impaired so Qi will be affected: blood no longer nourishes Qi, Qi becomes deficient and fails to move the blood. In this situation, when blood becomes vacuous so an individual's energy levels are similarly decreased. This is clearly reflected in the lethargy signs and symptoms that manifest when Blood vacuity occurs. However, the accompanying Qi vacuity needs to be carefully differentiated from a primary Qi vacuity. This is important, as primary Qi vacuity with primary Blood vacuity often result in pulses with reduced tension in the arterial wall. When Qi vacuity is a consequence or secondary response to Blood vacuity, then arterial wall tension is often increased.

The causes of Blood vacuity are many and varied. They range from impaired blood production processes affecting the quality of blood through to the simple loss of blood from the body as occurs with trauma so affect-ing the volume of blood. Other causes of Blood vacuity include:

- Poor nutritional intake affecting blood production
- Malabsorption of nutrients (due to inflammatory conditions affecting the small intestine, other inflammatory disease such as arthritis, genetic conditions, dietary-related such as alcoholism)
- Impaired blood production processes
- Blood loss (trauma, surgery, intestinal bleeding, menstruation, childbirth, tissue loss/destruction from burns or toxins) whether acute (haemorrhage) or chronic (insidious), and the blood loss is greater than that for which the body can replace it
- Increased demand for blood (growth, tissue repair/ replacement, pregnancy and nursing)
- Destruction of blood through disease processes (e.g. malaria).

In addition to the cause of Blood vacuity, the physiologic response of the body to Blood vacuity varies depending on two additional factors. The first factor relates to the degree of Blood vacuity, whether mild or severe. The second factor is temporal, whether Blood vacuity develops acutely or chronically. For example, sudden severe loss of blood volume will cause the body to go into shock causing a Faint pulse or Stirred pulse (from a CM perspective) or a pulse termed the weak and thready pulse (from a biomedical perspective). In contrast, mild to moderate Blood vacuity that develops over a long time can present with few symptoms as the body's physiological response adapts to cater to a reduced functional capacity of blood as it becomes vacuous (Rodak 2002: p. 208). In this situation, while the quality of the blood is affected, the maintenance of the arterial volume is balanced by the proportional increase in fluid to compensate. The pulse may present with an increase in arterial tension and be relatively easy to occlude.

Blood vacuity can also arise secondary to other pathological processes and so the pulse will not present discretely as one of the traditional pulse qualities. As with the formation of damp in the body, the underlying cause of Blood vacuity will dominate the clinical presentation of the pulse and Blood vacuity may only be apparent in the pulse because it is easy to occlude.

With this in mind, the range and severity of the underlying causes of Blood vacuity mean that patients with Blood vacuity arising from all causes will not be seen in general CM clinical practice; obvious examples include acute trauma-related blood loss, burns or toxic reactions. The traditional pulse qualities associated with these conditions will therefore not necessarily be

---

Box 8.3

Blood vacuity signs and symptoms

- Dizziness on rising from a seated or lying position
- Lethargy/tiredness
- Shortness of breath
- Palpitations
- Cold extremities: nose, hands, feet
- Poor PRR
- Dryness of skin, hair, eyes
- Difficult going to sleep and/or dream-disturbed sleep
- Pulse:
  - Rate is often increased above the normal resting rate when severe
  - Pulse is relatively easy to occlude (normal or wide width pulses)
  - Decrease in pulse force

seen unless the CM practitioner is working within a mainstream health system.

8.3.1.1 Anaemia

In biomedical practice the term *anaemia* is used broadly to describe Blood vacuity. Rodak (2002) states that anaemia results 'when red blood cell production is impaired, red blood cell life span is shortened, or there is frank loss of cells' (p. 212). A diagnosis of anaemia is made when blood chemistry indices, whether in combination or alone, fall outside a standard accepted reference range for normal healthy function and production of blood. The cause of anaemia is further differentiated through either visual examination of the red blood cells, with distinctive changes in their size and shape being diagnostic important indicators, or through further blood tests. Assessment of the patient's signs and symptoms is also used to help identify anaemia and determine the cause.

Anaemia can be classified as either morphologic or pathophysiologic. Morphologic classification of anaemia refers to the morphology or the size and shape of the red blood cells. The pathophysiologic classification of anaemia relates to the mechanism associated with discrete pathology causing decreased production, destruction or loss of red blood cells (Rodak 2002). Using this classification system there are many forms of anaemia arising from illness, impaired metabolism, environmental, genetic and other external causes; for example, iron-deficiency anaemia. (Reference should be made to appropriate biomedical texts for in-depth discussions on this topic and for detailed classification methods used to identify the causes and subsequent differential diagnosis of types of anaemia.)

Iron-deficiency anaemia
Iron-deficiency anaemia occurs when the intake of iron is inadequate to meet the body's requirements. It has three causes:

- Inadequate intake of iron
- Chronic loss of iron through bleeding
- Increased demand for iron.

An inadequate intake of iron requires time to affect the actual production of blood, because the body has excess iron in storage and when the circulating level of iron decreases more is released from the stored iron levels. It is only when these stored iron levels are depleted that morphological changes become apparent and anaemia results. Inadequate dietary intake of iron, growth and development, pregnancy, insidious loss of blood, heavy menstrual bleeding, stomach ulcers, nursing mothers and other pathology in which blood is lost all lead to iron-deficiency anaemia (Box 8.4).

Iron is metabolised into ferritin, a form usable by the body, and this is used for the formation and function of

---

Box 8.4

Diet and iron absorption

- Vitamin C assists the absorption of iron
- Caffeine inhibits the absorption of iron
- Alcohol consumption can cause folate deficiency

Box 8.5

Drumskin pulse and a Cold EPA

The Drumskin pulse is not necessarily about diagnosing blood vacuity, rather its main indication is that relating to Cold EPA. Clinically, treatment should be aimed at addressing the Cold EPA, not Blood vacuity. Herbs required for treating Cold EPA differ from those for Blood vacuity. If Blood-tonifying herbs are used, they may aggravate or cause a delay in resolution of the Cold EPA. Once the Cold EPA is expelled then the Drumskin pulse is likely to resolve into a pulse whose parameters are more typical of Blood vacuity.

---

red blood cells. When ferritin levels fall, red blood cell morphology is affected. The moisturising and nutritive functions attributed to blood by CM begin to be compromised.

Ferritin is also used for the production of *haemoglobin*. Haemoglobin is the part of the red blood cell that binds with oxygen and carbon dioxide and transports these molecules throughout the body; oxygen is transported to tissue cells for metabolic use and carbon dioxide, a metabolic by-product, is transported to the lungs for excretion. Individuals with iron-deficiency anaemia who physically exert themselves get tired easily and have shortness of breath because of the reduced oxygen-carrying capacity of the blood.

Iron-deficiency anaemia also affects energy metabolism by the mitochondria, the cell components in which energy is produced. Adamson (2001) describes iron as a 'critical element in iron-containing enzymes, including the cytochrome system in mitochondria' and states that 'without iron, cells lose their capacity for electron transport and energy metabolism'.

As described in previous chapters, the Qi is said to move the blood, which is made apparent in our discussions of the different pulses and theory. The blood nourishes the Qi and so it is now apparent that when Blood vacuity manifests, iron stores in the body are affected and so energy production is reduced.

From a CM perspective all iron-deficient individuals would probably be classified as blood vacuous. However, the converse does not hold: not all individuals diagnosed with Blood vacuity from a CM perspective would be considered anaemic. This is because the CM definition of Blood vacuity is determined by a specific group of signs and symptoms, and is reflective of the individual's body to maintain functional capacity associated with healthy levels of blood; it is not determined by a specific measurement. Individuals who are considered 'normal' in terms of the measured iron and haemoglobin can still manifest these Blood vacuity signs and symptoms in spite of blood chemistry indices being within the standard normal levels of measurement.

8.3.1.2 CM pulse qualities associated with Blood vacuity

Eight traditional pulse qualities are associated with Blood vacuity:

- Scallion Stalk pulse – Blood vacuity
- Vacuous pulse – Qi and Blood vacuity
- Faint pulse– Sudden acute blood loss
- Fine pulse – Fluid or blood loss (and Damp)
- Soggy pulse– Fluid or blood loss (and Damp)
- Drumskin pulse – Blood vacuity complicated by Cold EPA
- Rough pulse– Blood vacuity and Essence vacuity
- Weak pulse – Blood vacuity and Yang vacuity

Of these eight traditional pulse qualities, the Fine pulse, Soggy pulse, Faint pulse and Weak pulse all present with a decrease in arterial width. In contrast, the Scallion Stalk pulse, Vacuous pulse and Drumskin pulse all present with no change or an increase in arterial width. The Rough pulse is characterised by variation in the pulse contour and blood flow.

The traditional pulse qualities associated with blood vacuity fall into three broad categories. The first category is those pulses occurring due to primary Blood vacuity:

- Scallion Stalk pulse
- Vacuous pulse
- Faint pulse
- Fine pulse
- Soggy pulse.

The second category is for pulses that are also associated with primary Blood vacuity but are, or can be, complicated by the addition of a pathogenic factor:

- Drumskin pulse: Seen as the Scallion Stalk pulse combined by a complication of Cold EPA. Pulse reflects primary deficiency.
- Fine pulse (section 6.13.1)
- Soggy pulse (section 7.7.6).

The third category includes those pulses that reflect secondary Blood vacuity, arisen as a consequence of other pathological processes. The pathology involves internal problems of the organs related to blood production, the extraction of nutrients for blood formation or the catalytic conversion of blood; that is, the Kidneys and the Spleen. These pulses include:

- Rough pulse (section 7.9.2)
- Weak pulse (section 7.7.5).

8.3.1.3 Pulse parameters

The presentation of pulse parameters that represent Blood vacuity are broad (Table 8.2). The parameters changes that occur with pulses that reflect Blood vacuity are a consequence of the pathogenesis.

The common pulse parameter changes occurring with all Blood vacuous pulse include:

- Occlusion: Easy to occlude. Reduced blood concentration in the arterial volume causes a reduction in the density of blood and blood pressure reduces. The pulse is consequently easier to occlude.
- Force: Force is decreased as the density of blood decreases so the pressure wave does not propagate as strongly.

As previously noted, temporal factors of Blood vacuity development affect the physiological response of the body. This is particularly apparent in the development of Blood vacuity occurring over time, in which the body's physiology adapts to the apparent decrease in blood. Thus in addition to changes in pulse parameters associated with the pulses listed under this rubric, there will be additional changes:

- Rate: Increases in heart rate and respiratory rate. This increases the circulation rate of blood. In this way, although there is a decrease in blood, the functional capacity of blood is maintained as it moves around the body faster.
- Strength of cardiac contraction: This increases, moving a larger amount of the remaining blood throughout the circulatory system.

To comprehend the reason for the manifestation of different CM pulse qualities with Blood vacuity it is necessary to consider two factors. The first is the interrelationship between body fluids and blood. The second concerns the distinction between blood, that which circulates in the blood vessels, and blood (referred to in the following discussion as red blood cells), as a vital substance within the CM context.

8.3.1.4 Body fluids and Blood

The relationship between blood and fluids is apparent in dehydration, or where fluid moves from the blood

Table 8.2 ● Comparison of pulse parameters and the traditional CM pulse qualities associated with Blood vacuity

	Vacuous	Scallion Stalk	Drumskin	Rough	Weak	Faint	Soggy	Fine
Rate								
Tension	✓	✓	✓					
Contour Force				✓				
Superficial Depth	✓	✓	✓				✓	
Middle or deep					✓	✓		
Length								
Width narrow					✓	✓	✓	✓
Width not thin	✓	✓	✓					
Occlusion	✓	✓	✓					

to replenish tissue fluids. The movement of fluid in this way does not affect the actual number of red blood cells. That is, although arterial volume is affected, there is no change in actual iron levels or oxygen-carrying capacity of the red blood cells. When fluid moves out of the vessels to replenish the tissue fluids, likely changes in pulse parameters include a decrease in arterial width.

Hypothetically, if this situation occurred, and the individual was actually deficient in red blood cells (Blood vacuity), then additional changes to pulse parameters would include a decrease in pulse force and the pulse would be easy to occlude. This happens because when red blood cell concentration falls, arterial pressure also falls and the blood becomes less viscous. This probably gives rise to the Blood vacuity pulses that are characterised by a decrease in arterial width. These include the Soggy pulse, Fine pulse, Faint pulse and Weak pulse. These four pulses are additionally complicated by other factors contributing to their formation.

This is reversed in the case of haemorrhage, where fluids move from the tissues in order to maintain a functional arterial volume for continuing blood supply to the vital organs. In this situation, there is an actual loss of red blood cells and iron levels are affected, because blood has been lost from the body. When fluid moves into the vessels to compensate, this further dilutes the remaining red blood cells and so the blood becomes vacuous – even though actual volume of fluids in the vessels has been restored. This also occurs over time as fluid moves into the blood vessels in an attempt to maintain blood pressure, as blood production processes are no longer able to maintain a normal concentration of red blood cells in circulation. This probably gives rise to the Blood vacuity pulses that are charac-

terised by an increase in arterial tension and width. (The width of the pulse may become a little wider reflecting the relative Yang excess.) The Scallion Stalk pulse and Drumskin pulse each reflect this, especially with the increase in arterial tension, with the Drumskin pulse being additionally complicated by a Cold pathology (as discussed in section 8.2.2).

8.3.1.5 Increase in arterial tension: Blood heat arising from Liver hyperactivity due to vacuous Blood

In CM the blood, when not circulating, is stored in the Liver. (This has some relationship to the biomedical understanding of the liver's biological role in recycling iron from old or damaged red blood cells.) Blood, being Yin in nature, has a consequential cooling affect on the Liver. As the Liver is prone to hyperactivity, this is a complementary outcome. When blood levels decrease or the functional aspect of blood is impaired, then the liver may become hyperactive. Hyperactivity of the Liver produces heat. As the blood is stored in the Liver, heat is transferred to the blood and blood heat arises.

Liver hyperactivity additionally affects the free flow of both Qi and blood. If the circulatory movement is affected then substances can stagnate and this can additionally give rise to Phlegm-Damp.

The effect on the pulse is an increase in arterial tension. This may present as the traditional Stringlike (Wiry) pulse quality or eventually go on to form the Scallion Stalk pulse or the Fine pulse. Alternatively, the pulse parameters need not necessarily combine into a recognisable pulse quality and the pulse will simply present with an increase in arterial tension.

Blood vacuity presenting with Liver hyperactivity is often accompanied by hot signs and symptoms related to the liver, in addition to the usual Blood vacuity signs and symptoms. These include:

- Easy to anger
- Disturbed sleep
- Dry red eyes
- Headaches, especially occipital, and worse in the afternoon
- Stress and tension
- Erectile dysfunction (men)
- Amenorrhoea (women)
- Acne.

Additionally, muscles and tendons 'dry', becoming sinewy and can give rise to or become prone to inflammatory conditions such as overuse injuries (tendonitis, for example).

Dietary-related factors are often an underlying cause in the manifestation of this type of Blood vacuity.

8.3.1.6 The Vacuous pulse

Like the other Blood vacuity pulses, the Vacuous pulse is easily compressed, but it differs from the other Blood vacuous pulses in that there is not necessarily a decrease in width nor a noticeable increase in arterial tension. This is because the pulse is also diagnostic of a primary Qi vacuity. If Qi is vacuous then the ability to maintain tension in the arterial wall is also compromised. This indicates that the underlying pathogenesis is likely to lie with the Spleen processes affecting both Qi and blood production. An EPA of Summer Heat is said to specifically cause the Vacuous pulse.

8.3.1.7 Shock and severe acute blood loss

Severe trauma-related blood loss may result in shock: a potentially life-threatening cascade of events as the circulatory system shuts down. Shock can also occur in chronic organ dysfunction involving the heart. Heart failure is associated with myocardial cell disease leading to premature cell death resulting in reduced cardiac output (Katz 2000: p. 3). A reduction in the heart organ's capacity to maintain circulation causes blood pressure to fall. The heart continues to compensate by increasing heart rate, further stressing the heart. This can lead to shock (see section 7.4.2.1).

As blood volume decreases, the body compensates by shutting down the broader circulatory system (via sympathetic vasoconstriction) in an attempt to maintain cardiac output and blood flow in cardiac and cerebral circulatory systems.

In addition to loss of blood volume from trauma, conditions causing dehydration (diarrhoea, vomiting, sweating), and heart attack (acute onset) and cardiac failure (chronic onset) can lead to shock.

8.3.1.8 CM traditional pulses qualities indicating shock

The Stirred (Spinning Bean) pulse and the Faint pulse are the equivalent 'shock' pulses in CM associated with severe blood loss (in biomedicine this is termed the weak and thready pulse). The Skipping pulse may also present in shock but is more likely to manifest as a result of chronic pathology. Similarly with the Bound pulse; heart disease or disruption to the heart's normal conduction system causing severe bradycardia (Slow pulse) can lead to shock.

The Spinning Bean pulse is characterised by one other factor; it is also a short pulse, presenting only in one of the three pulse positions. In the Chinese medical literature, the Guan positions is often stated as the position where this pulse presents. The consensus arises for two reasons. Firstly, much of the pulse literature source and reiterate their pulse definitions from the *Mai Jing*, a single literature source, so there is similarity between different sources of information in the contemporary literature. The other reason has a physiological basis, relating to the support the arterial structure receives. Severe blood loss causes a decrease in blood pressure, making it difficult to palpate a clear pulse image. As the radial artery at the Guan position has support from the styloid process, a pulse might still be detectable there, although imperceptible at the Cun and Chi positions.

In CM the term 'shock' also encompasses emotional conditions in which the person may be easily frightened, timid, or manifest anxiety conditions such as panic attacks.

8.3.2 Blood stagnation

The term *Blood stagnation (stasis)* evokes images of an inability of the blood to circulate or a blockage in the normal free flow of blood. The term can be applied generically to fixed localised pain, used as a descriptive term when bruising is observed, or used diagnostically for chronic and serious conditions of organ impairment and degeneration (involving kidney/heart/liver), tumours (growths or 'masses') or infertility (Box 8.6). As such, it is the degree of 'stagnation' that dictates the relative severity of a Blood stagnation condition and hence prognosis and treatment application. All Blood stagnation conditions are characterised by fixed pain and the quality of the pain is usually described as boring, penetrative, deep or stabbing.

Blood stagnation has both external and internal causal factors. Externally, it can arise from acute impact trauma producing visible bruising. Internally, it arises from obstructive causal factors involving the organs and/or interruption to the smooth, free flow of Qi and blood. Both are termed Blood stagnation, yet obviously

Blood stagnation signs and symptoms

- Fixed localised pain
- Stabbing or boring pain
- Interruption to the free flow of Qi and Blood
- Bleeding that is clotted and dark
- Purple tongue

the diagnostic and prognostic seriousness of the stasis will differ.

When occurring with internal causes, Blood stagnation can either be diagnosed as a primary problem or it may be a secondary consequence or sequela of other pathological processes. For example, when Qi becomes vacuous (deficient) then blood is said to stagnate, as the Qi is too weak to move the blood. Conditions affecting the warming function and outward movement of Yang can also result in Blood stagnation. An EPA of Cold is such a factor, affecting Yang in this way. Cold in this sense is classified as an obstructive agent and a causal factor in the development of Blood stagnation. Obstructive agents also causing Blood stagnation include food; whether this is because Cold counters the body's digestion of food by countering the Yang function and so food remains undigested, or whether food literally obstructs the movement of blood, the end result is a diagnosis of Blood stagnation. That is, there are symptoms of fixed and stabbing pain.

8.3.2.1 Pulse qualities reflecting Blood stagnation (stasis)

Blood stagnation can be an extension of Qi stagnation and for this reason all five traditional pulse qualities associated with Blood stagnation are equally indicative of Qi stagnation. Interestingly, in spite of the number of conditions that can be classed under this heading, only three traditional pulse qualities are listed in the literature as relating to primary Blood stagnation:

- Tight pulse (section 7.5.2)
- Firm pulse (section 7.7.2)
- Rough pulse (section 7.9.2).

Two additional pulse qualities are also associated with Blood stagnation due to secondary causes:

- Bound pulse (section 6.7.2)
- Short pulse (section 6.11.2).

There are three reasons for the limited range of Blood stagnation pulses:

- Blood stagnation always causes the same cascading affect on the body system, irrespective of

the cause or individual traits. Hence the similarity in causal factors associated with the Tight pulse and Firm pulse, ranging from EPA through to food retention.
- Blood stagnation is often secondary to other conditions. As in all situations, the pulse reflects the primary condition rather than the secondary manifestation.
- Blood stagnation is associated with pain. Pain will inevitably produce an epinephrine (adrenaline)-mediated response from the sympathetic nervous system, causing arterial tension to increase. The increase in arterial tension imparts its signature on the pulse, which overrides more subtle changes in other pulse parameters and so limiting the formation of other pulses when Blood stagnation occurs.

8.3.2.2 Pulse parameters

Two pulse parameters demonstrate distinctive changes when Blood stagnation occurs:

- Arterial tension: This is increased
- Pulse contour: There is a loss of the smooth and regular contour shape of the flow wave.

An increase in arterial tension is not an unexpected effect on the pulse when Blood stagnation occurs. There are two ways of viewing this parameter change:

- Blood stagnation is characterised by fixed pain conditions. Pain always causes a sympathetic nervous system response from the body. Sympathetic nervous system responses cause increased contraction of the arterial smooth muscle, and so the arterial wall is felt distinctly palpable from the surrounding tissue. In this situation, the arterial tension is not reflecting stagnation of blood, but rather the pain the individual is feeling that has arisen from Blood stagnation.
- The arterial tension reflects the obstruction in the smooth flow of Qi that has occurred in the body region affected by Blood stagnation. Obstruction in the Qi's smooth flow affects the Liver, and Yang Qi is agitated. Arterial tension increases as a result.

The change in pulse contour with Blood stagnation can also be viewed in two ways:

- The constraining effect that an increase in arterial tension has on the ability of the pulse wave form to expand the vessel.
- An obstructive condition affecting blood flow means there is a constant barrier to the regular unimpeded volume flow of blood. This also occurs if the heart is not contracting in a regular and smooth fashion. Severe pain can also cause heart

Box 8.7

Pulse parameter differences between Blood vacuity and Blood stagnation

- Blood vacuity: Associated with compensatory changes in the width of the arterial structure
- Blood stagnation: Associated with changes in the blood flow contour

irregularities, further contributing to the circulatory impairment.

Whatever the cause, propagation of the arterial pressure wave and blood flow is impaired and so the contour of the pulse is not constant or it is constrained (Box 8.7).

8.3.2.3 Firm pulse and Tight pulse

The Firm pulse and the Tight pulse both occur in the presence of Cold pathogens and can also reflect the retention of food; both Cold and food retention can cause stagnation of blood and Qi. Each is accompanied by changes in the width, force and arterial tension parameters that are increased above normal. In terms of severity, the Firm pulse is the more serious of the two and is often described in the classical literature as occurring in the presence of severe pain. The Firm pulse also occurs in the deep level of depth and indicates an additional affect arising from either internal causes or constraint of Yang from expanding the pulse.

The Firm pulse could be argued to be a progression of the Tight pulse. As the obstructive nature of the Blood stagnation continues and becomes chronic, or as the Yang Qi begins to be affected by the causal factor of obstruction, notably Cold in this case, so Yang's innate warming function is affected. If pain is severe, then the Firm pulse rather than the Tight pulse would form, reflective of the greater degree of stagnation.

The Tight pulse and Firm pulse can also be categorised with pulses that form when Cold pathogens invade the body. Accompanying signs and symptoms are therefore required to determine whether Blood stagnation is symptomatic of the Cold pathogen or whether the stagnation is arising from another process.

8.3.2.4 Bound pulse and Rough pulse

The Bound pulse represents blood and Qi stagnation that is specifically affecting the heart. Like the Firm pulse and Tight pulse, the Bound pulse may be the result of a Cold EPA affecting the free flow of Qi and blood. Food retention is noted in the pulse literature as a causal factor for the Rough pulse; it can constrain the flow of blood and Qi, leading to Blood stagnation. In this

sense, the food is literally seen as compressing the arterial structures in the gut, exerting pressure from within the intestines and stomach, and physically obstructing the normal free smooth flow of blood. There would be a corresponding change in the parameter of pulse force if the Blood stagnation were arising from an obstructive factor. Yet, both the Bound pulse and Rough pulse can occur as a result of underlying vacuities also leading to Blood stagnation.

The Bound pulse occurs as a result of impairment of the heart organ's rhythm function. As the organ is affected, Blood stagnation is better viewed as arising from Qi vacuity. The Rough pulse also has a likely vacuity component in its formation arising from an internal depletion of Kidney Essence. Both pulses in their basic form would present with decrease in pulse force and/or occur at the deeper levels of depth.

8.3.3 Blood Heat

Blood Heat arises from several other factors, often involving conditions causing heat in the body, whether this be intrinsic from dysfunctional problems or external from diet and pathogenic agents. There are three traditional CM pulse qualities associated with Blood Heat:

- Stringlike (Wiry) pulse (section 7.5.1)
- Long pulse (section 6.11.1)
- Replete pulse (section 7.7.1).

All three pulses are associated with an increase in pulse length being palpable beyond the Chi positions, and if severe, also beyond the Cun positions. As with any Heat condition, the increase in pulse length arises from the agitating nature of Heat on the Qi and blood causing the pulse to become prominent beyond the usual three pulse positions. With the Stringlike (wiry) pulse, there is an additional factor of agitation arising from the hyperactive nature of the Liver Yang.

There will likely be accompanying increases in pulse rate, with EPA Heat causal factors having a greater change in pulse rate, probably forming the Rapid pulse, whereas internal-related Heat may simply be an increase in rate above the individual's normal resting rate.

As in any situation, if there is pain accompanying the Blood Heat, then an increase in arterial tension will result, irrespective of the Blood Heat arising from internal or external causes.

8.4 Qi

Qi is viewed as the motive force behind the movement and circulation of substances in the body. In this sense, Qi is broadly seen as 'function' in a CM health context, so any change in normal circulatory and physiological function is Qi related.

When viewed in clinical practice, Qi is further differentiated on the basis of two factors: Qi location and related physiological function.

- Qi differentiation based on location broadly relates to the tissue and organ structures and their related functions. For example, lung-related function is termed Lung Qi. When lung function is compromised and breathing is laboured, then the Lung Qi is seen as being affected. This can arise from internal causes, where the actual Qi physiology and production is impaired, or can result from external illness due to EPAs interfering with the normal function of Qi in the lungs.

- An example of differentiation based on physiological function is the classification of the body's immune or defensive mechanisms as Defensive, antipathogenic or Wei Qi. An individual who is constantly sick is diagnosed as Wei Qi vacuous. The normal healthy functioning of the organs relies on Yuan Qi. When the organs become impaired and their physiological function declines, whether through illness or age, so the Yuan Qi is implicated. (The topic is discussed in greater detail in relevant CM textbooks.)

8.4.1 Qi and the pulse

To revisit a previous concept, within the traditional pulse qualities, Qi and blood are inextricably bound within the same continuum; what affects one will affect the other. This is bound in the idea of Blood nourishing Qi and Qi moving blood. For example, when blood is vacuous, so Qi is not nourished, and feelings of fatigue with exertion may manifest. When blood stagnates so Qi stagnates; sometimes Qi stagnation can lead to Blood stagnation.

The interrelationship of Qi and blood is reflected in the traditional pulse qualities; the same pulse can present when either Qi or blood is affected. This is exemplified in the Vacuous pulse, occurring when both Qi and blood are vacuous. Differentiation of the Vacuous pulse as either a primary Qi vacuity or a primary Blood vacuity depends on which signs and symptoms are dominating (whether Qi or blood), and is assessed against aetiological factors.

In assessing Qi by the pulses there is an additional factor to keep in mind. Qi cannot be quantifiably measured. As such, assessment of the Qi by the pulse is not about measuring Qi. Rather, the pulse is about assessing normal organ function and body processes and the relationship these have to the formation of the pulse wave. When the pulse changes then the related organ or processes associated with that change is implicated and so it is then inferred that the related Qi process is

---

> ## Box 8.8
>
> ### Rhythm and the heart
>
> Changes in rhythm always infer that the heart organ, and heart Qi, is affected.

dysfunctional. This is based on theoretical, conceptual and physiologic models used within the CM paradigm. For example, if an arrhythmia is present then it is inferred that the heart Qi is affected; we are not feeling the actual heart Qi but rather inferring information about it from the change detectable in the pulse wave (Box 8.8).

In this context, when there is compromised body function, whether internal or external, then Qi pathology is diagnosed. There are four categories of Qi pathology:

- Qi vacuity
- Qi stagnation
- Qi sinking
- Rebellious Qi.

Kaptchuk (2000) arranges these into two broad categories of pathology, Qi vacuity and Qi stagnation, with Qi sinking a subcategory of the former and Rebellious Qi a subcategory of the latter.

8.4.2 Qi vacuity

There are four traditional pulse qualities associated with primary Qi vacuity. There are several other traditional pulses that also represent Qi vacuity, however, Qi vacuity is a consequence of other pathological processes with these pulses. For example, it often accompanies Blood vacuity pathologies (as has been discussed).

These four pulse qualities and their associated Qi aspects are:

- Vacuous pulse: Primary Qi vacuity (postnatal)
- Scattered pulse: Yuan Qi/Ancestral Qi (prenatal) vacuity – postnatal replenishment
- Intermittent pulse: Heart Qi vacuity
- Short pulse: Qi vacuity causing obstruction (or vice versa) – forceless and forceful versions.

The four Qi vacuity pulses can be further classified by the particular Qi type affected. In this sense, they are used as a guide to the general severity of the Qi vacuity and thus are used as a prognostic indicator. In order of increasing severity, they are:

- Vacuous pulse: Primary Qi vacuity develops; blood is also equally vacuous

- Intermittent pulse: This is strictly related to the vacuity of heart Qi and is defined by interruptions to the heart's normal regular rhythm. (Severity is determined by the frequency of interruptions. The Bound pulse and Skipping pulse may also develop when the heart Qi is vacuous but are complicated by additional aetiological and pathological processes.)
- Short pulse: The Short pulse occurs with Qi vacuity when the Qi is no longer sufficient to expand the pulse across the three pulse positions and is felt at one or two positions only
- Scattered pulse: The Scattered pulse occurs when the body's Yuan Qi is depleted. It can occur at the end stage of heart failure. There may be accompanying changes in pulse rate but the pulse usually is a poor prognosis.

Each of these four pulses is distinct in its presentation, with only the Vacuous pulse and Scattered pulse having some temporal relationship to each other in the relative severity of the Qi vacuity they reflect.

8.4.2.1 Vacuous pulse and Scattered pulse

The Vacuous pulse and the Scattered pulse both reflect Qi vacuity. They are similar in their presentation with a decrease in arterial force. The Scattered pulse is differentiated from the Vacuous pulse by additional changes in arterial tension. In particular, in the Scattered pulse arterial tension is absent; the Yang Qi's ability to hold tension in the artery is diminished as Qi becomes dangerously vacuous, unable to move blood to expand the arterial wall. The Scattered pulse occurs with vacuity of Yuan Qi. In this sense, the Scattered pulse is probably a natural progression of the Vacuous pulse occurring over a long period of time. If underlying Qi and Blood vacuity are not addressed then organ function becomes affected. The heart is prone to such effects, with physiological changes that can eventually damage its efficient functioning.

8.4.2.2 Pulse parameters

In the context of pulse diagnosis, the Qi is the motive force that moves the blood. This manifests as:

- The regular forward motion of blood
- Longitudinal expansion of the pulse along the arterial length.

As such, Qi vacuity effects changes in the following pulse parameters:

- Rhythm: Qi is seen as a motive force, giving rise to and ensuring the regularity of the movement of both Qi and blood in the vessels. Vacuity of Qi, especially relating to the heart, will affect rhythm

- Length: Qi, in the form of the pulse pressure wave, activates the movement of blood causing it to expand across the pulse positions as it flows through the arteries. In this sense, vacuity of Qi affects the pulse ability of the pulse to expand along the length of the artery
- Force: The strength of Qi is inferred in the functional ability of the cardiac muscle to contract. Variations in Qi result in variations of pulse strength.

8.4.3 Qi stagnation

Any pathological process or external pathogenic factor can potentially cause obstruction and/or lead to, stagnation of Qi. In this sense, many of the traditional pulse qualities can be associated with this pattern. For example, the Short pulse is also associated with Qi stagnation but occurs usually as a result of obstructive factors or secondary to Qi vacuity. However, there is one pulse in particular that primarily reflects Qi stagnation. This is the Stringlike (Wiry) pulse (see Chapter 7 for further detail).

8.4.3.1 Pulse parameter

There is a change in one pulse parameter that primarily reflects stagnation of Qi (and even then the change is not specific to Qi but can occur with any form of stagnation). This is arterial tension: specifically, an increase in arterial tension.

As such, any pulse that presents with an increase in arterial tension is potentially associated with pathology affecting the free flow of Qi and hence, concurrently or consequently, blood. Liver-related conditions involving stress, frustration, tension or anxiety are associated with an increase in arterial tension. Pathogenic factors such as Cold and internal phlegm similarly affect the free flow of Qi and so arterial tension is similarly raised.

Pain is considered to be a symptom of stagnation generally, whether this is Qi or blood related. As such, an increase in arterial tension is a likely response when pain is present (Box 8.9).

Box 8.9

Arterial tension

Pain, whether physical, emotional or psychological in origin, causes an increase in arterial tension, irrespective of the initial cause.

8.5 Yin vacuity

Three traditional CM pulse qualities are associated with Yin vacuity (Yin deficiency):

- Fine pulse: Fluid related
- Floating pulse: Functional ability of Yin to counter Yang
- Soggy pulse: Fluids and functional Yin.

The three pulses are related; the thin width of the Fine pulse and the superficial level of depth of the Floating pulse combine to form the Soggy pulse. In this way, it is understandable that all three relate to the diagnosis of Yin vacuity as they overlap in the mechanisms associated with their formation.

As previously discussed, the Fine pulse is the prototype of the Soggy pulse. They are both defined by a narrow arterial width, reflecting the loss of 'fluid' volume from within the arteries.

The Floating pulse occurs at the superficial level of depth, as does the Soggy pulse. Indeed, if the pulse is only felt strongest at the superficial level of depth and is accompanied by decreases in width and force, then this is the Soggy pulse. A pulse felt strongest at the superficial level of depth occurs during Yin vacuity because Yang floats, no longer adequately anchored by Yin.

The occurrence of any of the three pulses in a patient is not a definitive diagnosis of Yin vacuity as all three pulse qualities can occur during other pathological processes so other signs and symptoms should be taken into account (see below). From a pulse diagnosis perspective the parameter of pulse force is an ideal parameter to distinguish Yin vacuity from these other pathological processes.

When these three pulse qualities occur as a consequence of Yin vacuity the pulse force is often diminished, reflecting the vacuous nature of the process occurring. This also means that Yin vacuous pulses are often not detectable at the deep level of depth. Pulse rate also provides a further diagnostic indicator as to the process occurring. As Yin is vacuous then there is a relative excess of Yang and the activity of Yang is no longer restrained. Therefore, increases in pulse rate are likely to accompany Yin vacuity when heat signs also occur.

From a pulse parameter perspective the three pulse parameters that are most associated with conditions of Yin vacuity are:

- Arterial width: Decreased
- Level of depth: Superficial level of depth is strongest (but overall forceless)
- Rate: Increased when Yin vacuity is accompanied by heat signs.

Other associated signs and symptoms of Yin vacuity include:

- Night sweats
- Malar flush
- Insomnia
- Restlessness
- Five hearts hot (hands, feet and chest)
- Tidal fever
- Bright red tongue with no coat.

8.6 Yang vacuity

Four traditional CM pulse qualities may be associated with Yang vacuity:

- Sinking pulse (section 6.8.2)
- Hidden pulse (section 6.8.3)
- Faint pulse (section 7.7.4).
- Weak pulse (section 7.7.5)

In their vacuity form, the Sinking pulse, Hidden pulse and Weak pulse are all strongest at the deep level of depth, but are overall forceless at this level. This is because Yang is vacuous and so is unable to lift the pulse to the superficial levels of depth, while the strength of heart contraction (functional Yang) is not occurring.

The Faint pulse also represents Yang vacuity but is often described as occurring at any level of depth. This is because the Faint pulse also occurs with other vacuity patterns, especially Blood vacuity, and so it is difficult to definitively state its 'normal' level of depth. Depending on what vacuity is dominating, then the level of depth will vary. However, if Yang vacuity is dominating then this pulse may also be felt at the deep level of depth due to the same mechanisms as occurs in the vacuity forms of the Sinking pulse and Hidden pulse.

The four pulses can be arranged in order of the relative severity and chronicity of the Yang vacuity. The Sinking pulse is a relatively mild Yang vacuity while the Weak pulse being moderate to severe and the Faint pulse always a severe form of Yang vacuity when it presents in this form. The Hidden pulse represents an extreme vacuity of Yang (Fig. 8.5).

From a pulse parameter perspective the two pulse parameters that are most associated with conditions of Yang vacuity are:

- Level of depth: The deep level of depth is strongest (but overall forceless)
- Rate: Decreased.

There are additional changes in pulse amplitude (force), which becomes decreased, and so the pulse is often interpreted as forceless. This indicates that Yang's warming and expansive function has been compromised.

With this in mind, pulse force should be used to identify the Yang vacuity forms of the Sinking pulse and Hidden pulse. Both these pulse qualities also occur

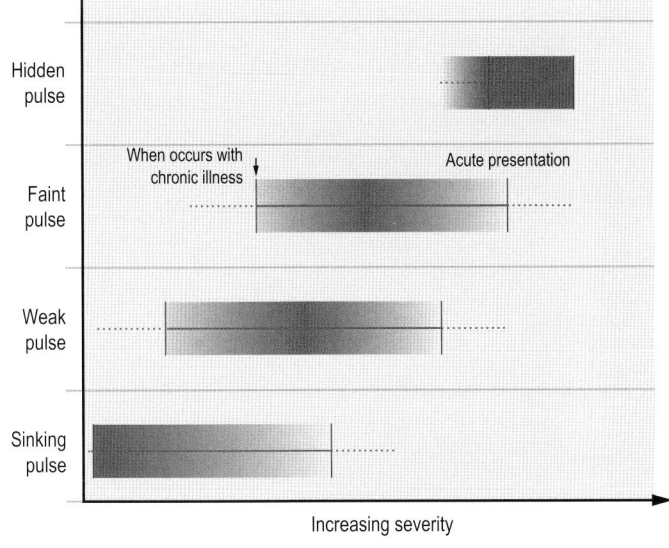

Hidden
pulse

When occurs with
chronic illness

Acute presentation

Faint
pulse

Weak
pulse

Sinking
pulse

Increasing severity

Figure 8.5
Schematic representation of the relative
severity of the four Yang vacuity pulses.

as a result of obstructive factors impeding the normal expansion of Yang (usually related to an EPA of Cold or Food retention). Obstruction (stagnation/stasis) is associated with a relative *increase in force only*, whereas Yang vacuity is associated with a *decrease in force and pulse rate*.

Other associated signs and symptoms of Yang vacuity should be used for making a definitive diagnosis. These include:

- Aversion to Cold
- Poor peripheral circulation – Cold limbs
- Fatigue
- Preference for heat
- Loose stools
- Clear profuse urine
- Swollen tongue and white coat.

8.7 Health

In a pulse context, health is defined by sufficient circulation of blood and nutrients to meet the functional and hence metabolic demands of the body. This requires an appropriate volume of blood combined with good heart function and a clear unobstructed circulatory pathway. An unobstructed circulatory pathway refers to the absence of pathological changes in the arterial wall, such as plaques, as well as sufficient dilatation of all blood vessels to allow the movement of blood into the periphery. In CM this relationship is viewed as the interaction of function with form and depends on sufficient blood to fill the vessels and nourish the organs including the heart, along with sufficient Qi to ensure a regular heart contraction and therefore provide an impetus to moving blood.

The pulse as an expression of health manifests distinctly in two pulse parameters:

- Pulse length: Sufficient blood and Qi means the pulse is felt along the entire length of the arterial segment at the wrist
- Contour and flow wave: Sufficient blood and Qi means the pulse wave contour is expressed freely.

When Qi and blood are abundant, and in the absence of an EPA, the CM literature notes the appearance of three pulse qualities related to these two listed parameters:

- Slippery pulse: Qi and blood fill the artery and are expressed clearly in the pulse contour and flow wave
- Moderate pulse: Qi and blood fill the artery and are expressed clearly in the pulse contour and flow wave. Heart Qi maintains heart contraction at 60 bpm. (This could also be the Slippery pulse appearing as 60 bpm.)
- Long pulse: Qi and blood expand along the pulse length.

All three pulses are interrelated, having a common mechanism in their formation: good cardiac contraction with large ejection duration. That is, abundant Qi and blood. All three are also associated with pathologies of Heat and/or Damp and therefore need to be carefully differentiated on the basis of presenting signs and symptoms.

The Slow pulse is also associated with health. The association also relates to appropriate Qi and blood levels and probably arises from the pulse's appearance in individuals who exercise regularly (see section 6.4). That is, appropriate blood levels mean that the heart maintains a steady rate, whereas if blood is vacuous the rate often increases to compensate for the depleted oxygen-carrying capacity. In this way, a Slow pulse can be a healthy pulse.

8.8 The Unusual or Death pulses

Apart from the 27 or so traditional CM pulse qualities there are a number of references in the classical CM literature to specific pulses associated with severe illness usually leading to death. These are called the Unusual or Death pulses and descriptions appear in the *Mai Jing*, *Nei Jing* and *Bin Hue Xue Mai*. Although these are often included in modern CM texts, it is usually noted that these are not expected to be commonly seen in general clinical practice. Rather, from their various descriptions, it is expected that they would be more likely to be seen in severely ill patients, reflective particularly of cardiovascular disease, and as such would more likely to be seen in the intensive care units or other hospital settings.

Wiseman & Ye (1998) list and describe the 'ten strange pulses' as follows:

1. Pecking sparrow pulse: 'An urgent rapid pulse of irregular rhythm that stops and starts, like a sparrow pecking for food' (p. 527)

2. Leaking roof pulse: 'A pulse that comes at long and irregular intervals, like water dripping from a leaky roof' (p. 527)

3. Flicking stone pulse: 'A sunken replete pulse that feels like flicking a stone with a finger' (p. 527)

4. Untwining rope pulse: 'A pulse described as being now loose, now tight, with an irregular rhythm like an untwining rope. Damage to a hemp rope made of tightly twined strands can cause local slackening of the twine, so that it is tight is some places and loose in others; hence the image used to describe this pulse' (p. 527)

5. Waving fish: A pulse that seems to be yet seems not to be present, like a fish waving in the water' (p. 527)

6. Darting shrimp pulse: 'A pulse that arrives almost imperceptibly and vanishes with a flick, like a darting shrimp' (p. 527)

7. Seething cauldron pulse: 'An extremely rapid floating pulse that is all outward movement with no inward movement, like water seething in a cauldron' (p. 527)

8. Upturned knife pulse: 'A pulse like a knife with the blade turning upward, i.e., fine, stringlike, extremely tight' (p. 606)

9. Spinning bean pulse: 'A pulse that comes and goes away elusive like a spinning bean. Also called a spinning pill pulse' (p. 606)

10. Frenzied sesame seed pulse: 'A pulse that feels like sesame seeds under the finger, extremely fine and faint, and urgent, skipping and chaotic' (p. 606)

Some of these unusual pulses match descriptions of the 'decaying Zang pulses' in the *Nei Jing*, associated with each of the five Yin organs and said to indicate impending death (Ni 1995: Chs 18, 19). These are also termed 'true visceral pulses' (Deng 1999), an extreme manifestation of the defining parameter characteristic of each organ's pulse. For example, the description of the decaying liver pulse encompasses the description of the 'upturned knife pulse' while the description of the decaying spleen pulse is likened to that of the 'leaking roof pulse'. Elsewhere in the *Nei Jing* there are numerous references to varying manifestations of pulse as prognostic indicators of death, ranging from death being imminent, to being days or months away.

The *Mai Jing* also discusses at length the prognosis of pulse changes in certain disease states or illness. Although some pulses are indicative of death, the appearance of another pulse quality in the same illness may signify recovery. Book 5, Chapter 5 discusses 'the various incongruous, inconsistent and death pulses'. The Death pulse Qi takes a number of different forms, described using various analogies such as 'like a flock of birds gathering (described in a footnote as 'tremendously scattered'), a tied horse galloping to and fro by the side of the water ('terribly swift and agitated'), or a rock falling from a precipice ('rising with momentum but falling abruptly'). The pulse may appear over the sinews or hide itself under the sinews as if inside an invulnerable fortress' ('very deep and barely perceptible') (Wang, Yang (trans) 1997: p.142). Other descriptors include the 'swimming shrimp pulse' that rises slowly but disappears very quickly and then rises again after a long break (two systolic peaks?); the 'hovering fish pulse' that is described as 'a fish staying (in one place) which only moves its tail and waves its head and trunk, staying where it is a long time'; 'like a rope drawing up a curtain . . . like the edge of a knife . . . if it gurgles continuously without intervals . . . if it comes and goes suddenly, returning after a (long) pause'. Deng describes all the unusual pulses as lacking 'stomach, spirit or root' (p. 145).

The unusual pulse qualities are characterised by a lack of regularity of normal blood flow, many featuring distinctive changes in rate or in rhythm. Some are differentiated by their lack of force, others by their distinctive contours or greatly increased tension. The interruption to rhythm usually indicates involvement of the heart, and as such these pulses are usually seen in conditions of heart damage or heart failure.

The unusual CM pulses have some equivalents in biomedicine. For example, the pulse described as a 'rock falling from a precipice' aptly describes the water-hammer or collapsing pulse which occurs with increased stroke volume resulting in rapid left ventricular ejection of blood flow followed by a rapid fall in ejection or an abnormally rapid run-off of blood. This may be caused by aortic regurgitation, a back-flow of blood returning along the arteries to the heart during diastole due to aortic valve problems. This may also occur due to a congenital defect such as patent ductus arteriosus, where some blood pumped into the aorta flows back into the pulmonary artery and back to the lungs.

The 'frenzied sesame seed' pulse is probably similar to ventricular fibrillation and/or tachycardia which causes a very irregular and rapid pulse heart rate, usually between 125 and 150 bpm, or could reflect pulses occurring with two distinct systolic peaks or two distinct pulse crests for every heartbeat (cardiomyopathy's). This arises from specific types of cardiomyopathy's or problems with heart conduction. The 'leaking roof' pulse, which comes at long and irregular pauses, is probably similar to that experienced in Stokes–Adams syndrome, where conduction through the heart from the atria to the ventricles is sometimes blocked anywhere from a few seconds up to weeks. This initially causes the ventricles to stop contracting until another part of the heart takes over as the pacemaker, usually at a much slower rate (15–40 bpm). If the length of time that the ventricles stop contracting is too long, this can result in death. Such a condition would once have been considered to be inevitably fatal, but can usually now be rectified by the implantation of an artificial pacemaker.

Two of the main 24 pulse qualities described by Wang, the Bound pulse and Intermittent pulse (regularly interrupted pulse), are also purported to signify death in certain circumstances. The Bound pulse is described as 'floundering like a rolling hemp seed' while the regularly interrupted pulse, in its critical form, is defined as having a consistent pattern of five beats followed by a pause. A worsening of the condition, leading to a pattern of seven beats and one interruption occurring in one respiration, strongly prognosticates death.

In this context, the unusual pulses could be considered to be the extreme continuum of some of the various 27 CM pulse qualities. For example, the description of the 'upturned knife pulse' is very similar to that of the Stringlike (Wiry) pulse but the increase in arterial tension occurs in an exaggerated form.

References

Adamson J 2001 Iron deficiency and other hypoproliferative anaemias. In: Braunwald E, Fauci A, Kasper D et al (eds) 2001a Harrison's principles of internal medicine, Volume 1, 15th edn. McGraw-Hill, New York, Ch 105, p. 660

Clavey S 2003 Fluid physiology and anthology. In: Traditional Chinese medicine, 2nd edn. Churchill Livingstone, Edinburgh

Deng T 1999 Practical diagnosis in traditional Chinese medicine. Churchill Livingstone, Edinburgh

Dinarello C A, Gelfand J A 2001. Fever and hyperthermia. In: Braunwald E, Fauci A, Kasper D et al (eds) Harrison's principles of internal medicine, Volume 1, 15th edn. McGraw-Hill, New York, Ch 17

Kaptchuk T 2000 Chinese medicine: web that has no weaver, revised ed. Rider Books, London

Katz A 2000 Heart failure pathophysiology, molecular biology and clinical management. Lippincott Williams and Wilkins, Philadelphia

Lyttleton J 2004 Treatment of infertility with Chinese medicine. Churchill Livingstone, Edinburgh

Maciocia G 2004 Diagnosis in Chinese medicine: a comprehensive guide. Churchill Livingstone, Edinburgh

Ni M (translator) 1995 The Yellow Emperor's classic of medicine: a new translation of the neijing suwen with commentary. Shambala, Boston

Rodak B 2002 Hamatology: clinical principals and applications. WB Saunders, Philadelphia

Unschuld P 2003 Huang di nei jing su wen. University of California Press, Berkeley

Wang S H, Yang S (translator) 1997 The pulse classic: a translation of the mai jing. Blue Poppy Press, Boulder, CO

Wiseman N, Ye F 1998 A practical dictionary of Chinese medicine, 2nd edn. Paradigm, Brookline, MA

Other systems of pulse diagnosis

9

Chapter contents

9.1 Qi and Blood balance 203
9.2 The Three Jiao 207
9.3 Eight Principle pulse diagnosis 212
9.4 Five Phase (Wu Xing) pulse diagnosis 214
9.5 Nine Continent pulse system 222

Chinese medicine is a diverse practice and this is apparent in the range of extant approaches used in assessing the radial arterial pulse. The subject of this book has focused on one of these approaches; the Cun Kou system. Although without a doubt one of the most regularly used and popular pulse diagnostic systems, it is by no means the only pulse assessment system used in clinical practice.

Similarly, the diversity of CM practice is also apparent in the clinical context where individual practitioners may utilise more than one system of pulse assessment. In this situation, the choice of pulse assessment used stems from two key factors:

- The style of CM practised by the individual practitioner
- The patient's cause for treatment: some pulse assumption systems are best used in assessing clinical dysfunction and overt illness whereas others are suited to the assessment of specific types of illness or even for health management. As such, not every pulse assessment system is necessarily relevant to all aspects of CM practice.

For these reasons, this chapter outlines five other pulse assessment systems that are clinically relevant to CM practice. These also use the radial arterial pulse positions, Cun, Guan and Chi, and or aspects of parameter assessment as discussed in Chapters 6 and 7. The five pulse assessment systems discussed in this chapter include:

- Qi and Blood balance
- San Jiao (Three Heaters)
- Eight Principles (Ba Gang)
- Five Phase (Wu Xing)
- Nine Continent.

9.1 Qi and Blood balance

In the First Difficult Issue of the *Nan Jing*, the pulse is discussed as the interaction of the 'constructive' with the 'protective' or the tangible fluid form called Blood and interaction with the body's Qi (Unschuld 1986: p. 66). Both Qi and Blood and the relative function and quality of these are inseparable from the understanding of pulse in CM. It is not surprising, then, that in addition to specific pulse qualities that assess the relative quality and interaction of Qi and Blood, there is also a distinct approach to assessing the relative balance of these substances as well. This is termed the Qi/Blood balance. Theory dictates that the overall pulse in the left wrist corresponds to Blood, while the right-hand pulse correspondingly relates to Qi (Box 9.1).

9.1.1 Relationship of the Qi and Blood to the Zang organs

Similar to the other systems of pulse diagnosis, the conceptual basis of assessing the Qi/Blood balance is based loosely on the *Nan Jing* arrangement of the Zang (Yin) organs at the Cun, Guan and Chi pulse positions on each side (Table 9.1). From this arrangement, the three zang associated with the left pulse positions relate to the strength of Blood and the three Zang associated with the right pulse positions relate to the strength of Qi.

9.1.1.1 The right side pulse and the Zang organs

The relationship between the organs represented at the three pulse positions on the right side and Qi is as follows:

- The Cun position relates to the lungs and its function of deriving *Da Qi* from the air and storing *Zheng Qi*. The lungs are considered the 'governor of Qi' (*Nei Jing*).

- The Guan position relates to the Spleen and Stomach, which are responsible for deriving the nutritive or Gu Qi, with digestion playing an integral part of the Qi transformation process.

- At the Chi position the Triple Heater and Pericardium have theoretical connections to the Kidneys and are consequently viewed as an extension of Kidney Yang, the foundation of Qi in the body.

Box 9.1

Relative strength of left and right pulses

The system probably derives from both actual and theoretical claims associated with gender-related pulse differences. The Qi represents Yang and so within the theoretical construct of Yin and Yang the Qi side pulses should feel stronger on the right side for women to balance their inherently Yin nature. For men this is reversed. The Blood represents Yin, so the Blood side pulses should feel stronger in men to balance their inherently Yang nature.

Clinically, the theoretical construct in relation to gender-related differences between the left and right pulses does not appear to be supported. King et al (2006) found that differences do occur between left and right hand pulses, but these are not gender dependent, with the majority of individuals being stronger on the right-hand side or having pulses of equal strength on both sides. Further research into this area is required to substantiate the clinical relevance of this pulse assumption theory.

Table 9.1 ● Zang organ arrangement at the left and right Cun, Guan and Chi pulse positions and their relationship to Qi and Blood

Left side pulses		Right side pulses
Blood		**Qi**
Heart (Moves Blood)	Cun	Lung (Da Qi/Zheng Qi/Air)
↑		↑
Liver (Stores Blood)	Guan	Spleen (Gu Qi/food)
↑		↑
Kidney (Kidney Yin–Blood matrix)	Chi	Pericardium (Kidney Yang–Motive force)
Prenatal Qi		**Postnatal Qi**
Constitution		Digestion

Table 9.2 ● An example of findings from pulse assessment using the Qi/Blood system

Left side (Blood)	Right side (Qi)	Interpretation of findings
+ (+1)	+ + (+2)	This means Qi is stronger than Blood, which is of normal strength. This may signify hyperactivity of Qi or Qi stagnation
– (–1)	– – (–2)	This means that both Qi and Blood are weak, however, Qi is more deficient than Blood
+ + (+2)	– (–1)	This means that Qi is weaker than normal, while Blood is stronger than would be expected. This could possibly mean Qi vacuity (deficiency) leading to Blood stasis (stagnation)
– – (–2)	– – (–2)	This signifies that both Qi and Blood are equally very deficient
+ ✓	+	This means that both sides are of 'normal' strength, however the Blood side is slightly stronger. This can reflect simple variations in normal strength of Qi such as that associated with hunger or fatigue at the day's end

+ = 'normal' strength; ++ = stronger than 'normal'; – = weaker than 'normal'; – – = very weak; ✓ = relatively stronger side.

Hence the right represents the body's Qi. This is very similar to, if not the same as, the Shen system in which the right side pulse represents postnatal Qi/digestion.

9.1.1.2 The left side pulse and the Zang organs

A similar relationship is noted for the associated Zang represented at the pulse sites on the left wrist.

• The Cun position is associated with the Heart which 'rules the blood', circulating it through the circulatory system.
• The Liver, which is associated with the Guan position, stores the Blood (and to some degree is responsible for the quality of the blood after production. For example, Liver heat produces Blood heat). It also plays a role in the distribution of Blood throughout the body, as needed via its role in enabling the smooth flow of Qi.
• At the Chi position are the Kidneys pulse, and in particular Kidney Yin, which stores the essence and has a relationship with the production and nutritive function of blood. Kaptchuk (2000) additionally recognises the role of the Kidneys to 'store the essence, rule birth, development and maturation – the stuff of life and development' (pp. 83–84). This represents the constitutional aspect of the individual.

Hence the left-hand pulse represents the Blood. The Blood pulse could be described as also representing the prenatal Qi. Consequently, the left side in Chinese medicine also has some relationship to the concept of 'constitution' proposed by the Shen system. The relationship is shown in Table 9.2.

9.1.2 Applying the Qi/Blood pulse assumption system

This Qi/Blood pulse assumption system is founded on the precept of sufficient Qi to move the Blood volume and sufficient Blood to nourish the Qi. This symbiotic relationship ensures that there is good circulation of nutrients to all parts of the body, maintaining balance and good functioning.

This approach can be used in three ways:

• As a preventive health measure: When the individual, for all intents and purposes, is healthy; there are often no overt signs of illness. The approach is used to address any disharmony or imbalance of Qi or Blood before pathology presents, ideally addressing the imbalance to prevent disease.
• For assessing the Qi and Blood balance during illness: This is particularly relevant for conditions that are chronic in nature, especially when both Qi and Blood may be deficient, providing further diagnostic information to pinpoint the focus of treatment.
• For its prognostic value: If signs of distinct or absolute differences in strength are present, this system is also useful as a prognostic gauge of the severity of the illness. In this way, the greater the strength divergence between the left (Blood) and right (Qi) pulses, the more severe the illness. In this situation, the practitioner would be best served by using a more appropriate pulse assessment approach, such as the parameters or overall pulse qualities.

9.1.3 Application and diagnostic interpretation

The process for evaluating the pulse in this system entails four stages:

Step 1 Assess the overall pulse strength within each side's pulse

Assessment of the Qi/Blood balance primarily focuses on the parameter of strength, similar to assessment of the force of overall pulse qualities described in Chapter 7. Separately on each side, all three radial pulse positions are palpated simultaneously at each of the three levels of depth. For example, at the superficial level an 'assessment' is made by the practitioner as to the overall strength of the pulse palpating the Cun, Guan and Chi positions simultaneously. This procedure is repeated at the middle and deep levels of depth. The strength at all three levels of depth is then averaged to arrive at the overall strength for that side's pulse. The procedure is repeated for the other side's pulse.

Step 2 Assess the relative strength of the overall pulse between the two sides

Once a baseline 'measure' for each side's overall pulse strength is obtained, the system, as with all comparative applications of pulse assessment, requires the strength between the two sides to be compared (that is, the relative difference in pulse strength between the sides). In this way, irrespective of whether both left and right side pulses are overall weak or overall strong, one side is compared to the other side to determine which of the two is relatively stronger or weaker. For example, both the left and right pulses may equally be assessed as 'weak' – lacking in strength –, yet of the two sides, the left pulse may be weaker than the right. Thus the right pulse is assessed as been relatively stronger, but need not be a definitively 'strong' pulse. It is only relatively stronger because the left pulse is weaker.

During the assessment the practitioner should try and maintain a similar amount of finger strength when palpating the left and right sides. To confirm that this is the case, always ask for feedback from the patient about whether the strength being applied is perceived by them as being similar.

Step 3 Assess whether any relative strength differences are due to vacuity (deficiency) or repletion (excess)

This step involves the subsequent evaluation of any perceived relative strength differences found in Step 2. This includes evaluating the pulse strength in both relative and absolute terms, to determine the presence of vacuity or replete patterns.

Relative strength differences

For health of the circulatory system Qi and Blood must be relatively balanced. Relative differences in pulse strength between the two sides indicate that the Qi and Blood are unbalanced. (This is in spite of whether both pulses are overall/absolute weak (that is forceless), of normal strength or have an increase in strength (forceful).)

Differences in relative strength imply that while the individual may be 'healthy' the identified imbalance represents a potentially impending imbalance/illness if not addressed. Accordingly, treatment attempts to address the rebalancing of the body's Qi and Blood.

Absolute strength differences

If there is a significantly noticeable difference in pulse strength between the two sides a judgement needs to be made by the practitioner about whether:

- One side is weaker and the other is of 'normal' strength, or
- One side is stronger and the other is of 'normal' strength.

Thus the practitioner is also required to determine the 'absolute' strength within each side's pulse: that is, is the pulse forceful or is it forceless? This is required to determine whether the 'weaker' pulse is reflecting a 'vacuity/deficiency' or whether it is of 'normal' strength but feels weaker because the other side's pulse is stronger than usual. Thus:

- An increase in pulse strength above 'normal' in the left or right pulse indicates replete disturbance of the Qi or Blood, depending on which side the pulse was stronger
- A decrease in pulse strength below 'normal' in the left or right pulse indicates vacuity of the Qi or Blood, depending on which side the pulse was weaker.

In either situation, the Qi/Blood balance is viewed as imbalanced and pathology already manifested. (Interpretation of the pulse via another pulse assumption system is preferred in this situation, as more appropriate and clinically useful information for informing about the nature of the pathology can be gained. For example, examining the pulse using pulse parameters and overall pulse qualities.)

If the left and right pulses are similar in strength then the Qi and Blood are balanced, irrespective of both being stronger or weaker in strength than is normal for that patient. As such, other pulse assumption systems such as overall pulse qualities or the Five Phase approach may be of more value in interpreting the pulse wave for diagnostic purposes and informing treatment.

Other pulse parameters in the determination of Qi/Blood balance

Additionally, the pulse parameters of arterial wall tension and ease of pulse occlusion can be utilised to provide further information about the quality of Qi and Blood:

- An increase in arterial tension in the left pulse indicates Blood vacuity.
- A decrease in arterial tension in the right pulse indicates Qi vacuity.
- A pulse which is easy to occlude indicates Qi and Blood vacuity irrespective of which side it is located on.

Step 4 Select appropriate acupuncture points, herbs or other therapeutic interventions to address the findings

Once it has been determined whether there are any differences in strength between the left and right pulses, relative or absolute, and if the differences are due to vacuity or repletion of the Qi or Blood, the practitioner needs to select appropriate acupuncture points, herbs or other therapeutic interventions to address the disharmony. Acupuncture and herbs would either supplement or drain, depending on the nature of the identified disharmony. Additionally, the patient's diet may need to be addressed.

9.1.4 Extraneous variables affecting the assessment of Qi/Blood balance

9.1.4.1 Practitioner handedness

The problem with comparing assessments of inter-arm differences, from the practitioner's perspective, is the consistent application of finger pressure. A difference in finger strength being applied by the practitioner between left and right sides would cause the pulse sensations to be perceived differently and the results interpreted incorrectly. For example, if a practitioner is right-hand dominant, they would have better discrimination in adjusting their fingers on the right hand when feeling for the different levels of depth as compared to their left hand. This may cause a bias in the assessment of inter-arm differences in pulse strength.

Solution to the problem
Palpating both pulses simultaneously helps to limit and control any bias in finger strength discrimination introduced by being left- or right-hand dominant. Either as a beginner to the technique, or as a seasoned practitioner, receiving feedback from the patient concerning finger strength will provide valuable feedback for:

- Learning to discriminate strength/finger pressure between the two hands
- Continuing to ensure that strength/pressure discrimination is similar

- Limiting extraneous variables and subsequent interpretation within a diagnostic framework.

As such, simultaneous palpation ensures that:

- Finger palpation is being applied accurately
- The technique is being applied reliably
- Any findings are valid within the conceptual framework being used.

9.1.4.2 Subject handedness

Further concerns with the system relate to the dominant hand of the subject or patient being assessed. For example, the individual's dominant hand usually has a greater muscle bulk, requiring a greater blood supply. Accordingly, the arteries will have remodelled to deliver the blood and nutrients required for healthy function. This may be felt as a wider artery. Thus assessment of the Qi/Blood balance maybe skewed in someone with a noticeable difference in arm use and muscle bulk. This may also apply to individuals with injuries such as sprains or broken bones in which the arm has been in a period of immobilisation. Thus pulse difference may be reflecting localised changes in blood flow requirements rather than being a systemic indicator of Qi or Blood balance.

Solution to the problem
Also look at other pulse parameters such as arterial tension. Often if Blood is deficient then arterial tension will be increased. When Qi is deficient then the arterial tension may be decreased.

9.2 The San Jiao: Three Heaters

The view that the individual's physiology is a microcosmic reflection of the macrocosm, the world in which the individual resides, is a recurring theme in CM. The best-known application of this theme in pulse diagnosis is the Five Phases (Wu Xing), but another is the San Jiao pulse system. In particular, the San Jiaos is an application of the Heaven–Earth–Humanity theme. It relates specifically to the thoracic, abdominal and pelvic cavities of the torso; these are known as the Three Jiaos (See Box 9.2). Each cavity has an association with certain organs and their association with the distribution and metabolism of Qi and fluids.

In this context, the Chinese cosmological perspective on the function and nature of Heaven, Earth and Human is reflected respectively within these three regions of the torso (Table 9.3):

- The Heart and Lungs are located in the thoracic cavity and are ascribed to Heaven and production of Qi (movement and function)
- The Spleen and Stomach are located in the abdominal cavity and are ascribed to the Earth and are responsible for the separation of the pure from the impure – (transportation and transformation –

Box 9.2

Translations of the term 'Jiao'

The term 'Jiao' can be translated in two ways:

- The first translation relates to its common conceptualization as 'burners' or 'heating' action. In this context Jiao literally means charcoal. In many English CM texts, Jiao has been taken to mean that the three torso cavities are distinctly related to a warming or heating action.
- The second translation relates to the concept of water channels. This refers to the CM San Jiao concept of relating the Jiaos to fluid metabolism: as conduits for both the movement and transformation of fluids. Traditional descriptions of the form of the San Jiao often describe the organ as being composed of a network of channels for fluid distribution (Qu & Garvey 2001).

Box 9.3

The application of the San Jiao in CM

This system has a number of different variations and names within the literature, but is primarily assessing the functional integrity of the San Jiao (Triple Heater) via the organs located within each of the respective cavities or Jiaos of the torso.

Table 9.3 ● Relationship of the organs to the Jiaos

	Left Position			Right Position
Cun	Heart	Upper Jiao	Lung
Guan	Liver	Middle Jiao	Spleen
Chi	Kidney Yin	Lower Jiao	Kidney Yang

---

digestion) and Gu Qi, nutrients and fluids. The Liver also has a relationship with digestion.

- The pelvic cavity contains the Kidneys and Intestines. These are ascribed to Humanity, and besides excretion (liquid and solid waste), are considered to be the foundation of Yin and Yang in the body.

9.2.1 San Jiao organ

The San Jiao or Triple Heater (Triple Energiser) organ is a concept unique to CM. Rather than being a distinct organ, it is a synergy of the three distinct regions, the three cavities which are often described as defining the San Jiao. Physiologically it is attributed to fluid metabolism, hence its definition as a curious Fu. In addition to the interaction with the fluid the San Jiao can be also classified as a curious Fu for the 'storage' of the organs Zang and Fu which are enclosed within the respective torso cavities. In this way, the San Jiao is described as both a Fu or hollow organ as well as a curious Fu; for both the cavity-like structure that it is and the interaction that it has in the metabolism and distribution of fluid, one of the three treasures

(San Bao) and storage of the organs. Even in CM the conceptual 'organ' that is the San Jiao is unique (Box 9.3).

9.2.2 Association of the pulse to the San Jiao

The logic of this pulse system lies with the location of the organs within the three cavities or Jiao in the torso. In this way, if a Jiao becomes dysfunctional then everything that it encloses or stores would additionally be affected, including the organs: and this is reflected in the related organ's pulse at the radial arterial.

In using this San Jiao pulse system, the corresponding pulse positions on each wrist are paired and associated with a Jiao (Table 9.3). These are:

- Upper Jiao: Paired Cun pulse positions
- Middle Jiao: Paired Guan pulse positions
- Lower Jiao: Paired Chi pulse positions.

Therefore, in this context, the zangfu organ pulses reflect the functional capacity of the related Jiao in which the organs reside. However, Jiao related dysfunction presents with simultaneous changes in two of the pulse positions; the two pulse positions relate to the two organs which the Jiao encloses (Table 9.4).

For example, if the heart is dysfunctional then resultant changes in pulse rhythm or strength may occur, or alternatively, the Heart pulse at the left Cun position may present with a decrease in strength. Similarly, if the patient presents with shortness of breath then the Lung would be indicated and the pulse at the right Cun position would reflect this. In both these situations, the individual organ is dysfunctional, not the Jiao because only a single pulse position was affected; the pulse that related to that specific organ. However, in the situation where the individual presents with both Lung and Heart symptoms described, this could be described as an Upper Jiao dysfunction or illness. In this sense, it is the poor functioning of the Upper Jiao distribution of fluids and nutrients that has caused the associated organs, (the heart and lungs), in this cavity to become dysfunctional. In terms of pulse diagnosis, this should

Table 9.4 ● The Three Jiaos and related cavities and functions

Combined pulse positions/sites	Related cavity	Organs within cavity	Division	Organ function
Cun	Thoracic cavity	Heart and Lungs	Heaven: Yang/intangible/function	Ruler of Blood – Visible movement of blood and Master of Qi – breathing
Guan	Abdominal cavity	Spleen and Stomach, Liver	Earth: Yin/solid	Transformation and transportation – (ripen and rot). Smooth flow of Qi
Chi	Pelvic cavity	Kidneys and intestines	Humanity: interaction of Yin and Yang – water/liquid	Excretion – Yin and Yang

be reflected bilaterally in the wrist pulses relating to the Upper Jiao. In the case just described, then there should be a similar pulse quality or change in pulse parameter manifesting simultaneously at the left and right side Cun positions: the organ dysfunction inferred from the pulse is secondary to the related Jiao dysfunction. In a clinical context, rather than directing treatment at the Lung or Heart separately, treatment is directed towards the Upper Jiao instead: the cavity in which the Lungs and Heart are housed (Box 9.4). Conversely, if a pathological pulse quality is presenting in only one of the paired pulse positions, then that respective organ is considered to be dysfunctional rather than the Upper Jiao and, as such, treatment focuses on that particular organ (Box 9.5).

9.2.3 Application and assessment

This system of pulse diagnosis uses the Zang organ arrangement in the *Nan Jing* to imply the functional integrity of the related cavity, or Jiao in which the organs reside (see Box 9.4 for a discussion of Cou Li).

San Jiao pulse diagnosis makes use of the paired pulse positions of each arm. For example, left Cun is matched with right Cun (upper Jiao), right Guan with left Guan (middle Jiao) and right Chi with left Chi (lower Jiao). Both positions are palpated simultaneously; the practitioner's right index finger is placed on the left Cun and the left index finger on the right Cun. The paired pulse positions are palpated simultaneously to identify possible common changes in pulse parameters (excluding pulse rate, which should be consistent across all positions) or the CM pulse quality that is manifesting within each arm's pulse (Box 9.5).

Although pulse assessment in the San Jiao pulse system focuses primarily on the parameter of pulse force, other changes in additional pulse parameters – for example, pulse occlusion or depth – may also be utilised, as long as they occur in both corresponding pulse positions in the Jiao in question. But for purposes of demonstrating the system we focus here on the parameter of force and the related assessment of relative strength.

There are five stages to the assessment process for interpreting pulse findings in the San Jiao pulse assumption system:

Step 1 Assess the overall pulse strength at each pair of pulse positions

Starting at the Cun positions, the overall strength is assessed at the paired pulse positions respectively on each arm. (Paired pulse positions refer to the left and right Cun, left and right Guan and left and right Chi, hence three paired pulse positions.) Assessment focuses on the parameter of strength. An assessment of strength at each of the three levels of depth, (superficial, middle and deep), is taken and then averaged to arrive at the overall strength for the respective pulse position on the left and right side of each pulse pairing.

Alternatively, assessment of strength can be undertaken at the middle level of depth only, for the respective pulse position on the left and right side of each pulse pairing. (There is little information in the literature regarding which approach to use)

Step 2 Assess the relative strength of the overall pulse between the left and right sides for each pair of position

Once an assessment of the pulse strength is obtained for each side of the paired pulse positions, it must be determined whether the pulse information is suitable for interpretation in the San Jiao approach. The logic of use for this pulse assumption system is based on the premise that when a Jiao is dysfunctional then both organs within the Jiao, and their related pulses, are similarly affected.

Box 9.4

Three Jiaos and the Cou Li

In their discourse on the classical medical location, shape and structure of the San Jiao, Qu & Garvey (2001) proposed that rather than the distinct organ entities, it is the lining or distribution network of actual cavities/spaces between tissue linings that constitutes the San Jiao. These are termed the *Cou Li. Cou* refers to cavities. The largest of these are the thoracic (chest), abdominal and pelvic cavities. Additionally, the San Jiao Cou concept also encompasses smaller spaces in the extremities and muscles. All these spaces are connected via a distributing network of tubes. These are termed the *Li*. Based on classical descriptions of the San Jiao in the Ling Shu (Chapter 18), they propose that the San Jiao is constituted from the cavities rather than actual organs. The San Jiao is described by Kaptchuk (2000: p. 96) as having 'a name but no shape', attributed to its 'formless' nature.

Some interesting recent published research papers indirectly supports the Qu & Garvey discourse. Lee et al (2004), Shin et al (2005) and Lee et al (2005) report on the histological identification of threadlike structures on the surfaces of internal organs, in the blood and lymphatic vessels, and under the skin. These are termed the Bonghan ducts after Bonghan Kim who reported first observing them in 1963. Lee et al (2004) describes the Bonghan ducts as a 'circulatory system that was completely different from the blood vascular, nervous and lymphatic systems' (p. 27). As a circulatory system, it is reported a distinct and observable liquid flow within these vessels with a hypothesized large mitochondrial count and nerve-like properties (p. 6, Lee et al, 2005).

Just as the San Jiao is a radical concept to a physiologist, Shin et al (2005) describe the Bonghan ducts similarly as a radical challenge to modern anatomy. Lee et al (2005) state:

Whatever the eventual outcome of deeper investigations of these claims, the finding of the novel structure inside lymphatic vessels is not mere curiosity but rather a herald of a breakthrough in establishing the third circulatory system that consists of the Bonghan ducts inside blood vessels, on the organ surfaces and under the skin. Further studies of its histological aspects and physiological functions suggest the possibility of new insights in both biology and medicine as well as acupuncture theory (p. 6).

While speculative (as is much of the discussion on the San Jiao), if these structures are as reported, it is not inconceivable that they occur throughout the lining of the cavities and interstitial spaces of the muscles, as explained in the concept of the Cou Li or San Jiao. Further investigations are required to establish certain claims about the ducts reported by Kim (1965) 'the lymphatic intravascular threadlike structures . . . related to immunological and hematopoietic function' (Kim 1965, as reported in Lee et al, 2005).

It is the immunologic claim that is of most interest to the concept of the San Jiao as the distributions of Cou via the Li within the muscle and skin also have an immunologic function against external pathogens (Qu & Garvey, 2001).

Box 9.5

Relation of the San Jiao to anatomical and physiological structures

The literature relates the San Jiao to a range of anatomical and physiological structures, including:

- Cou Li
  - Organs
  - Cavities
  - Lining of cavities
  - Water channels
- Burners
  - Heat and metabolism.

Accordingly, it is important to determine whether pulse strength is presenting at a similar intensity for the left and right components of the paired pulse positions. In this way, stage 2 requires the strength of the left side and right side to be compared; for example, comparing strength as assessed at stage 1 for left Cun and right Cun. That is, irrespective of whether each position's pulse is overall weak, of 'normal' strength or overall strong, do each of the paired pulse positions manifest a similar strength intensity? If they are, then the pulse is reflective of the functioning of the Jiao to which it relates. However, if there are noticeable differences in strength between the left and right sides of each paired pulse position, then the San Jiao pulse assumption system is not the most suitable approach for interpreting the pulse findings. (Rather, Five Phase, Eight Principles or qualitative interpretation is a more appropriate system to use.)

Step 3 Assess the relative strength between each of the three pulse pairings

Once it is established that each of the three pairs of pulse positions (that is, within each Jiao) has a similar strength, the three Jiaos must be compared. The paired pulse positions are compared to determine whether there is a similar strength occurring between the three paired positions or not; remembering that each pair of positions reflect the functioning of the related Jiao. Thus the paired Cun positions reflect the Upper Jiao and consequently the functioning of that Jiao is inferred from the strength of the combined Cun positions. In this way, the functional integrity of each Jiao is compared against the function of the other Jiao. This comparison assessment assesses both relative differences in strength as well as absolute differences in strength, as described below.

Transitory changes in strength

Transitory differences in strength may indicate normal circadian rhythms of the body. For example, relatively stronger Guan positions may reflect the fact that the patient has just eaten, thus the Blood is in the digestive tract. Relatively weaker Chi positions pulse may occur at the end of the day. However, if such differences are not associated with any circadian cycles then this may indicate an actual or established underfunctioning (rather than dysfunction) of that particular Jiao.

Established differences in strength

Established differences in strength are likely to occur when there are actual physiological problems or dysfunction in the related Jiao. Established differences refer to paired pulse positions that are classified either as 'weak', a pulse lacking strength, or 'strong', a pulse with strength greater than normal and for which transitory variables affecting strength have been excluded.

In the diagnostic interpretation, any region that is comparatively stronger than the other two regions indicates an excess or fullness. For example, the paired Cun positions are stronger than usual or as expected would indicate a condition affecting the upper Heater or the Cou Li. As the Cou Li are affected, so the organs in the region will be affected. Conversely, any region with less force than usual indicates a region of vacuity or deficiency. For either occurrence, treatment should address the Jiao rather than the individual organs affected.

Step 4 Determine whether any differences are relative strength differences or are distinct differences in force

The practitioner attempts to determine the overall relative strength of each of the Jiaos. If there are rela-tive differences in strength between Jiaos, then we need to determine whether these differences are due to pulse strength that is stronger than usual or weaker than usual. This is done in assessing the force of cardiac contraction with other related factors, as described under the parameter of pulse force in section 7.6.

Step 5 Selecting an appropriate treatment intervention

Once it has been determined whether any strength differences between positions are relative strength related or absolute force differences, the practitioner next needs to select appropriate acupuncture points, herbs or other therapeutic interventions, including dietary and activity advice, to best address the findings.

9.2.4 Interpreting the San Jiao pulse assessment information

There are two presentations of the paired pulse positions when dysfunction is present:

- Strong paired positions: Reflecting replete (excess/fullness), stasis or obstructive conditions
- Weak paired positions: Reflecting vacuity (deficiency/empty) conditions

9.2.4.1 Strong paired positions

There are two possible indications for increased pulse force in a particular Jiao:

- Replete or excess conditions: For example, acute respiratory infection may cause a stronger Upper Jiao pulse.
- Stasis or obstruction: Stagnation in the Middle Jiao or food stagnation may result in a forceful Middle Jiao pulse, due to the accumulation of undigested food. Alternatively, the paired Chi positions may present as strong with constipation due to the retention of waste products, impairing free flow of Qi. Damp heat in the Lower Jiao will similarly present with both paired Chi positions as being stronger, accompanied possibly by signs and symptoms such as thrush or cystitis.

9.2.4.2 Weak paired positions

Weakness in a particular Jiao may be due to:

- Vacuity patterns: Vacuity of the Middle Jiao pulses may indicate impaired production of Qi, blood and fluids and the subsequent distribution of these substances to the other Jiaos. Alternatively, the paired Chi positions may present as weak in the presence of diarrhea or vacuous Kidney Qi. Weakness in the paired Cun positions can denote a respiratory and/or circulatory dysfunctions.

- Stagnation: Stagnation in the Middle Jiao or food stagnation may result in the Upper and Lower Jiao both having relatively weaker pulses, as the Middle Jiao is not distributing Qi between the three regions.

9.3 Eight Principle pulse diagnosis

The Eight Principles system is based on the broad classification of signs and symptoms associated with illness into eight categories to arrive at an overall picture of the nature of an illness and how the body is responding, thus informing the treatment approach. The eight categories include heat, cold, excess, deficiency, external, internal, Yin and Yang.

The system is not meant to apply a precise name to a condition or disease but rather to provide an explanatory diagnosis with regard to the affect and response the body is going through. Accordingly, it is a useful system for any difficult-to-diagnose conditions, especially where there may be multiple patterns occurring, providing meaningful information to focus the treatment approach. For example, if fever presents then the condition can be broadly categorised as hot, and heat-draining herbs and acupuncture points are used.

9.3.1 Using the Eight Principles to identify changes in pulse

The Eight Principles is a relatively simple approach to pulse diagnosis that can be of assistance in the overall diagnostic process, especially if you have difficulty identifying the pulse quality as it relates to the 27 specific CM pulse qualities.

As the experienced clinician realises, rarely does a pulse quality occur alone: it is usually in combination with at least one other quality or a combination of many parameters and this can make identification of overall pulse qualities difficult. In fact, often, there is no overall 'traditional pulse quality' to be felt, as described in the CM literature.

By using the Eight Principles pulse diagnosis you may be able to recognise a pattern emerging, with a combination of basic pulse parameters that defines one of the CM specific pulse qualities. As such, the Eight Principles may help with the pulse parameter system, identifying specific CM pulse qualities by simplifying recognition of the pulse changes.

The Eight Principles approach uses three general pulse parameters. These are:

- Pulse rate
- Level of depth
- Pulse force

Information obtained during pulse examination is categorised based on the relative changes occurring in these pulse parameters. For example, pulse rate can be increased or decreased from normal and thus is divided simply into Rapid or Slow. If the pulse is Rapid, then this is seen as a heat condition manifesting in the individual. Similarly, if the pulse is Slow then this indicates Cold. Both the level of depth and the pulse force similarly tell us something about the effect a condition is having on the body.

9.3.2 Using the pulse parameters within the Eight Principles concept

In the context of pulse diagnosis, the basic pulse parameters used in this system are the level of depth, pulse rate and strength. Each parameter as a standalone 'diagnostic' imparts only limited information about the condition. For example, an increase in pulse rate (perhaps the Rapid pulse) can be categorised as representing heat. However, whether the heat is due to an external pathogen or internal causes cannot be determined from this parameter alone (see Box 9.6). For this reason two other pulse parameters, pulse force and depth, are used in addition to rate (Table 9.6). It is the use of all three sets of parameters together that allows the practitioner to correctly identify the condition and inform treatment intervention within an Eight Principles context (Box 9.7). If a Rapid pulse also presents with a lack of force, it can therefore be categorised as vacuity heat (or empty heat, deficiency

Box 9.6

Exceptions to the rule

The appearance of a superficial and forceful pulse at the start of an acute EPA is generally a sign of strong immune system, with Zheng Qi and blood rushing to the surface to fight off the pathogenic factor. However, the pulse may not be felt either strongest at the superficial level or forcefully in acute conditions if the individual is already Qi or Yang deficient. In the case of Yang deficiency, the pulse may be felt relatively strongest at the deep level, due to a lack of Yang Qi to raise it to the surface.

The parameters in an Eight Principles context

Depth

- Depth indicates the location of the condition. Is it occurring at the exterior level of the body, for example if the body is fighting off an illness? Or is the illness due to internal factors or has it progressed into a deeper level within the body (interior)?
- Alternatively, a pulse felt relatively strongest at the superficial level may indicate that Yin is weak (and therefore cannot be felt at the deep level where it is usually represented), while a pulse that cannot be felt at the superficial level may be seen as vacuous Yang (insufficient Yang to lift it to the surface)

Rate

- The rate parameter reflects the response effect on cellular function and reveals the nature of the condition – is it heating? (increase in pulse rate) or is it cooling? (decrease in pulse rate).

Force

- The force indicates the chronicity of the process occurring, whether it is arising from an excess condition or from a vacuous condition.

heat). If the Rapid pulse presented with excessive force then it can be categorised as Excess heat.

To determine the nature or source of Excess (replete/full) heat, further differentiation of the pulse would be required. Where is the pulsation felt most forcefully, at the superficial or deep level of depth? If superficial, this would then appear to indicate an EPA of Heat. If the pulse is strongest at the deep level then the heat could be seen as either arising internally, or an EPA has now progressed to the internal level. The acuteness or chronicity of the condition can help provide further clues as to which case it may be.

Thus the basic pulse parameters can inform about the location, nature and duration of the condition. Treatment then aims to support ailing organs or correct Qi and Blood for vacuities; excess or repletion are drained, while EPAs are expelled (Box 9.7).

The Eight Principles system also encompasses a fourth category, Yin/Yang, which is used to describe the general nature of a condition. Whether a condition is described as Yin and Yang depends on the determination of the preceding three categories:

- Yin conditions are generally cold, vacuous (deficient) and internal and characterised by aversion to cold, tiredness, fluid retention, weak voice and dysfunction associated with organ related functions or with the Qi and Blood. Thus the pulse is likely to be slow, lack strength and be located at the deep level of depth.
- Yang conditions tend to be hot, replete (excess/full) and external and characterised by sudden appearance of symptoms or signs. Fevers, facial flushing, aversion to heat and a liking for cool drinks represent Yang type conditions. The pulse is likely to be rapid, forceful and be felt strongest at the superficial level of depth, in addition to the middle level of depth.

This categorisation approach using Eight Principles can also apply to chronic conditions such as rheumatoid arthritis that has a sudden acute flare-up, and hence Yang (heat) signs within a chronic Yin (Damp) condition. Similarly a Yin condition can have Yang signs. For example, vacuity of Yin may give rise to vacuity (empty/deficient) heat signs over time. Another common example is damp accumulation causing stagnation in the interior and eventually transforming to heat. This would be viewed as Yang signs within a Yin condition (in this case, accumulation of Yin fluids).

Thus the Eight Principles also can be used to identify:

- Vacuity heat/Yin vacuity conditions (heat conditions that arise from an inability of the body to slow or cool itself down – parasympathetic nervous system dysfunction), or
- Vacuity cold/Yang vacuity conditions (cold conditions that arise from an inability of the body to maintain metabolism or retain body warmth – sympathetic nervous system dysfunction).

213

9.3.3 Descriptive terminology must not be confused with the specific CM pulse quality names

Some literature sources use basic descriptive pulse qualities that relate to depth (Floating and Sinking), strength (Replete and Vacuous), and rate (Rapid and Slow) parameters, which can be used within the Eight Principles as demonstrated above. However, as distinct CM pulse qualities, there are other pulse parameters that define these CM pulse qualities beyond the Eight Principles system. (Refer to Chapters 6 and 7). For example the Floating pulse, while often described as strongest at the superficial level, is also defined by an incremental decrease in strength when finger pressure is applied. That is, the pulse can be felt at the superficial level but also at the middle level, to a lesser degree. As such, generic pulse parameter descriptors, as illustrated in Table 9.5, rather than specific CM pulse quality names, are best used in the Eight Principles system to prevent confusion with the overall CM pulse qualities.

Table 9.5 ● Eight Principles classification and diagnostic association

Eight Principles category	Pulse	Nature
Depth	Superficial Deep	Location: External (li) Internal (biao)
Rate (nature)	Fast Slow	Nature: Heat (re) Cold (han)
Force	Forceful Forceless	Chronicity: Replete (shi) Vacuity/deficiency (xu)
Yin/Yang		A generalised overall description of the above three categories: hot, excess, external, etc.

9.4 Five Phase (Wu Xing) pulse diagnosis

The Five Phases is a theoretical construct which arose from the writings of the *Nei Jing* and *Nan Jing*, organising natural phenomena in terms of Yin and Yang and recognising the cyclical relationships between them, for example seasonal changes reflected growth patterns in nature. Similar principles could also be applied to the human body, with organs assigned to each of the Five Phases, with each phase further differentiated into Yin and Yang.

Five Element acupuncture is a way of incorporating the system of correspondences or itemised lists of naturalistic phenomena attributed to each of the phases described in the *Nei Jing* (Chapters 4 and 5, Ni 1995). In this way, pathology or dysfunction can be categorised simply as the adverse interactions within and between the phases. The system and variations thereof are variably termed the 'five stages of change', 'five elements' (Rogers 2000), 'five-agents doctrines' (Unschuld 2003: p. 106) 'five element constitutional acupuncture' (Hicks et al 2004) or simply the Five Phases or movements.

In spite of the system's purported European origins and popularisation by Worsley and others in the West, Birch (2007) notes the system as originally derived from Japan and the interpretive teachings of the *Nan Jing* by practitioner scholars during the 1920s and 1930s with the development of 'Meridian Therapy'.

The system was 'exported' to Germany in the 1950s by a visiting German physician to Japan, whom returning to Germany was accompanied by Japanese teachers of the system. The following instructions on five phase pulse diagnosis stems primarily from the system as practiced in the 'West'.

9.4.1 Five Phase and pulse assessment

The diagnostic use of pulse assessment in this pulse assumption system is predicated on the notion that

Box 9.8

Sheng and Ke cycles

- Sheng cycle: Also termed the constructive or mother/son law, this cycle illustrates the relationship of organs and associated functions assigned to each element or phase support and assist with the functions of other organs. On a broader scale, it relates to the movement of the seasons. Hence Wood is associated with spring. Spring leads to summer, thus the Wood feeds Fire. The heat of summer turns to the humidity of long summer, associated with the Earth. Similarly, the human body (the microcosm) can be viewed as a reflection of the environment (the macrocosm) and so a similar relationship can be recognised in terms of organ function, with consecutive phases engendering the organ function of the next phase.
- Ke cycle: This is a controlling cycle, and represents the regulatory effect that certain organs have on others. It may also represent the adverse or pathological effect that an organ or phase would have on other organs and body functions if it became hyperactive or if the organ or phase it was regulating was under functioning. In this sense, particular organs or phases are normally considered capable of keeping other phases in check, but over-'checking' gives rise to illness.

disharmonies within the organ systems, whether emotionally, psychologically, physiologically or spiritually based, can be identified by certain changes occurring in the pulse. In this sense, disharmonies are caused by a disturbance affecting normal Qi function and consequently organ function.

Depending on the nature of the identified disharmony, acupuncture treatment aims to correct the identified disturbance through the movement, drainage or harmonisation of Qi between and within the organ groupings using the *Sheng* and *Ke* cycles (Box 9.8). A specific group of points termed Five Phase or elemental points located at the channel segments that transgress

Table 9.6 ● Common combinations of Eight Principles pulse characteristics

Pulse parameters and appropriate Eight Principles category			Diagnosis	Mechanism
Rate (Hot/Cold)	Depth (External/ internal)	Force (Replete/ vacuous)		
Increased			Heat/Fire	Increase in quantity or functioning of Yang Qi
Increased	Superficial		External Heat	
Increased	Superficial	Forceful	EPA Heat	Wei Qi meeting EPA – hence pulse rises to following the outflow of Qi to defence
Increased	Superficial	Weak	Vacuity of Yin	Yin can no longer anchor yang hence Yang floats or reverts to its nature of expanding and upward
Increased	Deep		Internal Heat	
Increased	Deep	Forceful	Internal Replete Heat	Wei Qi meeting EPA – hence pulse descends to follow the inflow to defend the internal organs, or obstruction internally causes heat because of the stasis – obstruction
Increased	Deep	Forceless	Internal Vacuity Heat	Likely arising from some form of obstructive disorder with an underlying vacuity
Decreased			Cold	
Decreased	Superficial		External Cold	
Decreased	Superficial	Forceful	EPA Cold	Wei Qi meeting EPA – hence pulse rises to following the outflow of Qi to defend the body
Decreased	Superficial	Forceless	Vacuity of Yang	Not a likely combination. If occurs, more likely to reflect blood vacuity
Decreased	Deep		Internal Cold	
Decreased	Deep	Forceful	Internal Replete Cold	Wei Qi meeting EPA – hence pulse descends to following the inflow of to defend the internal organs. EPA cold can ove dIrectly to the internal in ST, LI, uterus
Decreased	Deep	Forceless	Internal Vacuity Cold	Yang is vacuous and hence no longer expand the pulse against the contracting nature of Yin, hence a deep pulse. With Cold the arterial tension will increase because Cold causes pain but also due to the nature of Cold to contract. That is, the smooth muscle contracts

the distal portions of the limbs is needled for this purpose. There are additional point groupings that are also needled, including the Lou, Yuan, Mu and Back Shu points. This process of regulating Qi is termed the movement of energy and finds a use within Five Phase or elemental acupuncture.

9.4.2 Clinical use of Five Phase pulse diagnosis

In the Five Phase system, the pulse is used in two ways:

Box 9.9

The importance of pulse diagnosis in Five Phase versus other CM systems

The use of pulse diagnosis in Five Phase acupuncture differs distinctly from other CM systems/models in that the pulse findings play a pivotal or even solitary role in the selection of acupuncture points for treatment. In other CM systems/models, pulse assessment contributes to informing diagnosis but does not necessarily dictate point or herb selection. Thus the pulse findings in the Five Phase pulse assumption system are used to determine whether acupuncture points are selected to drain excess Qi, supplement vacuities, or harmonise the function of elemental/phase organ Yin Yang partners.

Box 9.10

Uses of pulse diagnosis in the Five Phase system

- Locate affected organs by assessing the changes in pulse strength at the related pulse position
- Identify the nature of the dysfunction; whether it is excess (hyperactivity or stagnation), vacuity (hypoactivity)
- Inform point selection to correct imbalances by the movement of energy
- Inform treatment affect via subsequent changes in the patient's Qi as reflected in the pulse.

9.4.2.1 For health maintenance

By evaluating the subtle changes within the pulse, disturbance in any of the Five Phases or elements can be addressed. This is done through the assessment of differences in pulse strength within and between several pulse positions at the wrist. Strength differences in the pulse reflect the functional integrity of the organ, so if the organ function is compromised then the pulse would concomitantly be affected. In this sense, the pulse is used as a predictive sign of potential or impending illness. The system finds use as a construct for health maintenance, identifying potential organ and Qi imbalances via the pulse and correcting these with acupuncture before physical signs manifest (Box 9.9). According to Rogers (2000), the aim therefore is to 'supply energy to those areas that are weak and to calm the energy of those areas that are over-active' (p. 47).

The assessment of relative strengths derives from the Nan Jing's view on the interconnectedness of the channels, and hence Qi, reflected in the pulse. Accordingly then, Birch (2007, prs. comm.) states 'the core model of practice in the *Nan Jing* is to apply supplementation to the channels that are vacuous and drainage to the channels that are replete in order to restore yin–yang and five-phase balance'. This includes the distribution of Qi and its flow among the twelve channels. Assessment of the relative strength of the individual pulse positions are used to this end.

9.4.2.2 For identification of Qi imbalances

The second way that pulse diagnosis is used is assessing the relative level of Qi within and between organs if accompanying signs and symptoms indicate that the organ or phase is the problem. Rogers notes:

Five element system strives to balance the energy flow and levels of Qi, and it is therefore somewhat less effective in the presence of a strong perverse energy, or a physical blockage of Qi
(Rogers 2000: p. 46).

Accordingly, as a system, its strength is said to lie in the treatment of diseases with an emotional or psychological origin, (irrespective of whether there are physical signs and symptoms are manifest), which respond more favourably than conditions of a primary physical cause alone (Rogers 2000).

It is also a useful approach for identifying internal imbalances deriving from impaired organ function and Qi movement identified through signs and symptoms such as lethargy, oedema, insomnia, gastric reflex, migraine and hot flushing, (as opposed to actual organic organ disease). It can additionally be useful for assessing the relative balance of Qi between the Yin and Yang partner channels of an associated phase (Box 9.10).

9.4.3 Application of the Five Phase pulse assumption system

This pulse assumption system is used specifically to identify imbalances reflected by relative and absolute differences in strength between and within the Zang and Fu organs via the wrist pulses. The system uses the three pulse sites Cun, Guan and Chi on each wrist at two levels of depth: superficial and deep (Box 9.11). Thus there are 12 positions, six located superficially and 6 located at the deep level of depth, with each position associated with a Zang or Fu organ.

The assignment of organs and associated phase or element characteristic to each of the 12 pulse positions is based on the arrangement presented in the *Nan Jing* (Table 9.7, Fig. 9.1, Box 9.13). Thus the six Zang or Yin organs are assigned to the deep level positions and their related Fu or Yang organs to the superficial level of the same corresponding position. For example, the left Cun position has the Heart assigned to the deep level of depth and its related Yang organ, the Small Intestine, is assigned to the superficial level of depth. The Heart and Small Intestine are assigned to the Fire element.

Thus the system assesses the relative and absolute strength of balance between the two levels of depth within a pulse site, the superficial and deep, comparing the balance of the Yin and Yang organ partners, as well as assessing the strength between other pulse sites and related organs.

Box 9.11

Utilising three levels of depth within Five Phase pulse diagnosis

As noted, the Five Phase pulse assessment usually uses two levels of depth: superficial and deep. However, when palpating the radial pulsation, the pulse is often felt strongest in the middle level of depth. If using the Zang Fu (organ) approach to assessing the pulses then this would likely result in a pulse interpreted as being both Yin and Yang deficient or vacuous (not to be confused with the Vacuous pulse). That is, the individual would be assessed as being in a constant state of ill health and continuously requiring treatment to address the pulse findings.

However, another way to view this is to consider the Yin and Yang in balance when the pulse occurs strongest in the middle level of depth for the associated phase. When the pulse is felt strongest at the superficial level of depth or the deep level of depth then the phase is considered out of harmony. Whether this is Yin or Yang related depends on the level of depth that the pulse is felt strongest or weakest.

9.4.4 Pulse assessment method

Assessment of pulse using this system primarily focuses on comparative differences in strength. This occurs discretely within each of the pulse positions when assessing relative differences in strength between the superficial and deep levels of depth. Comparative differences in strength are also required in comparing the strength of one phase to another by comparing the strength difference between the pulse positions. This generates a lot of data, so it is it is useful to use a paper-based recording method to note your assessment results. This assists in making diagnostic judgements on your findings and subsequent selection of acupuncture points.

The 'normal' pulse is used as a gauge to determine whether pulse strength, of the pulse generally, is appropriate or not. Physique, age, gender and level of activity are important variables in this process, assisting in determining what is normal or abnormal for the individual having their pulses assessed. With this in mind, these variables provide a range of normal pulse presentations and are always considered against the 'normal' pulse as described in Chapter 5 and 6. (Never subjectively assume what the 'normal' pulse for a patient should be.)

The five stages of the Five Phase pulse assessment method are as follows:

Step 1 Evaluation of overall pulse strength at the superficial and deep level at each pulse site

Assess each position at both the superficial and deep level of depth. Start by palpating each pulse site separately. Feel for the pulse strength at the superficial level of strength, that which corresponds to the related phase's Yang organ, and at the deep level of depth for the Yin organ. It is best to be methodical so start at the Cun position, next feel the Guan and finally the Chi. (Refer to Chapter 5 for the location of these sites and pulse depths.) Repeat this process for the other side.

Table 9.7 ● Five Phase organ arrangement at the Cun, Guan and Chi positions (*Nan Jing* arrangement)

Left side			Right side	
Superficial	**Deep**		**Deep**	**Superficial**
Small intestine	Heart	Cun	Lung	Large Intestine
Gallbladder	Liver	Guan	Spleen	Stomach
Bladder	Kidney	Chi	Pericardium	Triple Heater
Yang	**Yin**		**Yin**	**Yang**

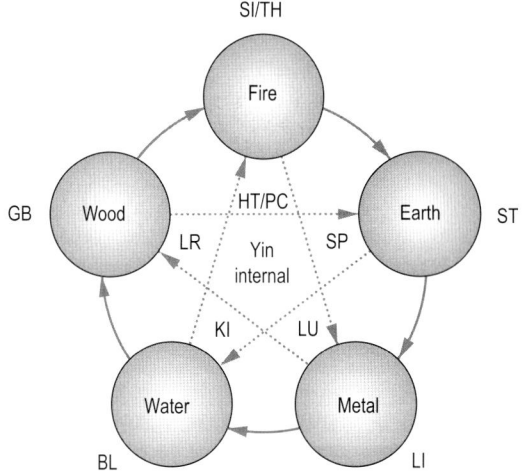

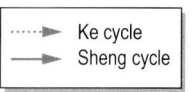

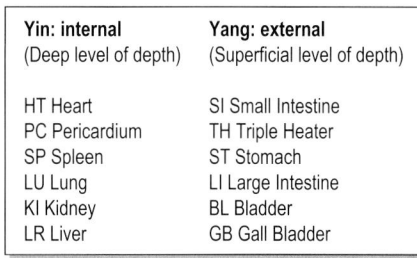

Yin: internal	Yang: external
(Deep level of depth)	(Superficial level of depth)
HT Heart	SI Small Intestine
PC Pericardium	TH Triple Heater
SP Spleen	ST Stomach
LU Lung	LI Large Intestine
KI Kidney	BL Bladder
LR Liver	GB Gall Bladder

┈┈► Ke cycle
───► Sheng cycle

Figure 9.1
The Five Phases (Wu Xing) and their related Yin and Yang partner organs. The Sheng cycle follows each consecutive phase in a clockwise direction as indicated (solid circular line). The Ke cycle also moves in a clockwise direction moving between every second phase as indicated (dashed line in star formation).

When palpating the pulse you are attempting to ascertain whether:

- A pulse is present at each of the superficial and deep levels of depth for that pulse site
- The overall pulse strength, if a pulse is present at that site. Is it strong, of appropriate strength for that individual (considering their age, gender, exercise, physique) or is it weak?

For example, starting at the left Cun pulse site, the superficial level of depth is found and the strength of the pulse assessed. This position relates to the Small Intestine pulse. This is repeated at the deep level of depth. This pulse relates to the Heart. This procedure is repeated for the other positions.

Additionally, an assessment also needs to be made on whether the Yang and Yin pulses are of a similar strength for that phase/position, irrespective of whether the pulse strength is overall forceless or overall forceful. That is, are they in balance?

Step 2 Assessment of the strength between each phase

This step requires the pulse strength of one phase to be compared with the pulse strength in other phases to further identify any actual or relative differences in strength.

Step 3 Concurrently recording your pulse findings

It is recommended that you write your findings down as there are twelve different 'pulses' that need to be assessed. Two possible methods of recording the pulse information are described here as examples: other methods are available in the relevant CM literature.

Method 1: Tabular form

Information derived in the comparative pulse assessment can be easily presented in a table format for evaluation (an example is shown in Table 9.8). This is used for diagnostic and treatment purposes, where a plus sign (+) indicates pulse strength, a minus sign indicates pulse weakness (−), and a tick (✓) indicates appropriate pulse strength. This strength assessment is undertaken separately for both the superficial and deep levels at each of the pulse positions on each wrist. More than one sign can be used to indicate a position of great strength or weakness (for example +++ or +3). Such multiple notation adds a further level of usefulness to the pulse information as it notes 'degrees' or difference in strength, where as the use of a single sign simply denotes a difference.

Note that the positive and negative notation is unique to the practitioner that assessed the pulse. Because of this, inter-practitioner interpretation of

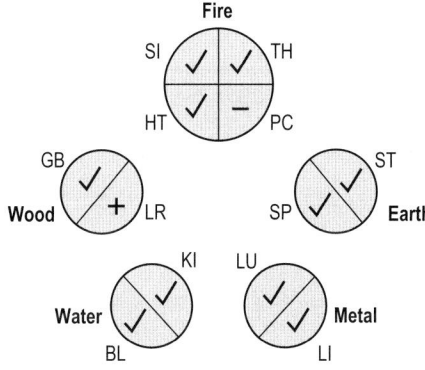

Table 9.8 ● Five Phase pulse assessment. Example of method 1. Although not precise in terms of actual qualities, it is a useful visual guide to recording the assessment of differences in strength felt. The example illustrated shows excess in the Liver and a deficiency in the Pericardium

Left hand					Right hand			
Superficial		Deep			Deep		Superficial	
Yang		Yin			Yin		Yang	
SI	✓	HT	✓	Cun	LU	✓	LI	✓
GB	✓	LV	+	Guan	SP	✓	ST	✓
BL	✓	KD	✓	Chi	PC	−	TH	✓

✓ = appropriate strength; − = decreased strength (relative deficiency); + = increased strength (relative excess).
After Rogers (2000: p. 89), with the author's permission.

Figure 9.2
Wu Xing diagram for recording pulse assessment findings. (From Rogers 2000, with the author's permission.)

Method 2: Five Phase diagram
The information can be transferred into a Five Phase or Wu Xing diagram to assist with the interpretation of the pulse findings and appropriate point selection (Fig. 9.2).

Step 4   Interpretation of findings
The pulse findings can be examined in a number of ways:

Within phases
Differences in strength between the Yin and Yang organs within a phase usually reflect dysfunction of the organs of the associated phase. For example, a strong Stomach pulse and weak Spleen pulse indicate the phase is imbalanced. As such treatment requires the use of the Luo points to transfer energy from the Stomach to the Spleen.

Thus a stronger pulse strength at the superficial level of depth could mean either Yin is relatively weak or Yang is in excess. Similarly, a stronger pulse strength at the deep level of depth may indicate that the Yang is weaker and the Yin is in excess.

A similarity in strength at the deep and superficial levels of depth indicates that the phase is in balance. If however the pulse overall is weak or stronger than would be expected at both levels then this is interpreted as the whole phase being deficient or in excess.

A weaker Yang pulse is considered a better prognosis than a weaker Yin, as Yin is seen as the foundational energy of the phase in the body and the Yang is an extension of the phase function. Thus a weak Yin usually indicates weak Yang but Weak Yang does not necessarily indicate weak Yin.

Yang is also more responsive to circadian rhythms, and other variables such as a poor night's sleep or a missed meal may cause a transient decrease in pulse

another's Five Phase assessment tables needs to be approached with caution so as to not misinterpret the significance of a positive or negative notation, as the notation is generally used to denote relative, not absolute, strength differences. However, this does not exclude the practitioner from undertaking assessment of absolute strength differences, although one factor must be kept in mind: Five Phase pulse assessment is also used for assessing the relative balance of the phases and is often used for health maintenance, so changes in absolute strength (that is, force) may not be apparent. (If force changes are occurring then the Cun Kou approach to pulse assessment is likely to be more appropriate.)

The notation and subsequent pulse record generated is a subjective approach to pulse diagnosis. Because of this, it is important that the same strength notation is consistently used to note degrees of relative strength, to maintain the reliability of the method (if only for a particular practitioner).

strength; such transient changes may be expected to occur and need not necessarily indicate any concerns.

Between phases or organs
- Positive: Move the excess into the deficient region
- Negative: Area of deficiency. If a single organ is affected, use the Yuan point
- If positive and negative: Move the excess to tonify the vacuity
- If single positive: Drain or control.

Sheng cycle
The Sheng cycle is known as the engendering or generating cycle and this is responsible for ensuring the smooth flow of Qi between the successive phases. If obstruction or stasis occurs in one phase this can impact on the next phase, reducing its access to the flow of Qi. This should be reflected in the relevant pulse positions as an excessive strength in the obstructed phase and accordingly deficient pulse strength in the subsequent phase (Fig. 9.2).

Ke cycle
As noted earlier, the Ke cycle helps to regulate the function of the organs. When this regulation becomes over rigorous, this can impact adversely on the organ or phase being controlled. This may occur when the organ being regulated is itself deficient, therefore allowing the controlling organ to affect its functions. A common example of this is the pattern of Wood attacking Spleen. This may occur when the Liver Qi becomes hyperactive, through stagnation or a result of pathogenic heat or fire. This overflows into the Earth phase, impairing the normal functioning of the Earth organs (Spleen and Stomach) resulting in a mixture of both Wood and Earth pathological signs and symptoms such as alternating constipation and loose stools, flatulence, intestinal pain and bloating. This may be reflected in the pulse as a strong Wood phase pulse with a weak Earth phase pulse.

Within an organ
Sometimes a single pulse position at either depth may be weak within a phase, without a concomitant increase in the pulse for the partner organ. This indicates deficiency within that particular organ only which has not yet begun to impact on its partner. In this case, treatment of the affected organ could be addressed by the use of the Yuan points to tonify the Qi of the deficient organ.

Step 5 Acupuncture point selection

The Five Phase system of treatment uses the command or elemental points. For the upper limb, these are located between the elbow and finger tips and for the lower limb, from the knees to the toe tips. They fall into five categories:

- Luo points: Transfer between the Yin and Yang channel partners
- Horary points: Same as the channel. For example, Wood on Wood, Earth on Earth
- Tonification points: Promote Qi
- Sedation points: Drain Qi
- Yuan points: Promote Qi in the related channel.

Generally, only the Luo points and tonification points are used to achieve the balance of energies within the Five Element system. Tonification helps to supply energy to an organ or area via the channels, while sedation in this context means to draw energy away from a hyperactive organ or area. (Rogers 2000: pp. 46–47). (For more details on the use of the Five Phase system, see Rogers 2000.)

9.4.5 Chinese clock and Five Phase pulse diagnosis

Five Phase pulse diagnosis has a few idiosyncratic variations not normally considered in other systems of pulse diagnosis. For example, the movement of the Qi ebbs through the channels with respective times of the day – the Chinese Clock or the Law of Midday–Midnight. This in effect produces a two-hourly 'high tide' zone of Qi, termed the *horary flow*, reflected in a relatively stronger pulse at the wrist for which the position correlates to the organ. Concurrently, there is also a 'low tide' ebb and the pulse position of the corresponding organ would be expected to have a relatively weaker pulse at that two-hourly time of the day. As such, the Zang and Fu organ positions show whether the energy flow to its particular functional area is normal, excessive or deficient. For example, at midday the Heart is said to be at its 'strongest' with the Qi ebb at its maximum. Concurrently, the gallbladder is at its weakest. The GB is strongest at midnight, at which time the Heart is at its lowest Qi ebb point.

The normal strength variations with the ebb and flow of Qi as described by the Chinese Clock may also be useful in identifying deficient and excess conditions during the horary flow time for the related organ. For example:

- When palpating the corresponding pulse of a organ/channel at high tide, yet the organ is weak or of 'normal' strength, then this can indicate vacuity
- If the organ/channel is of strong strength during low tide, than this can indicate an excess.

This approach to pulse diagnosis has relevance to the system which uses 'open hourly points' (*na zi fa*) (Fig. 9.3).

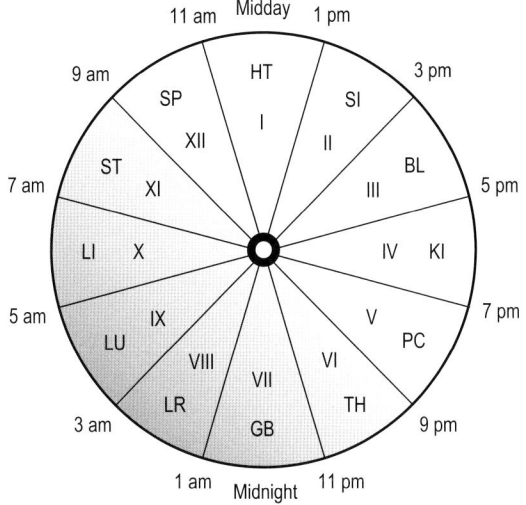

Yin: internal	Yang: external
(Deep level of depth)	(Superficial level of depth)
HT Heart	SI Small Intestine
PC Pericardium	TH Triple Heater
SP Spleen	ST Stomach
LU Lung	LI Large Intestine
KI Kidney	BL Bladder
LR Liver	GB Gall Bladder

Figure 9.3
The Chinese Clock, and related organs. The Roman numerals stem from a European attempt to standardise the channels by number, rather than by name. (From Rogers 2000, with the author's permission.)

221

9.4.6 Pulse qualities

There are variations in the available literature on the Five Phase approach which incorporate pulse qualities in addition to simply assessing differences in strength. Such approaches are derived from the traditional descriptions of overall pulse qualities found in the *Mai Jing* and grafted on to assessment of channels using Five Phase pulse diagnosis. For example, such an approach proposes that a Stringlike (wiry) pulse can simultaneously occur at one position while at another position the pulse is a Short pulse, complicated by a Replete pulse in yet a third position and a Slippery pulse in the deep level at a fourth position. There are assumptive and practical problems with this approach, the most obvious of which is the manifestation of pulse 'qualities' forming simultaneously within the same individual's pulse but which in fact are mutually exclusive, both by definition and by each pulse's respective underlying formation mechanisms (see Box 9.12).

9.5 Nine Continent pulse system

The Nine Continent pulse system is one of the central methods of pulse diagnosis in the *Nei Jing* and has been included for discussion in this chapter because it still

receives some coverage in the contemporary literature and is probably still used by some practitioners. The topic has been approached from a discussion perspective rather than as a prescriptive guide to its application, as with the other pulse systems covered in this chapter.

The *Nei Jing* is generally regarded as the earliest reference documenting the Nine Continent pulses as a distinct system of diagnosis. Although it was not the only method of pulse diagnosis, the extensive coverage it received in assessing health and illness indicates it was an important pulse system at the time. Chapter 20 of the *Su Wen*, 'Treatise on the three regions and the nine subdivisions', is central to the discourse between Huang Qi and Qi Po and the revealing of this regional pulse assessment system. The system is premised on the microcosmic arrangement of the macrocosm reflected within the body. In particular, the Nine Continent system is another application of the Heaven–Earth–Humanity theme.

To apply this pulse system the body is first divided into three portions. In this way, components of Heaven, Earth and Humanity are simultaneously assigned to the upper, middle and lower portions or regions of the body. (Note, however, that the division is different from that used in the San Jiao system where the thoracic cavity containing the lungs and heart is the upper Heater, whereas in this system the thoracic cavity con-

Box 9.12

Terminology within the Five Phase context

- Avoid using the terms 'vacuous' and 'replete' as these have connotations associated with the traditional CM pulse quality system and as such have a differing definition to that in the Five Phase system
- This system also uses the terms 'excess' and 'deficient' simply as generic descriptors which have no relationship to the overall pulse qualities Vacuous (empty) or Replete (full).

Box 9.13

Channel versus organ

The Five Phase system uses the *Nan Jing* arrangement of organs with the Small Intestine and Large Intestine located at the Cun positions, reflecting the location of these channels in the upper regions of the body (in spite of the organs being located in the lower abdomen). The Pericardium and Triple Heater are represented on the Chi position of the Lower Jiao or pelvic cavity in spite of the pericardium being located around the heart. These two 'channels' have theoretical and functional linkages to the Kidneys. As such this model is also termed a functional model and has a direct association with the layout of the channel network in acupuncture.

Maciocia (2004: p. 439) notes Li Shi Zhen's arrangement of the organs and channels to the Cun, Guan and Chi pulse positions as a herbalist model. The herbalist arrangement has the SI and LI organs respectively placed at the left and right Chi positions, reflecting the anatomical layout of the body rather than the channel layout. Hence this would be called an anatomical model.

Box 9.14

Nine Continent pulses and heavenly perfection

For the practitioner of the *Nei Jing* era, numerology formed an important part of medicine. Three subdivisions within three regions arrived at the number nine, and nine in Chinese medicine numerology represented the pre-heavenly state, the idea of perfection and absolute Yang. It is likely that the idea of nine subdivisions was not developed from clinical practice alone, but also driven by intellectual requirements of 'harmony' dictated by the tenants of 'medical' numerology. The exclusion from the system of important pulse sites that which were in common usage at the compilation of the *Nei Jing* provides support for this view. The most notable exclusion is the Ren Ying (Man's prognosis) pulse site in the neck, otherwise known as the carotid artery. This in turn could indicate that the Nine Continent pulse system came from a teaching tradition associated with the cosmological premises of health underlying the teachings of the *Nei Jing*.

Perfection to the authors of the *Nei Jing* required an aspect of both Heaven (Yang) and Earth (Yin) to be residing within Humanity, in each of the three regions. As such, each region is further divided into three subdivisions also correspondingly associated with the cosmological Heaven, Earth and Humanity. For example, this means there is an aspect of Heaven within Heaven, Earth within Heaven and Humanity within Heaven within the upper region. This arrangement is similarly repeated with the other two regions. It is the consequent nine subdivisions that name the Nine Continent pulse system (Table 9.9, Fig 9.4).

Interestingly the number nine had important auspicious connotations in Chinese numerology and probably influenced the system's development, as numerology did for so many of the earlier theoretical clinical constructs in CM (Box 9.14).

9.5.1 Application of the Nine Continent pulse system

In using contemporary theory and extant systems of practice as a reference to interpret the description of the Nine Continent pulses in a clinical context, it would be easy to make the mistake of associating the pulses with specific acupuncture points or anatomical sites reflecting blood flow. Before the Han era the artery and pulse were synonymous with the channel, and as such it was the pulsating length of the palpable artery that correspondingly inferred the strength of the channel Qi and

stitutes the central region.) The three regions in the Nine Continent system are:

- Upper (Heaven): From the shoulders to the head. Associated with the Qi of the head and senses: expression of the Shen
- Middle (Earth): The thoracic cavity and the upper limbs: Associated with the Lungs and Heart: movement of Qi and Blood
- Lower (Humanity): From the diaphragm to the feet. Associated with the abdominal and pelvic cavities; includes the Liver, Spleen Kidneys and Stomach organs.

Table 9.9 ● Assignment of the body area and related pulse site to each of the nine subdivisions according to different literature sources

Regions	Subdivision	Pulse location	Reflection
Nei Jing according to Veith (1972: pp. 187–188)			
Upper (Heaven)	Upper (Heaven)	Arteries on either side of forehead	Corners (temples) of the head and brow
	Middle (Earth)	Arteries within both cheeks (jaw)	
	Lower (Humanity)	Arteries in front of ears	Corners of the mouth and the teeth
			Corners of the ears and the eyes
Middle (Earth)	Upper (Heaven)	Great Yin within hands	Lungs (Po)
	Middle (Earth)	Region of 'sunlight' within hands	Breath within the breast (Zheng Qi)
	Lower (Humanity)	Region of lesser Yin within hands	Heart (Shen)
Lower (Humanity)	Upper (Heaven)	Region of absolute Yin within the feet	Liver (Hun)
	Middle (Earth)	Region of lesser Yin within the feet	Kidneys (Jeh)
	Lower (Humanity)	Region of the Great Yin within the feet	Force of life of the spleen and the stomach (Ji)
Nei Jing according to Unschuld (2003: p. 254)			
Upper (Heaven)	Upper (Heaven)	Moving vessels on the two sides of the forehead	Qi at the corners of the head
	Middle (Earth)	Moving vessels on the two sides of the cheeks	Qi of mouth and the teeth
	Lower (Humanity)	Moving vessels in front of the ears	Qi of ears and the eyes
Middle (Earth)	Upper (Heaven)	Major Yin [locations] of the hands	Lungs
	Middle (Earth)	The Yang brilliance [locations] of the hands	Qi in the chest
	Lower (Humanity)	Minor Yin [locations] of the hands	Heart
Lower (Humanity)	Upper (Heaven)	Ceasing Yin [locations] of the feet	Liver
	Middle (Earth)	Minor Yin [locations] of the feet	Kidneys
	Lower (Humanity)	Major Yin [locations] of the feet	Qi of spleen and the stomach
Nine Continent according to Maciocia (2004: p. 434)			
Upper (Heaven)	Upper (Heaven)	Taiyang	Qi of the head
	Middle (Earth)	ST 3	Qi of the mouth
	Lower (Humanity)	SJ 21	Qi of ears and eyes
Middle (Earth)	Upper (Heaven)	LU 8	Lungs
	Middle (Earth)	LI 4	Centre of thorax
	Lower (Humanity)	HR 7	Heart
Lower (Humanity)	Upper (Heaven)	LR 10: Alternative LR 3	Liver
	Middle (Earth)	KD 3	Kidneys
	Lower (Humanity)	SP 11, Alternative ST 42	Spleen and Stomach

223

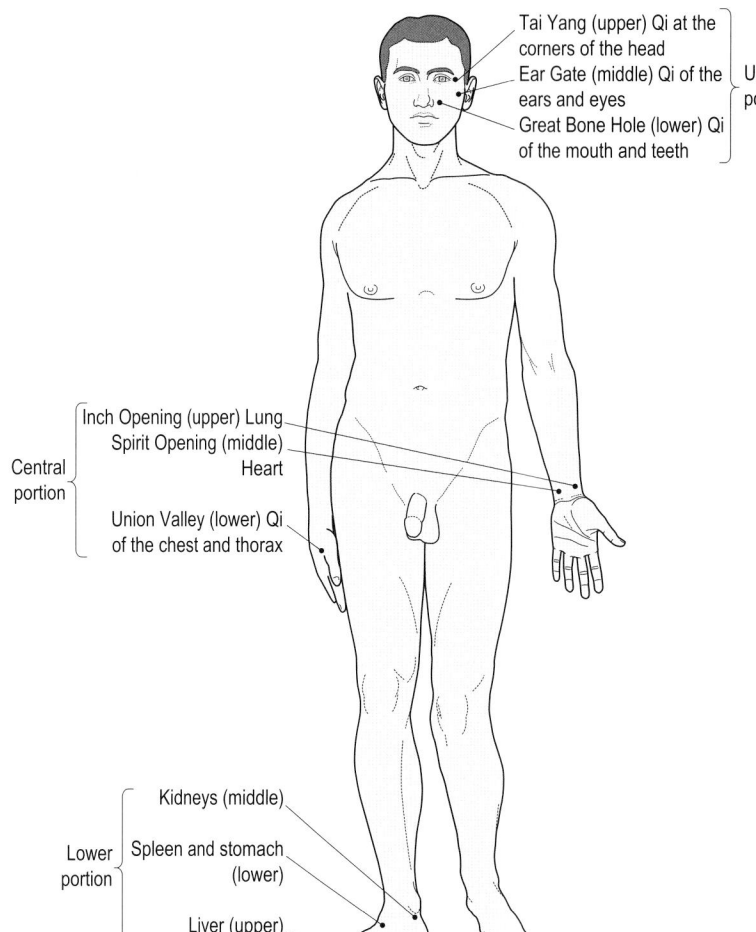

Tai Yang (upper) Qi at the corners of the head ⎫
Ear Gate (middle) Qi of the ears and eyes ⎬ Upper portion
Great Bone Hole (lower) Qi of the mouth and teeth ⎭

Inch Opening (upper) Lung
Spirit Opening (middle) Heart
Central portion
Union Valley (lower) Qi of the chest and thorax

Kidneys (middle)
Lower portion
Spleen and stomach (lower)
Liver (upper)

Figure 9.4
Location of the Nine Continent pulse sites.

the region for which it transgressed. The arteries were simply extensions of the channels.

> It has become common in popular Western acupuncture texts to distinguish between tangible and therefore morphologically visible blood vessels and deep-lying conduit vessels that are considered mere theoretical constructs. Such a distinction, however, did not exist in Chinese antiquity. All vessels, conduits, and conduit vessels were considered morphologically present.
> (Unschuld 2003: p. 170).

This is confirmed in the writings of the *Jia Yi Jing* (*The Systematic Classic of Acupuncture and Moxibustion*). It is written that 'three vessels pulse around the large toe and their state of repletion or vacuity should be examined' in determining the nature of an illness affecting the associated channels to which the pulses related (Mi 1994: p. 306). The three vessels are allocated by the translators as arterial segments:

• ST 45–ST 42 (dorsalis pedis artery)
• LR 1–LR 3
• KD 1–KD 3 (tibial artery).

Depending on the state of the blood vessels, the indication for using acupuncture to supplement or drain depends on whether the pulse is replete and racing or vacuous and slow.

Interestingly, Veith's (1972: p. 189) translation of the *Nei Jing* relates the Nine Continent pulse to the five spiritual resources (controlled by the five Zang: Lungs (Po), Liver (Hun), Heart (Shen), Spleen (Ji), Kidneys (Jeh); Qi relating to the temples, ears and eyes, mouth and teeth; and the space within the breast (the expression of the organ's spiritual aspect and the body's upright Zheng Qi).

However, identifying the nature of a disease may not have been the primary use of the Nine Continent pulse system. Rather, it was identifying the *location* of the disease (Unschuld 2003: pp. 254–255). It is the 'physical appearance and the treatment of the vessel to 'regulate depletion and repletion and to eliminate evil and disease' that is important. For example, a pulse that was different in strength from other pulses indicated the presence of a pathogen. The nature of the pathogen didn't particularly matter, as treatment often involved bleeding points to release pathogens from the channels.

The *Nei Jing* also provides extensive coverage on the prognostic use of the Nine Continent pulses and includes extensive discourses on determining the appropriateness of the body's response in the presence of illness from these as well. This is based on changes in the pulse parameters within each of the nine positions and also by comparing the pulses between positions. For example, the following points regarding the determination of health or illness by the Nine Continent pulse are derived from the *Nei Jing*.

Health is indicated when:

- The pulses correctly reflect the nature of an illness
- Pulses within the three subdivisions in a region are similar (relative similar rhythm and strength)
- Pulses between the nine subdivisions are similar (similar rhythm and strength)
- All pulses are synchronised in terms of strength, depth and rate.

Illness is indicated when:

- The regions of the pulses are not synchronised in strength, rhythm, depth, rate
  - If one of the pulses is not synchronised then illness arises
  - When two pulse are not sychronised then this indicates a grave illness will occur
  - When three pulses are affected then it is seen as a dangerous illness.
- All subdivision pulses should respond in accordance to illness
- Death is indicated when the three subdivision pulses within a region are not congruent.

It is strange and somewhat ironic that to understand the potential uniqueness of the regional pulse system for diagnostic purposes, it is best to look at the biomedicinal system for guidance. For biomedicine, regional pulse palpation forms a small but important aspect of assessing the circulatory integrity of blood perfusion into the skin, muscle and limbs – conditions quite distinct from organ function as posited in the *Nan Jing*. In this way, simultaneous comparison of the strength in the dorsalis pedis and femoral arteries can determine whether blockages are impeding the arterial blood flow, while simultaneous pulsation in the femoral and radial pulses indicate potency of systemic blood flow.

References

Hicks A, Hicks J, Mole P 2004 Five elemental constitutional acupuncture. Churchill Livingstone, Edinburgh

Kaptchuk T 2000 Chinese medicine: web that has no weaver, revised edn. Rider Books, London

King E, Walsh S, Cobbin D 2006 The testing of classical pulse concepts in Chinese medicine: left- and right-hand pulse strength discrepancy between males and females and its clinical implications. Journal of Alternative and Complementary Medicine 12(5):445–450

Lee B, Baik K, Johng H et al. (2004) Acridine orange staining method to reveal the characteristic features of an intravascular threadlike structure. Anatomical Record 278B:27–30

Lee B, Yoo J, Baik K et al 2005 Novel threadlike structures (Bonghan ducts) inside lymphatic vessels of rabbits visualized with a Janus green B staining method. Anatomical Record 286B:1–7

Maciocia G 2004 Diagnosis in Chinese medicine: a comprehensive guide. Churchill Livingstone, Edinburgh

Mi H F, Yang S & Chance C (translators) 1994 The systematic classic of acupuncture and moxibustion. Blue Poppy Press, Boulder, CO

Ni M S (translator) 1995 The Yellow Emperor's classic of medicine. Shambhala, Boston

Qu L, Garvey M 2001 Location and function of the san jiao. Journal of Chinese Medicine 65:26–32

Rogers C 2000 The five keys: an introduction to the study of traditional Chinese medicine, 3rd edn revised. Acupuncture Colleges Publishing, Syndey

Shin H, Johng H, Lee B et al 2005 Feulgen reaction study of novel threadlike structures (Bonghan ducts) of the surface of mammalian organs. Anatomical Record 284B:35–40

Unschuld P (trans) 1986 Nan-ching: the classic of difficult issues. University of California Press, Berkeley

Unschuld P 2003 Huang di nei jing su wen. University of California Press, Berkeley

Veith I (translator) 1972 The Yellow Emperor's classic of internal medicine. University of California Press, Berkeley

Index

A

acupuncture, 2, 25, 36, 58, 112
    Five Phase (Element) system,
        214–15, 216, 220
acute illness, 169–70, 200–1
    see also haemorrhage
adrenaline (epinephrine), 78, 82, 109
age
    physiological changes, 75, 78,
        120, 142
    pulse differences, 67–8, 151
aldosterone, 109
anaemia, 122, 123, 130–1, 133,
    190–1
anatomy of radial artery and forearm,
    11–12, 47–9, 50
antidiuretic hormone, 109
anxiety *see* stress
aorta, 7
aortic valve insufficiency, 16, 17, 201
apprenticeships, 1–2
arrhythmia, 83, 84, 85–7, 136, 200–1
    see also rhythm (pulse parameter)
arterial physiology, 7–13
arterial wall tension (pulse parameter),
    62, 116–23
    assessment techniques, 105, 117–
        18, 123–4, 127, 130, 134
    biomedical factors, 11, 118–20
    Blood pathologies and, 126, 192,
        194
    EPAs and, 183, 185–6, 188
    Liver and, 102, 118
    normal, 57, 118
    pulse qualities and, 123–38, 153,
        171
    Qi imbalance, 118, 197
    Qi/Blood balance, 207
    see also occlusion
arteriosclerosis, 13, 120, 158
assessment techniques *see* methodology
athletes, 75
atrial fibrillation, 82, 86, 201
atrial flutter, 86
atrioventricular node, 77, 85
autonomic nervous system, 77–8,
    118–19, 142

B

bigeminal pulse, 18
Bin Hue Mai Xue (*Lakeside Master's
    Study of the Pulse*) (Li Shi-Zhen)
    on gender differences, 66
    on the organs, 29, 58
    on pulse diagnosis, 27, 30
    pulse quality definitions
        by arterial wall tension, 124,
            129, 130, 134, 137
        by depth, 99
        by flow wave, 159, 164
        by force, 143, 145
        by length, 102
biomedicine
    blood loss and anaemia, 122–3,
        132–3, 190–1
    fever, 169
    gastrointestinal distension, 129
    pregnancy, 67, 76, 158, 161
    pulse diagnosis, 13–17, 30
    pulse parameters, 73
        arterial wall tension, 11, 118–20
        depth, 94
        flow wave/pulse contour, 68,
            157–8, 166, 167
        force, 140–2, 144, 149–50
        length, 101
        occlusion, 122–3
        rate, 77–8, 80, 81–2, 170
        rhythm, 85, 88, 89, 91
        width, 109
    shock, 123, 137–8, 149–50
bisferiens pulse, 18
Bladder, 58
Blood (in CM), 188
    Blood Heat, 195
    body fluids and, 108, 111, 191–2
    organs and, 108, 111
        Liver, 192–3
    pulse parameters and
        arterial wall tension, 126, 130–
          2, 135, 137, 192, 194
        flow wave, 165–6, 194–5
        force, 140, 145–6, 147, 149,
          152, 191
        occlusion, 121–2, 191

        rate, 191
        rhythm, 89, 195
        width, 107, 110–11
    Qi and, 25, 109, 155, 189, 196
        Qi/Blood balance, 203–7
    stagnation (stasis), 89, 145–6,
        166, 193–5
    vacuity, 107, 121–2, 140, 188–93
        Drumskin pulse, 135, 191
        Faint pulse, 149, 191
        Fine pulse, 110–11, 191
        Rough pulse, 165–6, 191
        Scallion Stalk pulse, 130–2, 191
        Scattered pulse, 137
        Soggy pulse, 152, 191
        Stirred pulse, 193
        Stringlike pulse, 126
        Vacuous pulse, 147, 191, 193
        Weak pulse, 150, 191
blood (in biomedicine), 10–11
    anaemia, 122, 123, 130–1, 133,
        190–1
    loss of, 82, 122–3, 132–3, 193
blood pressure, 7, 9, 141
    hypertension, 119–20
body fluids, 106–8, 121, 155–6
    Blood and, 108, 111, 191–2
    loss of, 111, 121–2, 131, 135, 165
body temperature
    force and, 142, 148
    hypothermia, 89
    rate and, 76, 81
    seasonal differences, 69, 76, 93
    width and, 106
    see also fever
body type, 68, 69, 106, 152
Bonghan ducts, 210
Bound pulse, 88–9, 90, 113, 195,
    201
bounding pulse, 122
bradycardia, 80
    see also Slow pulse

C

cardiac output, 10, 76
carotid artery, 8, 11, 25

227

Chi pulse position
    association with body regions/
        organs, 26, 51, 204, 205, 209,
        217
    finger position, 19, 49, 50
    gender differences, 65
    length and, 100, 103
    pulse qualities and, 27
children, pulse rate in, 67, 75, 80
Chinese clock, 220–1
Chinese medicine (CM)
    in classical texts, 23–31
    contemporary, 2–4, 6, 17–20,
        30–1, 64
Choppy (Rough) pulse, 35, 162–8,
        192, 195
chronic illness, 72, 132, 133, 135,
        149, 151, 169
circulation in classical CM, 24, 25,
        100–1
circulatory system in biomedicine,
        5–13, 67, 93, 118–20
Classic of Difficult Issues see *Nan Jing*
CM *see* Chinese medicine
Cold, 94, 183–5
    Bound pulse, 89
    Drumskin pulse, 135, 185
    Firm pulse, 145, 146, 185
    Hidden pulse, 100
    Rough pulse, 166
    Slow pulse, 79, 184–5
    Tight pulse, 129, 185
collapsing (water hammer) pulse, 16,
        200–1
complex pulse parameters, 115–16,
        171–2, 174–5
    see also arterial wall tension; flow
        wave; force; occlusion
constitutional weakness, 151
consultations, when and how to use
        pulse diagnosis, 4, 46, 59–63
coronary heart disease, 120, 170
cortisol, 126
Cou Li, 210
Cun Kou pulse site, 19, 25–6, 48
Cun pulse position
    association with body regions/
        organs, 26, 51, 100, 204, 205,
        209, 217
    finger position, 19, 49, 50
    gender differences, 65
    length and, 100, 103
    pulse qualities and, 27

D

Damp, 109, 180–3
    Fine pulse, 111, 181–2
    Moderate pulse, 82–3, 182
    Rough pulse, 166
    Slippery pulse, 160, 182

Soggy pulse, 152, 181–2
Stringlike (Wiry) pulse, 125,
        182–3
Death (Unusual) pulses, 169–70,
        200–1
deep pulse depth, 54–6, 91, 93, 94,
        97, 98
dehydration, 108, 131, 148
depression, 76
depth (pulse parameter), 55–6, 58–9,
        62, 69, 91–4
    assessment methods, 42, 53–5, 91,
        92, 95, 97, 98–9
    Eight Principles diagnosis, 213
    EPAs and, 94, 96, 183, 186
    Five Phase diagnosis, 215, 217
    normal, 57, 91, 92–3
    number of levels, 29, 53
    organ associations, 26
    pulse qualities and
        complex, 124, 129, 133, 136,
        153
        simple, 94–100, 170
    Yin/Yang and, 55–6, 58, 93–4,
        98, 99–100, 198
diameter waves, 7
diastole, 7, 142
diastolic pressure, 7, 141
dicrotic pulse, 18
diet, 129, 180
    see also food retention
dorsalis pedis pulse, 15, 25
Drumskin pulse, 119, 128, 133–5,
        185, 192

E

ectopic beats, 86–7
education and training, 1–2, 36–7
Eight Principles, 93, 212–14
ejection duration, 78, 142
elderly patients *see* age
emotional effects on pulse parameters,
        76, 118
Empty pulse *see* Vacuous pulse
endocrine system *see* hormones
endometriosis, 166
epinephrine, 78, 82, 109
Essence (Jing), 108, 111, 135, 166
exercise, 75–6
external pathogenic agents (EPA),
        179–80
    pulse depth and, 94, 96, 183, 186
    see also Cold; Damp; Heat; Wind

F

Faint pulse, 148–50, 153, 192, 198
females, 65–7, 69, 75
fever, 81, 119, 125–6, 168, 169

Fine pulse
    Blood vacuity, 192
    Damp, 111, 181–2
    width, 103–4, 110–12, 113
    Yin vacuity, 198
finger placement, 16, 19, 50, 51
fingernails
    patients', 56
    practitioners', 51
Firm pulse, 144–6, 153, 154
    arterial wall tension, 127–8
    Blood stagnation, 195
    Cold, 145, 146, 185
    length, 103
Five Phase diagnosis, 214–21
Floating pulse, 94–6, 113, 180, 188,
        198
flow wave (pulse parameter), 9–10, 63,
        154–7
    biomedical factors, 68, 157–8,
        166, 167
    Blood and, 155, 165–6, 194–5
    Heat and, 185
    normal, 57
    pregnancy, 161
    pulse qualities and, 158–70, 172,
        182
Fluctuating pulse, 38
fluid balance *see* body fluids
food retention, 129, 157, 160, 166,
        195
force (pulse parameter), 63, 69,
        138–42
    assessment techniques, 138–40,
        143, 145, 146–7, 149, 150,
        151–2
    biomedical factors, 140–2, 144,
        149–50
    Blood vacuity, 191
    Eight Principles diagnosis, 213
    Five Phase diagnosis, 215, 217–20
    Heat and, 185
    pulse qualities and, 128, 142–54,
        164, 171
    Qi vacuity, 197
    Qi/Blood balance, 206
    San Jiao assessment, 209–11
Four Levels pattern identification, 168
Fu organs, 217
Fu Yang pulse site, 25

G

Galen, 13–14
Gallbladder, 58, 125
gender, 65–7, 69, 75, 204
Guan pulse position
    association with body regions/
        organs, 26, 51, 204, 205, 209,
        217
    finger position, 19, 49–50

length and, 103
    pulse qualities and, 27
gynaecological conditions, 125, 135,
        161, 166
    see also pregnancy

H

haemorrhage
    biomedical consequences, 82,
        122–3, 132–3, 193
    CM consequences, 111, 121,
        131–2, 135
handedness, 59, 69, 207
Harvey, William, 30
health, 199
    Long pulse, 102, 199
    Moderate pulse, 82, 199
    in the Nine Continent system,
        225
    normal pulse parameters, 38–9,
        56–7, 74, 92–3, 106, 118
    Rapid pulse, 80
    Slippery pulse, 159, 199
    Slow pulse, 78, 199–200
Heart (in CM)
    Blood and, 108
    pulse positions and, 58, 205
    rhythm, 84, 85–6, 88, 89, 91
    San Jiao system, 207, 208
    Shen, 57, 84
heart (in biomedicine), 7, 9
    arrhythmias, 80, 84, 85
    vascular disease, 120, 170
heart rate, 10, 74–8, 80
    see also rate (pulse parameter)
Heat, 185–8
    Blood Heat, 195
    Long pulse, 102
    Rapid pulse, 186, 188
    Replete pulse, 143, 181, 188,
        195
    Skipping pulse, 88
    Slippery pulse, 160, 188
    Slow pulse, 80
    Surging pulse, 168, 186–7
    Vacuous pulse, 148, 186, 187
heat exhaustion, 148
Helicobacter pylori, 133
herbal medicine, 36, 58, 76
Hidden pulse, 98–100, 113, 198
history
    classical CM texts, 23–31
    pulses in biomedicine, 13–15, 30
horary flow of Qi, 220–1
hormones
    blood volume, 109
    heart rate, 78, 82
    menstrual cycle, 161
    stress, 126
hyperkinetic pulse, 18

hypertension, 119–20
hypokinetic pulse, 18
hypothermia, 89
hypovolaemic shock, 76, 123, 132–3,
        149–50, 193

I

immune system status, 96
inch opening pulse site *see* Cun Kou
        pulse site
Intermittent pulse, 89–91, 113, 197,
        201
iron deficiency, 123, 133, 190–1

J

jarring pulse, 14
Jia Yi Jing, 28
Jin body fluids *see* body fluids
Jing (Essence), 108, 111, 135, 166
Jing Qi, 91
jugular venous pulse, 15

K

Ke cycle, 214, 220
keiraku chiryo, 43
Kidney(s)
    Blood and, 108
    pulse positions, 58, 204, 205
    Qi and, 137
    Root, 57
    San Jiao system, 208
Kidney Essence (Jing), 108, 111, 135,
        166

L

Lakeside Master's Study of the Pulse see
        Bin Hue Mai Xue
Large Intestine, 58, 208
left and right hand pulses
    assessment methods, 51, 59, 206,
        207
    force, 140
    gender and, 65, 66, 67, 69, 204
    length, 103
    Qi/Blood balance, 203–7
    rhythm, 84
length (pulse parameter), 62, 100–1
    Heat and, 185
    pulse qualities and
        complex, 123, 127, 153, 169
        simple, 101–3, 170
    Qi vacuity, 197
Li Shi-Zhen *see Bin Hue Mai Xue*
lifestyle, 38, 89

Liver
    arterial wall tension, 102, 118
    Blood and, 108, 192–3
    disharmonies, 102, 124–5, 192–3
    pulse positions, 58, 205
    San Jiao system, 208
    Spleen and, 125
Long pulse, 101–2, 103, 113
    Blood Heat and, 102, 195
    as sign of good health, 102, 199
Lung
    Blood and, 108
    pulse positions, 58, 100, 204
    San Jiao system, 207

M

Mai Jing (Wang Shu-He)
    on gender differences, 66
    on pulse diagnosis, 26–7, 28, 29, 37
    pulse quality definitions
        by arterial wall tension, 128,
            130, 134, 136, 137
        by depth, 95, 98, 99
        by flow wave, 168, 169
        by force, 147, 149, 150, 152
        by rate, 78, 80, 82
        by rhythm, 88, 89, 90
        by width, 110
malaria, 125–6
males, 65–7, 69, 75, 204
Mawangdui scrolls, 24
medication, 36, 58, 76
men, 65–7, 69, 75, 204
menstrual cycle, 161
methodology
    in biomedical practice, 16
    consistency, importance of, 2–4,
        42–3, 45, 60–1
    decision to use pulse diagnosis, 4,
        59–60
    Five Phase method, 217–20
    left vs right comparison, 51, 59,
        206, 207
    palpation, 19, 46–51, 60–1
    parameter assessment, 51, 61–3,
        170–7
    arterial wall tension, 105,
        117–18, 123–4, 127, 130, 134
    depth, 42, 53–6, 91, 92, 95, 97,
        98–9
    flow wave, 155
    force, 138–40, 143, 145, 146–7,
        149, 150, 151–2
    length, 100, 101
    occlusion, 54, 117–18, 124
    rate, 74, 77
    rhythm, 83–4
    width, 104–5, 110
    Qi/Blood balance, 206
    San Jiao method, 209–11

middle pulse depth, 55, 56, 91
Moderate pulse, 82–3, 113, 162, 182, 199

N

Nan Jing, 25–6, 48, 58, 66
    commentaries on, 28–9, 29–30
Nei Jing
    on gender differences, 65–6
    Nine Continent system, 224–5
    on pulse diagnosis, 2–3, 23–5, 28
    pulse quality definitions
        by depth, 98
        by flow wave, 168
        by rate, 77, 79, 80, 82
    on seasonal differences, 64
    on sinus arrhythmia, 84
neurogenic shock, 137–8
Nine Continent system, 17, 24–5, 221–5
nitric oxide, 120
norepinephrine, 82, 109
normal pulse parameters, 24, 38–9, 56–7, 74, 92–3, 106, 118
    see also health

O

occlusion (pulse parameter), 63, 120–3
    assessment techniques, 54–5, 117–18, 124
    Blood vacuity, 191
    force and, 140
    healthy pulse, 57
    pulse qualities and, 123–6, 128, 136, 153, 171
    Qi/Blood balance, 207
    see also arterial wall tension
oedema, 157

P

pain, 91, 98, 125, 129, 146, 194
palpation methods
    in biomedicine, 16
    in CM, 19, 46–51, 60–1
    see also methodology
palpitations, 85–6
parasympathetic nervous system, 78, 142
patient positioning, 16, 46
Pericardium, 58, 204
peripheral systolic pressure (PSP), 122
pharmaceuticals, 76
Phlegm, 102, 125, 160, 182–3
physiology of the pulse, 5–13, 67
PMaxPdt, 122
polycythemia, 10, 166

postpartum haemorrhage, 135
Practical Jin's Pulse Diagnosis, 65
practitioners
    handedness of, 59, 207
    inter-rater reliability, 39–41
    position during pulse assessment, 46, 47, 51
pregnancy
    Drumskin pulse, 135
    haemodynamic changes during, 67, 76, 158, 161
    Nei Jing on, 65–6
    Rough pulse, 165–6, 166
    Scattered pulse, 137
    Slippery pulse, 67, 159–60, 162, 163
pressure waves, 7–9, 154
Pulse Classic see Mai Jing
pulse contour see flow wave (pulse parameter)
pulse force see force (pulse parameter)
pulse parameters, 71–3, 170–7
    assessment techniques see methodology, parameter assessment
    Blood vacuity and, 191
    complex, 115–16, 171–2, 174–5
        see also arterial wall tension; flow wave; force; occlusion
    normal, 24, 38–9, 56–7, 74, 92–3, 106, 118
    simple, 73, 112–13, 170, 174
        see also depth; length; rate; rhythm; width
pulse positions/sites
    association with different organs, 26, 51
    in biomedicine, 15–16
    locating, 47–51
    Nine Continent system, 24–5, 224
    on the radial artery (Cun Kou), 19, 25–6, 48
    regional pulse assessment, 24–5, 27–9, 224
        see also Chi, Cun and Guan pulse positions
pulsus alternans, 18, 167
pulsus tardus, 18

Q

Qi, 195–6
    Blood and, 25, 109, 155, 189, 196
        Qi/Blood balance, 203–7
    EPAs and, 180
    horary flow, 220–1
    Jing Qi, 91
    Kidney Qi, 137
    Liver and, 124–5
    pulse parameters, 108–9, 118, 197

stagnation (stasis), 145–6, 166, 197
    Stomach Qi, 57
    vacuity, 196–7
        Bound pulse, 89
        Faint pulse, 149
        Fine pulse, 110
        Intermittent pulse, 91, 197
        Scattered pulse, 137, 197
        Short pulse, 103, 197
        Sinking pulse, 98
        Soggy pulse, 152
        Vacuous pulse, 147, 196, 197
        Wei Qi, 94, 196
        Yang Qi see Yang Qi
        Yuan Qi, 91, 109, 137, 196, 197
        Zheng Qi, 96, 135, 143, 168
qie mai, 17
quality control see reliability of pulse measurement

R

Racing pulse, 81
radial artery, 11–12, 47–9, 50, 56
    see also Cun Kou pulse site
radius, 48, 50
Rapid pulse, 80–2, 113, 186, 188
rate (pulse parameter), 62, 73–8
    assessment methods, 74, 77
    biomedical factors, 77–8, 80, 81–2, 170
    Blood vacuity, 191
    in children, 67, 75, 80
    Eight Principles diagnosis, 212, 213
    EPAs and, 183, 185
    Five Phase diagnosis, 215
    normal, 24, 57, 74
    pulse qualities and, 78–83, 167, 169, 170
red blood cells
    in anaemia, 123, 190
    increased levels, 10, 166
reflective waves, 7
regional pulse assessment, 24–5, 27–9, 224
reliability of pulse measurement, 1–4, 33–43
    within/between-individual variables, 64–70, 74–6, 106
Ren Ying pulse site, 25
Replete pulse, 35, 142–4, 153, 154
    Heat and, 143, 181, 188, 195
respiratory method for measuring pulse rate, 77, 78
rhythm (pulse parameter), 62, 83–7
    pulse qualities and, 88–91, 167, 170
    Qi stagnation or vacuity, 89, 195, 197
    see also arrhythmia

right and left hand pulses
 assessment methods, 51, 59, 206,
  207
 force, 140
 gender and, 65, 66, 67, 69, 204
 length, 103
 Qi/Blood balance, 203–7
 rhythm, 84
Root, 57
Rough (Choppy) pulse, 35, 162–8,
 192, 195

S

San Jiao system, 103, 207–12
Scallion Stalk pulse, 116, 119, 127–8,
 129–33, 192
Scattered pulse, 116, 135–8, 154, 197
seasonal effects, 64–5, 69, 76, 92–3
sepsis, 144
Shen, 57, 84
Sheng cycle, 214, 220
shock, 193
 hypovolaemic, 76, 123, 132–3,
  149–50
 neurogenic, 137–8
Short pulse, 101, 102–3, 113, 194,
 197
simple pulse parameters, 73, 112–13,
 170, 174
 see also depth; length; rate; rhythm;
  width
Sinking pulse, 96–8, 113, 198
sinoatrial node, 77, 85
sinus arrhythmia, 84
sites for pulse palpation see pulse
 positions/sites
Six Division pattern identification,
 168
skin, appearance of, 56, 164
Skipping pulse, 35, 88, 113
Slippery pulse, 158–62
 EPAs and, 160, 182, 188
 in pregnancy, 67, 159–60, 162,
  163
 as a sign of good health, 159,
  199
Slow pulse, 78–80, 113, 184–5,
 199–200
Small Intestine, 58, 208
Soggy pulse, 96, 151–4, 181–2, 192,
 198
sphygmology, 8, 13–17
Spinning Bean (Stirred) pulse, 35, 103,
 169–70, 193
Spleen
 Blood and, 108
 Damp and, 180
 Liver and, 125
 pulse positions, 58, 204
 San Jiao system, 207

steel hammer pulse, 14
Stirred (Spinning Bean) pulse, 35, 103,
 169–70, 193
Stomach, 57, 58, 129, 204, 207
stress, 76, 81–2, 88, 126
Stringlike (Wiry) pulse, 103, 120,
 123–6, 127–8
 Blood Heat and, 195
 EPAs and, 125, 182–3, 188
 Qi stagnation, 126, 197
stroke volume (SV), 8–9, 10, 75–6,
 122
students, 41
superficial pulse depth, 54, 55, 91,
 93, 94
Surging pulse, 168–9, 186–7
sympathetic nervous system, 77–8,
 118–19, 142
systole, 7, 78–9, 142
systolic pressure, 7, 122, 141

T

tachycardia, 80, 81–2
 see also Rapid pulse
techniques see methodology
temperature
 force and, 142, 148
 hypothermia, 89
 rate and, 76, 81
 seasonal differences, 69, 76, 93
 width and, 106
 see also fever
tense pulse, 14
terminology
 Eight Principles system, 213–14
 Five Phases system, 222
 problems caused by ambiguity,
  34–7, 40, 41–2
 specific vs descriptive, 34, 138,
  147
thready pulse, 14
Three Five pulse, 164
Three Heaters, 103, 207–12
thrills, 15–16
thumb position, 50
thyroid disorders, 76, 82
Tibetan medicine, 100
Tight pulse, 126–9, 181, 185,
 195
timing of the pulse see rate; rhythm
training, 1–2, 36–7
treatment planning, 36
trigeminal pulse, 14
Triple Heater, 58, 143, 204, 208

U

Unusual (Death) pulses, 169–70,
 200–1

V

Vacuous pulse, 96, 146–8, 153
 Blood vacuity, 192, 193
 Heat and, 148, 186, 187
 Qi vacuity, 147, 196, 197
variability see reliability of pulse
 measurement
vascular (circulatory) system, 5–13,
 67, 93, 118–20
veins, appearance of, 56
ventricular contraction, 9
ventricular fibrillation, 86
viscosity of blood, 9, 10, 111, 121–2,
 131, 158

W

Wang Shu-He see Mai Jing
water hammer (collapsing) pulse, 16,
 200–1
Weak pulse, 150–1, 153, 154, 192,
 198
weather see seasonal effects
Wei Qi, 94, 196
weight, 68, 69
Western medicine see biomedicine
width (pulse parameter), 62, 103–9
 Damp and, 182
 pulse qualities and
  complex, 126, 129, 133, 136,
   153, 167, 168
  simple, 110–12, 170
Wind, 188
Wiry pulse see Stringlike (Wiry) pulse
women, 65–7, 69, 75, 204
Wu Xing diagrams, 219

Y

Yang, 64, 65
 Eight Principles diagnosis, 213
Yang Qi
 arterial wall tension, 118, 131
 blood loss and, 131, 149
 depth, 55–6, 58, 93–4, 98, 99–
  100, 198
 occlusion, 121, 131
 rate, 76–7, 79–80, 80–1
 rhythm, 89
 vacuity, 199
  Bound pulse, 89
  Faint pulse, 149, 198–9
  Hidden pulse, 99–100, 198–9
  Sinking pulse, 98, 198–9
  Slow pulse, 79–80
  Weak pulse, 150–1, 198–9
Ye body fluids see body fluids
Yellow Emperor's Classic of Medicine see
 Nei Jing

Yin, 64, 65
  arterial wall tension, 118
  depth, 55–6, 58, 94, 96
  Eight Principles diagnosis, 213
  flow wave/pulse contour, 155–6
  occlusion, 121–2
  rate, 81
  rhythm, 88

vacuity, 198
  Drumskin pulse, 135
  Floating pulse, 180, 198
  Rapid pulse, 81, 188
  Rough pulse, 165
  Soggy pulse, 152, 198
  Surging pulse, 168–9
  see also Blood, vacuity

width, 106–8
Yuan Qi, 91, 109, 137, 196, 197

Z

Zang organs, 204–5, 217
Zheng Qi, 96, 135, 143, 168